Practice*Planners*®

Arthur E. Jongsma, Jr., Series Editor

Helping therapists
help their clients...

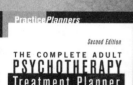

PracticePlanners

Second Edition

THE COMPLETE ADULT
PSYCHOTHERAPY
Treatment Planner

A new, fully revised edition of the bestselling *The Complete Psychotherapy Treatment Planner*, this invaluable resource features:

- Treatment plan components for 39 behaviorally based problems—including five completely new problem sets
- A step-by-step guide to writing treatment plans
- Over 500 additional prewritten treatment goals, objectives, and interventions
- Handy workbook format with space to record your own treatment plan options
- Over 100,000 **Practice Planners** sold

Arthur E. Jongsma, Jr., and L. Mark Peterson

PracticePlanners
Arthur E. Jongsma, Jr., Series Editor

Brief Therapy
HOMEWORK
PLANNER

- Contains 62 ready-to-copy homework assignments that can be used to facilitate brief individual therapy
- Homework assignments and exercises are keyed to over 30 behaviorally-based presenting problems from *The Complete Psychotherapy Treatment Planner*
- Assignments may be quickly customized using the enclosed disk
- Over 100,000 **Practice Planners** sold

Gary M. Schultheis

PracticePlanners®

The Clinical
DOCUMENTATION
SOURCEBOOK

Second Edition

A Comprehensive Collection of
Mental Health Practice
Forms, Handouts, and Records

FEATURES

- Contains ready-to-use forms for managing the mental health treatment process
- Covers every stage of the treatment process
- Includes customizable forms on disk
- Over 100,000 **Practice Planners** sold

Donald E. Wiger

PracticePlanners
Arthur E. Jongsma, Jr., Series Editor

The Adult Psychotherapy
PROGRESS NOTES PLANNER

This time-saving resource:

- Contains Progress notes components for 39 behaviorally based problems
- Covers the gamut of possible outcomes for every intervention as expressed in the best-selling *Complete Adult Psychotherapy Treatment Planner*, 2nd Edition
- Includes 1,000s of prewritten treatment and patient presentation descriptions
- Provides a handy workbook layout with space to record your own progress note options
- Over 100,000 **Practice Planners** sold

Arthur E. Jongsma, Jr.

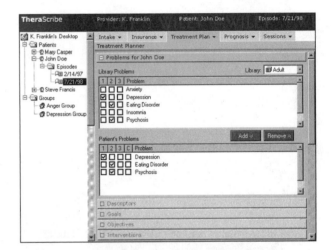
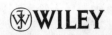

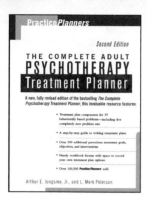

Treatment Planners cover all the necessary elements for developing formal treatment plans, including detailed problem definitions, long-term goals, short-term objectives, therapeutic interventions, and DSM-IV diagnoses.

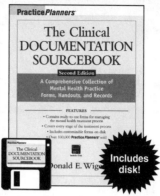

Documentation Sourcebooks provide a comprehensive collection of ready-to-use blank forms, handouts, and questionnaires to help you manage your client reports and streamline the record keeping and treatment process. Features clear, concise explanations of the purpose of each form—including when it should be used and at what point. Includes customizable forms on disk.

The Complete Adult Psychotherapy Treatment Planner,
Second Edition
0-471-31924-4 / $44.95

The Child Psychotherapy Treatment Planner, Second Edition
0-471-34764-7 / $44.95

The Adolescent Psychotherapy Treatment Planner,
Second Edition
0-471-34766-3 / $44.95

The Chemical Dependence Treatment Planner
0-471-23795-7 / $44.95

The Continuum of Care Treatment Planner
0-471-19568-5 / $44.95

The Couples Psychotherapy Treatment Planner
0-471-24711-1 / $44.95

The Employee Assistance (EAP) Treatment Planner
0-471-24709-X / $44.95

The Pastoral Counseling Treatment Planner
0-471-25416-9 / $44.95

The Older Adult Psychotherapy Treatment Planner
0-471-29574-4 / $44.95

The Behavioral Medicine Treatment Planner
0-471-31923-6 / $44.95

The Group Therapy Treatment Planner
0-471-37449-0 / $44.95

The Family Therapy Treatment Planner
0-471-34768-X / $44.95

The Severe and Persistent Mental Illness Treatment Planner
0-471-35945-9 / $44.95

The Gay and Lesbian Psychotherapy Treatment Planner
0-471-35080-X / $44.95

The Clinical Documentation Sourcebook, Second Edition
0-471-32692-5 / $49.95

The Psychotherapy Documentation Primer
0-471-28990-6 / $45.00

The Couple and Family Clinical Documentation Sourcebook
0-471-25234-4 / $49.95

The Clinical Child Documentation Sourcebook
0-471-29111-0 / $49.95

The Chemical Dependence Treatment Documentation Sourcebook
0-471-31285-1 / $49.95

The Forensic Documentation Sourcebook
0-471-25459-2 / $85.00

The Continuum of Care Clinical Documentation Sourcebook
0-471-34581-4 / $75.00

NEW AND FORTHCOMING

The Traumatic Events Treatment Planner
0-471-39587-0 / $44.95

The Special Education Treatment Planner
0-471-38873-4 / $44.95 p

The Mental Retardation and Developmental Disability Treatment Planner
0-471-38253-1 / $44.95

The Social Work and Human Services Treatment Planner
0-471-37741-4 / $44.95

The Rehabilitation Psychology Treatment Planner
0-471-35178-4 / $44.95

Name_____

Affiliation_____

Address_____

City/State/Zip_____

Phone/Fax_____

E-mail_____

To order, call 1-800-753-0655
(Please refer to promo #1-4019 when ordering.)
Or send this page with payment* to:
John Wiley & Sons, Inc., Attn: J. Knott
605 Third Avenue, New York, NY 10158-0012

❏ Check enclosed ❏ Visa ❏ MasterCard ❏ American Express

Card #_____

Expiration Date_____

Signature_____

*Please add your local sales tax to all orders.

www.wiley.com/practiceplanners

Practice Management Tools for Busy Mental Health Professionals

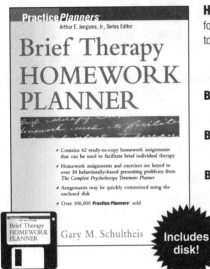
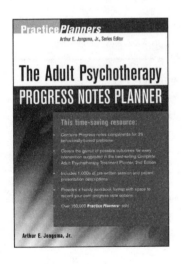
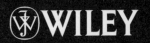

The Adult Psychotherapy
Progress Notes Planner

PRACTICE *PLANNERS*® SERIES

Treatment *Planners*

The Chemical Dependence Treatment Planner
The Continuum of Care Treatment Planner
The Couples Psychotherapy Treatment Planner
The Employee Assistance Treatment Planner
The Pastoral Counseling Treatment Planner
The Older Adult Psychotherapy Treatment Planner
The Complete Adult Psychotherapy Treatment Planner, 2e
The Behavioral Medicine Treatment Planner
The Group Therapy Treatment Planner
The Gay and Lesbian Psychotherapy Treatment Planner
The Child Psychotherapy Treatment Planner, 2e
The Adolescent Psychotherapy Treatment Planner, 2e
The Family Therapy Treatment Planner
The Severe and Persistent Mental Illness Treatment Planner
The Mental Retardation and Developmental Disability Treatment Planner
The Social Work and Human Services Treatment Planner
The Traumatic Events Treatment Planner
The Personality Disorders Treatment Planner
The Rehabilitation Psychology Treatment Planner

Progress Notes *Planners*

The Child Psychotherapy Progress Notes Planner
The Adolescent Psychotherapy Progress Notes Planner
The Adult Psychotherapy Progress Notes Planner

Homework *Planners*

Brief Therapy Homework Planner
Brief Couples Therapy Homework Planner
Chemical Dependence Treatment Homework Planner
Brief Child Therapy Homework Planner
Brief Adolescent Therapy Homework Planner
Brief Employee Assistance Homework Planner
Brief Family Therapy Homework Planner

Documentation *Sourcebooks*

The Clinical Documentation Sourcebook
The Forensic Documentation Sourcebook
The Psychotherapy Documentation Primer
The Chemical Dependence Treatment Documentation Sourcebook
The Clinical Child Documentation Sourcebook
The Couple and Family Clinical Documentation Sourcebook
The Clinical Documentation Sourcebook, 2e
The Continuum of Care Clinical Documentation Sourcebook

PracticePlanners®

Arthur E. Jongsma, Jr., Series Editor

The Adult Psychotherapy Progress Notes Planner

Arthur E. Jongsma, Jr.

JOHN WILEY & SONS, INC.

New York • Chichester • Weinheim • Brisbane • Singapore • Toronto

Library of Congress Cataloging-in-Publication Data:

Jongsma, Arthur E., 1943-
    The adult psychotherapy progress notes planner//Arthur E. Jongsma, Jr.
        p. cm. — (Practice planner series)
    ISBN 0-471-34763-9 (alk. paper)
        1. Psychotherapy—Handbooks, manuals, etc.   2. Medical records—Handbooks, manuals, etc.
3. Adulthood—Psychological aspects—Handbooks, manuals, etc.   4. Mental illness—Treatment—Planning—
Handbooks, manuals, etc.   I. Title. II. Practice planners.

RC480.5 .J663 2001
616.89'14—dc21
`   00-053370

Printed in the United States of America.

10 9 8 7 6 5 4 3 2 1

This book is dedicated to Marcia Berends, a faithful and loyal assistant who always goes the extra mile without being asked.

CONTENTS

PRACTICE PLANNERS SERIES PREFACE

The practice of psychotherapy has a dimension that did not exist 30, 20, or even 15 years ago—accountability. Treatment programs, public agencies, clinics, and even group and solo practitioners must now justify the treatment of patients to outside review entities that control the payment of fees. This development has resulted in an explosion of paperwork.

Clinicians must now document what has been done in treatment, what is planned for the future, and what the anticipated outcomes of the interventions are. The books and software in this Practice Planner series are designed to help practitioners fulfill these documentation requirements efficiently and professionally.

The Practice Planner series is growing rapidly. It now includes the second editions of the *Complete Adult Psychotherapy Treatment Planner,* the *Adolescent Psychotherapy Treatment Planner,* and the *Child Psychotherapy Treatment Planner.* Additional Treatment Planners are targeted to specialty areas of practice, including: chemical dependency, the continuum of care, couples therapy, employee assistance, behavioral medicine, therapy with older adults, pastoral counseling, family therapy, group therapy, neuropsychology, therapy with gays and lesbians, and more.

In addition to the Treatment Planners, the series also includes *TheraScribe®,* the latest version of the popular treatment planning, patient record-keeping software, as well as adjunctive books, such as the *Brief, Chemical Dependence, Couple, Child,* and *Adolescent Therapy Homework Planners, The Psychotherapy Documentation Primer,* and *Clinical, Forensic, Child, Couples and Family, Continuum of Care,* and *Chemical Dependence Documentation Sourcebooks*—containing forms and resources to aid in mental health practice management. Finally, the most recent additions to the Practical Planner series are the Psychotherapy Progress Notes Planners for adults, adolescents, and children, respectively. These books feature over 1,000 prewritten progress notes. Components are organized around presenting problems covered in the specific Treatment Planners written for adults, adolescents, and children. The goal of the series is to provide practitioners with the resources they need in order to provide high-quality care in the era of accountability—or, to put it simply, we seek to help you spend more time on patients, and less time on paperwork.

ARTHUR E. JONGSMA, JR.
Grand Rapids, Michigan

ACKNOWLEDGMENTS

No other book has been created with more struggle to get it done and get it right. It was only with the urging of Kelly Franklin and the encouragement of Peggy Alexander at John Wiley & Sons that this project eventually found successful completion. I also would like to thank Cristina Wojdylo at Wiley for her professional oversight of the manuscript in the production process.

The preparation of the manuscript was the work of Kendra VanElst and Susan Rhoda. Many thanks to them for their push to the finish line. But the coordination of the multitude of details to bring the manuscript to completion has rested in the competent hands of Jen Byrne, the project manager. Without her organization skills, we would all still be confused.

Finally, a warm thank you to my loving and supportive wife, Judy, who kept pumping me up whenever my motivation to continue this project wavered.

INTRODUCTION

INTENT AND FOCUS

The Adult Psychotherapy Progress Notes Planner is another step in the evolution of the Practice Planner series. This book is written as a companion to *The Complete Adult Psychotherapy Treatment Planner,* Second Edition, as it provides a menu of sentences that can be selected for constructing a progress note based on the "Behavioral Definitions" and "Therapeutic Interventions" from the Treatment Planner.

Our hope and desire is that both students and seasoned clinicians will find this resource helpful in writing progress notes that are thoroughly unified with the patient's treatment plan. In our progress note sentences, we have tried to provide a range of content that can document how a patient presented and what interventions were used in the session.

INTERFACE WITH TREATMENT PLANNER

Progress notes are not only the primary source for documenting the therapeutic process, but also one of the main factors in determining the patient's eligibility for reimbursable treatment. Although the books can be used independently, *The Adult Psychotherapy Progress Notes Planner* provides prewritten sentences that are directly coordinated with the symptom descriptions in the "Behavioral Definitions" section and with the clinical activity description in the "Therapeutic Interventions" section of *The Complete Adult Psychotherapy Treatment Planner,* Second Edition (John Wiley & Sons, New York, 2000). Used together, you'll find these books both a time saver and a guidepost to complete, integrated clinical recordkeeping.

ORGANIZATION OF THE PROGRESS NOTES PLANNER

Each chapter title is a reflection of the patient's potential presenting problem. The first section of the chapter, "Patient Presentation," provides a detailed menu of statements that may describe how that presenting problem manifested itself in behavioral signs and symptoms. The numbers in parentheses within the "Patient Presentation" section correspond to the number of the "Behavioral Definition" from the Treatment Planner. For example, consider the following two items from the chapter entitled "Antisocial Behavior" of this Progress Notes Planner:

8. Aggressive/Argumentative (7)
A. The patient presented in a hostile, angry, and uncooperative manner.
B. The patient was intimidating in his/her style of interaction.

C. The patient is trying to interact in a more cooperative manner within social and employment settings.

D. The patient is showing less irritability and argumentativeness within therapy sessions.

9. Authority Conflicts (7)

A. The patient acknowledged a history of irritability, aggression, and argumentativeness when interacting with authority figures.

B. The patient's history of conflict with acceptance of authority has led to employment instability and legal problems.

C. The patient is beginning to accept direction from authority figures, recognizing his/her need to resist challenging such directives.

In the preceding sample, the number 7 in parentheses refers to the seventh Behavioral Definition from the chapter, "Antisocial Behavior," in *The Complete Adult Psychotherapy Treatment Planner*, Second Edition. Within the "Patient Presentation" section of each chapter, the statements are arranged to reflect a progression toward resolution of the problem. The latter statements are included to be used in later stages of therapy as the patient moves forward toward discharge.

The second section of each chapter, "Interventions Implemented," provides a menu of statements related to the action that was taken within the session to assist the patient in making progress. The numbering of the items in the "Interventions Implemented" section follows exactly the numbering of "Therapeutic Intervention" items in the corresponding Treatment Planner. For example, consider the following two items from the chapter, "Antisocial Behavior," in this Progress Notes Planner:

8. Confront Responsibility for Broken Relationships (8)

A. The patient was firmly and consistently confronted with the reality of his/her own behavior that caused pain to others and resulted in their breaking of the relationship.

B. The patient was asked to identify how he/she was insensitive to the needs and feelings of others.

C. Role reversal techniques were used as an attempt to get the patient in touch with the pain that he/she has caused in others due to disrespect, disloyalty, aggression, or dishonesty.

9. Confront Self-Centeredness (9)

A. The patient was taught, through role playing and role reversal, the value of being empathetic to the needs, rights, and feelings of others.

B. The patient presented his/her attitude of "look out for number one" as the only way to live.

C. The patient justified his/her self-focused attitude as the way that he/she learned to live because of the abuse and abandonment suffered as a child.

D. Attempts were made to get the patient to view his/her own behavior from another person's perspective.

In the two preceding samples, the item numbers **8** and **9** correspond directly to the same numbered items in the "Therapeutic Interventions" section from the chapter, "Antisocial Behavior," of *The Complete Adult Psychotherapy Treatment Planner*, Second Edition. Within the "Interventions Implemented" section of each chapter, each set of statements under a keyword reflects an elaboration on the original Intervention statement from the Treatment Planner. Various ways to implement the intervention may be described and the patient's response to the intervention within the session or in a follow-up session may be described.

Finally, all item lists begin with a few keywords. These words are meant to convey the theme or content of the sentences that are contained in that listing. The clinician may peruse the list of keywords to find content that matches the patient's presentation and the clinician's intervention.

USING *THE ADULT PSYCHOTHERAPY PROGRESS NOTES PLANNER*

If the reader has not used *The Complete Adult Psychotherapy Treatment Planner,* Second Edition, to initiate treatment, then relevant progress notes can be found by finding the chapter title that reflects the patient's presenting problem, scanning the keywords to find the theme that fits the session, and then selecting the sentences that describe first how the patient presented for that session and then what interventions were used to assist the patient in reaching his/her therapeutic goals and objectives. It is expected that the clinician will modify the prewritten statements contained in this book to fit the exact circumstances of the patient's presentation and treatment. Individualization of treatment must be reflected in progress notes that are tailored to each patient's unique presentation, strengths, and weaknesses.

To maintain complete patient records, in addition to progress note statements that may be selected and individualized from this book, the date, time, and length of a session; those present within the session; the provider, provider's credentials, and a signature must be entered in the patient's record.

All progress notes must be tied to the treatment plan—session notes should elaborate on the problems, symptoms, and interventions contained in the plan. If a session focuses on a topic outside those covered in the treatment plan, the provider must update the treatment plan accordingly.

ANGER MANAGEMENT

PATIENT PRESENTATION

1. Explosive, Destructive Outbursts (1)

A. The patient described a history of loss of temper in which he/she has destroyed property during fits of rage.

B. The patient described a history of loss of temper that dates back to childhood, involving verbal outbursts as well as property destruction.

C. As therapy has progressed, the patient has reported increased control over his/her temper and a significant reduction in incidents of poor anger management.

D. The patient has no recent incidents of explosive outbursts that have resulted in destruction of any property or intimidating verbal assaults.

2. Explosive, Assaultive Outbursts (1)

A. The patient described a history of loss of anger control to the point of physical assault on others who were the target of his/her anger.

B. The patient has been arrested for assaultive attacks on others when he/she has lost control of his/her temper.

C. The patient has used assaultive acts as well as threats and intimidation to control others.

D. The patient has made a commitment to control his/her temper and terminate all assaultive behavior.

E. There have been no recent incidents of assaultive attacks on anyone, in spite of the patient having experienced periods of anger.

3. Overreactive Irritability (2)

A. The patient described a history of reacting too angrily to rather insignificant irritants in his/her daily life.

B. The patient indicated that he/she recognizes that he/she becomes too angry in the face of rather minor frustrations and irritants.

C. Minor irritants have resulted in explosive, angry outbursts that have led to destruction of property and/or striking out physically at others.

D. The patient has made significant progress at increasing frustration tolerance and reducing explosive overreactivity to minor irritants.

4. Harsh Judgment Statements (3)

A. The patient exhibited frequent incidents of being harshly critical of others.

B. The patient's family members reported that he/she reacts very quickly with angry, critical, and demeaning language toward them.

---

* The numbers in parentheses correlate to the number of the Behavioral Definition statement in the companion chapter with the same title in *The Complete Adult Psychotherapy Treatment Planner,* second edition (Jongsma and Peterson) by John Wiley & Sons, 1999.

C. The patient reported that he/she has been more successful at controlling critical and intimidating statements made to or about others.

D. The patient reported that there have been no recent incidents of harsh, critical, and intimidating statements made to or about others.

5. Angry/Tense Body Language (4)

A. The patient presented with verbalizations of anger as well as tense, rigid muscles and glaring facial expressions.

B. The patient expressed his/her anger with bodily signs of muscle tension, clenched fists, and refusal to make eye contact.

C. The patient appeared more relaxed, less angry, and did not exhibit physical signs of aggression.

D. The patient's family reported that he/she has been more relaxed within the home setting and has not shown glaring looks or pounded his/her fists on the table.

6. Passive/Aggressive Behavior (5)

A. The patient described a history of passive-aggressive behavior in which he/she would not comply with directions, would complain about authority figures behind their backs, and would not meet expected behavioral norms.

B. The patient's family confirmed a pattern of the patient's passive-aggressive behavior in which he/she would make promises of doing something, but not follow through.

C. The patient acknowledged that he/she tends to express anger indirectly through social withdrawal or uncooperative behavior, rather than using assertiveness to express feelings directly.

D. The patient has reported an increase in assertively expressing thoughts and feelings and terminating passive-aggressive behavior patterns.

7. Challenging Authority (6)

A. The patient's history shows a consistent pattern of challenging or disrespectful treatment of authority figures.

B. The patient acknowledged that he/she becomes angry quickly when someone in authority gives direction to him/her.

C. The patient's disrespectful treatment of authority has often erupted in explosive, aggressive outbursts.

D. The patient has made progress in controlling his/her overreactivity to taking direction from those in authority and is responding with more acts of cooperation.

8. Verbal Abuse (7)

A. The patient acknowledged that he/she frequently engages in verbal abuse of others as a means of expressing anger or frustration with them.

B. Significant others in the patient's family have indicated that they have been hurt by his/her frequent verbal abuse toward them.

C. The patient has shown little empathy toward others for the pain that he/she has caused because of his/her verbal abuse of them.

D. The patient has become more aware of his/her pattern of verbal abuse of others and is becoming more sensitive to the negative impact of this behavior on them.

E. There have been no recent incidents of verbal abuse of others by the patient.

INTERVENTIONS IMPLEMENTED

1. Identify Anger (1)

A. The patient was assisted in becoming more aware of the frequency with which he/she experiences anger and the signs of it in his/her life.

B. Situations were reviewed in which the patient experienced anger but refused to acknowledge it or minimized the experience.

C. The patient has acknowledged that he/she is frequently angry and has problems with anger management.

2. Assign Books on Anger (2)

A. The patient was asked to read *Of Course You're Angry* (Rosellini and Worden) or *The Angry Book* (Rubin) to increase his/her understanding and experiencing of anger.

B. The patient followed through and read the assigned material on anger, and key ideas from this material were processed within the session.

C. The patient has not followed through on reading the assigned material and was encouraged to do so.

D. The patient reported learning a lot from the material that was assigned, and he/she stated that he/she is more aware of the causes for and targets of his/her anger.

3. Assign Anger Journal (3)

A. The patient was assigned to keep a daily journal in which he/she would document persons or situations that cause anger, irritation, or disappointment.

B. The patient has kept a journal of anger-producing situations, and this material was processed within the session.

C. The patient has become more aware of the causes for and targets of his/her anger as a result of journaling these experiences on a daily basis.

4. List Targets of/Causes for Anger (4)

A. The patient was assigned to list as many of the causes for and targets of his/her anger that he/she is aware of.

B. The patient's list of targets for and causes of anger was processed in order to increase his/her awareness of anger management issues.

C. The patient has indicated a greater sensitivity to his/her angry feelings and the causes for them as a result of focusing his/her attention on these issues.

5. Confront Session Anger (5)

A. When the patient seemed to be experiencing anger during the session, but would minimize or deny it, he/she was confronted.

* The numbers in parentheses correlate to the number of the Therapeutic Intervention statement in the companion chapter with the same title in *The Complete Adult Psychotherapy Treatment Planner,* second edition (Jongsma and Peterson) by John Wiley & Sons, 1999.

B. The patient reacted with increased denial, minimization, and rationalization when confronted about his/her feelings of anger.

C. The patient has become more accepting of his/her feelings of anger being confronted.

D. The patient's anger, reflected back to him/her, has increased his/her awareness of feelings of anger.

6. Anger Management Group Referral (6)

A. The patient was referred to a group that teaches anger management and sensitivity to the feelings of others.

B. The patient has followed through with the referral to an anger management group and has attended consistently.

C. The patient has refused to follow the recommendation to attend an anger management class.

D. The patient has developed, through attending an anger management group, an increased awareness of his/her anger expression patterns and a means of anger control.

7. Identify Anger Expression Models (7)

A. The patient was assisted in identifying key figures in his/her life that have provided examples to him/her as to how to positively or negatively express anger.

B. The patient identified several key figures who have been negative role models in expressing anger explosively and destructively.

C. The patient acknowledged that he/she manages his/her anger in the same way that an explosive parent figure had done when he/she was growing up.

D. The patient was encouraged to identify positive role models throughout his/her life that he/she could respect for their management of angry feelings.

E. The patient acknowledged that others have been influential in teaching him/her destructive patterns of anger management.

8. List Own Hurtful Experiences (8)

A. The patient was assisted in identifying those painful and hurtful experiences from his/her past that have led to feelings of anger and revenge.

B. The patient reported a significant history of verbal and physical abuse, which fueled his/her anger toward others.

C. As the patient has shared experiences of pain and hurt from the past, he/she has become less reactive with anger in the present.

9. Empathize with Hurtful Feelings (9)

A. The therapist empathized with the patient's pain from past hurtful experiences and assisted him/her in clarifying reasons for this pain and the other feelings that were triggered by the pain.

B. The patient's traumas of the past were explored to help him/her clarify his/her feelings of hurt, disappointment, and suppressed rage.

C. As the patient has gained understanding and empathy within the therapy sessions regarding his/her feelings of pain from past traumas, his/her expressions of anger have diminished.

10. Assign Assertiveness Classes (10)

A. The patient was assigned to attend assertiveness training classes to gain a greater understanding of ways to express feelings directly, constructively, and in a controlled fashion.

B. The patient has followed through with attendance at assertiveness training classes and has learned more adaptive ways to express thoughts and feelings.

C. The patient has not followed through on the recommendation to attend assertiveness classes and was encouraged to do so.

D. The patient's attendance at assertiveness training has taught him/her increased skills at expressing himself/herself with control.

11. Process Recent Anger Outbursts (11)

A. Incidents of recent anger outbursts by the patient were processed, and alternative adaptive ways to express that anger were reviewed.

B. The patient has begun to implement alternative, positive ways to express anger in a controlled fashion.

C. The patient expressed feeling good about the fact that he/she was capable of expressing anger in a more controlled, assertive way that did not negatively impact others.

12. Role-Play Anger Control (12)

A. Role-playing techniques were used to teach the patient non-self-defeating ways of managing angry feelings.

B. The patient has learned to utilize assertive methods versus aggressive methods to express anger.

C. The patient has implemented assertive methods learned through the role-playing techniques and has reported success at managing anger more adaptively.

13. Assign Anger Management Exercise (13)

A. The patient was assigned an anger management exercise from a workbook.

B. The patient completed the assigned anger management exercise, and the material produced was processed.

C. The patient has learned to decrease the number and duration of his/her angry outbursts as a result of completing the workbook exercise.

D. The patient has not followed through with completing the assigned workbook exercise on anger management and was encouraged to do so.

14. Teach Relaxation Techniques (14)

A. The patient was taught deep-muscle relaxation, rhythmic breathing, and positive imagery as ways to reduce muscle tension when feelings of anger are experienced.

B. The patient has implemented the relaxation techniques and reported decreased reactivity when experiencing anger.

C. The patient has not implemented the relaxation techniques and continues to feel quite stressed in the face of anger.

15. List Negative Anger Impact (15)

A. The patient was assisted in listing ways that his/her explosive expression of anger has negatively impacted his/her life.

B. The patient identified many negative consequences that have resulted from his/her poor anger management.

C. The patient's denial about the negative impact of his/her anger has decreased, and he/she has verbalized an increased awareness of the negative impact of his/her behavior.

16. Identify Bodily Impact of Anger (16)

A. The patient was taught the negative impact that anger can have on bodily functions and systems.

B. The patient indicated an increased awareness of the stress of his/her anger on such things as heart, brain, and blood pressure.

C. The patient has tried to reduce the frequency with which he/she experiences anger in order to reduce the negative impact that anger has on bodily systems.

17. Empty-Chair Technique (17)

A. The empty-chair technique was used to approach the patient in expressing angry feelings in a constructive, non-self-defeating manner.

B. The patient identified several instances in his/her daily life in which the adaptive means of expressing anger, learned through the empty-chair technique, were able to be used.

C. The patient reported success at implementing constructive ways of expressing anger and terminating verbal and physical abusive ways of expressing anger.

18. Identify Anger Triggers (18)

A. The patient was assisted in increasing his/her ability to recognize triggers that lead to explosive expressions of anger.

B. The triggers for anger experience were listed, and coping mechanisms for each trigger were identified.

C. The patient has implemented effective coping mechanisms for his/her hot buttons for anger, and this has reduced aggressive anger expression.

19. Utilize Rational Emotive Therapy Techniques (19)

A. The patient was trained in the use of rational emotive therapy (RET) techniques for coping with feelings of anger, frustration, and rage.

B. The patient has implemented the techniques that he/she learned in managing anger.

C. The patient has successfully implemented rational emotive therapy techniques to reduce aggressive reaction to anger triggers.

20. Assign Anger Letter (20)

A. The patient was asked to write a letter expressing his/her feelings of anger toward the targets of those feelings, focusing on the reasons for his/her anger toward that person.

B. The patient has written an anger letter and his/her reasons for feeling anger were processed.

C. The patient reported that his/her feelings of anger have diminished since he/she wrote the anger letter and processed the causes for his/her anger.

21. Encourage Anger Expression (21)

A. The patient was encouraged to express and release his/her feelings of rage and violent urges that are felt toward others.

B. The patient was cautioned to exercise control over these feelings even though he/she was encouraged to express such angry feelings within the session.

C. The patient showed a high degree of rage and seemed to indicate little interest in trying to control it.

D. The processing of the patient's feelings of anger and rage have diminished these feelings and increased his/her sense of control over them.

22. Teach Forgiveness (22)

A. The patient was taught about the process of forgiveness and encouraged to begin to implement this process as a means of letting go of his/her feelings of strong anger.

B. The patient focused on the perpetrators of pain from the past, and he/she was encouraged to target them for forgiveness.

C. The advantages of implementing forgiveness versus holding onto vengeful anger were processed with the patient.

D. The patient has committed himself/herself to attempting to begin the process of forgiveness with the perpetrators of pain.

23. Assign *Forgive and Forget* (23)

A. The patient was assigned to read the book *Forgive and Forget* (Smedes) to increase his/her sensitivity to the process of forgiveness.

B. The patient has read the book *Forgive and Forget*, and key concepts were processed within the session.

C. The patient has not followed through with completing the reading assignment of *Forgive and Forget* and was encouraged to do so.

D. The patient acknowledged that holding onto angry feelings has distinct disadvantages over his/her beginning the process of forgiveness.

24. Assign Forgiveness Letter (24)

A. The patient was asked to write a letter of forgiveness to the target of his/her anger as a step toward letting go of that anger.

B. The patient has followed through with writing a letter of forgiveness to the perpetrator of pain from his/her past, and this was processed within the session.

C. The patient has not followed through with writing the forgiveness letter and is very resistive to letting go of his/her feelings of angry revenge.

D. Writing and processing the letter of forgiveness have reduced the patient's feelings of anger and increased his/her capacity to control its expression.

ANTISOCIAL BEHAVIOR

PATIENT PRESENTATION

1. Adolescent Antisocial History (1)

A. The patient confirmed that his/her history of rule breaking, lying, physical aggression, and/or disrespect for others and the law began when he/she was a teenager.

B. The patient reported that he/she was often incarcerated within the juvenile justice system for illegal activities.

C. The patient acknowledged that his/her substance abuse paralleled his/her antisocial behavior dating back to adolescence.

2. Dysfunctional Childhood History (1)

A. The patient described instances from his/her childhood in which severe and abusive punishment resulted whenever a parent laid blame on him/her for some perceived negative behavior.

B. The patient described a history of experiences in which he/she was unfairly blamed for others' behavior, leading to feelings of resentment of authority and a pattern of lying to avoid punishment.

C. The patient provided examples from his/her own childhood of instances where parent figures consistently projected blame for their behavior onto others, causing the patient to learn and practice this same behavior.

D. The patient began to verbalize some insight into how previous instances of pain in childhood are causing current attitudes of detachment from the concerns of others and a focus on self-protection and self-interest.

E. The patient began to understand how his/her own attitudes of aggression are the result of having learned to accept and normalize aggression during childhood abusive experiences.

3. Blaming/Projecting (2)

A. The patient showed an attitude of blaming others for his/her problems.

B. The patient refused to take responsibility for his/her own behavior and decisions; instead, he/she pointed at the behavior of others as the cause for his/her decisions and actions.

C. Interpersonal conflicts are blamed on others without taking any responsibility for the problem.

D. The patient is beginning to accept responsibility for his/her own behavior and to make fewer statements of projection of responsibility for his/her actions onto others.

E. The patient is gradually accepting more responsibility for his/her behavior and increasing the frequency of such statements.

4. Rule Breaking (3)

A. The patient's behavior pattern confirms his/her attitude of disregard for rules within academic, social, or employment settings.

* The numbers in parentheses correlate to the number of the Behavioral Definition statement in the companion chapter with the same title in *The Complete Adult Psychotherapy Treatment Planner,* second edition (Jongsma and Peterson) by John Wiley & Sons, 1999.

B. The patient verbalized that he/she sees rules as applying to others but not to himself/herself.

C. The patient is beginning to accept the need for rules within any society and to apply them to himself/herself.

D. The patient has not had a recent incident of breaking rules and is more compliant.

5. Reckless/Thrill Seeking (4)

A. The patient reported having engaged in reckless, adventure-seeking behaviors, showing a high need for excitement, having fun, and living on the edge.

B. The patient described a series of reckless actions but showed no consideration for the consequences of such actions.

C. The patient has begun to control his/her reckless impulses and reported that he/she is trying to think of the consequences before acting recklessly.

6. Lying (5)

A. The patient reported a pattern of lying to cover up his/her responsibility for actions with little shame or anxiety attached to this pattern of lying.

B. The patient seemed to be lying within the session.

C. The patient acknowledged that his/her lying produced conflicts within relationships and distrust from others.

D. The patient has committed himself/herself to attempting to be more honest in his/her interpersonal relationships.

7. Sexual Promiscuity (6)

A. The patient reported a history of repeated sexual encounters with partners with whom there is little or no emotional attachment.

B. The patient's described sexual behaviors are focused on self-gratification only and reflect no interest in the needs or welfare of the partner.

C. The patient acknowledged that his/her sexual behavior has no basis in respect or expression of commitment to a long-term relationship.

D. The patient reported that he/she would like to develop a relationship in which sexual intimacy was a reflection of commitment and caring, rather than merely sexual release.

8. Aggressive/Argumentative (7)

A. The patient presented in a hostile, angry, and uncooperative manner.

B. The patient was intimidating in his/her style of interaction.

C. The patient is trying to interact in a more cooperative manner within social and employment settings.

D. The patient is showing less irritability and argumentativeness within therapy sessions.

9. Authority Conflicts (7)

A. The patient acknowledged a history of irritability, aggression, and argumentativeness when interacting with authority figures.

B. The patient's history of conflict with acceptance of authority has led to employment instability and legal problems.

C. The patient is beginning to accept direction from authority figures, recognizing his/her need to resist challenging such directives.

10. Lack of Remorse (8)

A. The patient, after describing his/her pattern of aggression or disrespect for others' feelings, showed no remorse for his/her behavior.

B. The patient projects blame for his/her hurtful behavior onto others, saying there was no alternative.

C. The patient is beginning to develop some sensitivity to the feelings of others and recognizes that he/she has hurt others.

D. The patient reported feelings of remorse and guilt over previous behaviors that were hurtful to others.

11. Verbal/Physical Aggression (9)

A. The patient reported physical encounters that have injured others or have threatened serious injury to others.

B. The patient showed little or no remorse for causing pain to others.

C. The patient projected blame for his/her aggressive encounters onto others.

D. The patient has a violent history and continues to interact with others in a very intimidating, aggressive style.

E. The patient has shown progress in controlling his/her aggressive patterns and seems to be trying to interact with more assertiveness than aggression.

12. Legal Conflicts (10)

A. The patient maintained a disregard for laws, rules, and authority figures.

B. The patient reported engaging in illegal activities in his/her current life.

C. The patient has repeatedly engaged in illegal activities in the past.

D. The patient often minimized the seriousness of his/her offenses against the law and other people's rights.

E. The patient acknowledged that his/her disregard for the law has resulted in serious problems and has pledged to live within the rules of society.

13. Impulsivity (11)

A. The patient has a pattern of impulsive behavior, which is demonstrated in his/her frequent geographical moves, traveling with little or no goals, and quitting one job after another.

B. The patient's impulsivity has resulted in a life of instability and negative consequences for him/her and others.

C. The patient has acknowledged that his/her life of impulsive reactivity has had many negative consequences, and he/she has committed to an effort of control over these impulses.

D. The patient has shown progress in controlling impulsive reactivity and now considers consequences of actions before quickly reacting.

14. Employment Conflicts (12)

A. The patient reported that authority conflicts have erupted in the employment situation.

B. The patient described coworker conflicts where he/she does not trust others and does work as part of a team.

C. The patient's work history is very unstable, in that he/she has held many different jobs with little or no longevity to them.

D. The patient acknowledged a need to develop a tolerance for frustration within the work situation and accept authority that will give him/her direction within that setting.

E. The patient has maintained employment for the longest period of time in his/her life.

15. Irresponsible Parenting (13)

A. As the patient began to acknowledge a history of irresponsible parenting, he/she also tried to minimize the consequences and project blame for these actions onto others.

B. The patient described a feeling of love and devotion to his/her children, but, behaviorally, there is little evidence of it.

C. The patient has not paid child support on a regular basis nor shown consistent interest in the welfare of his/her children.

D. The patient acknowledged some guilt over his/her lack of responsible parenting and has committed to behaving in a more responsible and consistent manner to support them.

E. The patient has initiated responsible behavior toward the children in terms of financial support and consistent contact.

INTERVENTIONS IMPLEMENTED

1. Take History/Confront Denial (1)

A. The patient's history of illegal activities was collected.

B. The patient was confronted consistently on his/her attempts to utilize minimizations, denial, or projection of the blame onto others for which he/she was responsible.

C. The patient's history was explored for instances of unkind, insensitive behavior that trampled on the feelings and rights of others.

2. List Antisocial Consequences (2)

A. The patient was asked to list the negative consequences that have accrued to him/her due to his/her antisocial behavior.

B. The patient was confronted with the fact that his/her antisocial behavior results in others losing respect for him/her, loss of freedom for him/her due to legal consequences, and loss of self-respect.

C. The patient was consistently reminded of the pain that others suffer as a result of his/her antisocial behavior.

D. The patient was asked to list others who have been negatively impacted by his/her antisocial behavior and the specific pain that they have suffered.

E. The patient was confronted with the fear, disappointment, loss of trust, and loss of respect that results in others as a consequence of his/her lack of sensitivity and self-centered behavior.

* The numbers in parentheses correlate to the number of the Therapeutic Intervention statement in the companion chapter with the same title in *The Complete Adult Psychotherapy Treatment Planner,* second edition (Jongsma and Peterson) by John Wiley & Sons, 1999.

3. Identify Trust Loss (3)

A. The patient was reminded that his/her behavior of broken promises, insensitivity, and trampling on the rights of others results in broken relationships as others lose trust in him/her.

B. The patient was consistently reminded that any meaningful relationship is based on trust that the other person will treat you with kindness and respect.

C. The patient's behavior pattern was reviewed as to how he/she treated others with a lack of respect and a lack of kindness, and how these actions resulted in the loss of trust in the relationship.

4. Confront Lawlessness (4)

A. The patient's pattern of unlawful behavior was reviewed, and he/she was reminded that if everyone in society adopted his/her unlawful attitude, anarchy would result.

B. The patient was taught that respect for law and order and the rights of others is the only way that a civilized society can function.

5. Solicit Commitment to Lawfulness (5)

A. The patient was asked to give his/her commitment to living within the laws of society.

B. The patient was asked to give a rationale for a prosocial, law-abiding lifestyle being adopted.

C. The patient was asked to list 10 reasons why he/she would commit himself/herself to a law-abiding lifestyle.

6. Inhibit Future Lawlessness (6)

A. The patient was firmly and consistently reminded of the negative legal consequences that would accrue to him/her if continued lawlessness was practiced.

B. The patient was asked to list six future negative consequences of continued antisocial behavior.

7. Review Broken Relationships (7)

A. The patient was asked to list any and all relationships that have been lost due to his/her pattern of antisocial behavior.

B. As lost relationships were reviewed, the patient was confronted with his/her responsibility for the actions that resulted in the broken relationships.

C. As broken relationships were reviewed, the patient was asked to identify what behavior of his/her own led to the broken relationship.

8. Confront Responsibility for Broken Relationships (8)

A. The patient was firmly and consistently confronted with the reality of his/her own behavior that caused pain to others and resulted in their breaking of the relationship.

B. The patient was asked to identify how he/she was insensitive to the needs and feelings of others.

C. Role reversal techniques were used as an attempt to get the patient in touch with the pain that he/she has caused in others due to disrespect, disloyalty, aggression, or dishonesty.

9. Confront Self-Centeredness (9)

A. The patient was taught, through role playing and role reversal, the value of being empathetic to the needs, rights, and feelings of others.

B. The patient presented his/her attitude of "look out for number one" as the only way to live.

C. The patient justified his/her self-focused attitude as the way that he/she learned to live because of the abuse and abandonment suffered as a child.

D. Attempts were made to get the patient to view his/her own behavior from another person's perspective.

10. Teach the Value of Honesty (10)

A. The patient was asked to list the benefits of honesty and reliability for himself/herself and others.

B. The patient was taught the absolute necessity for honesty as the basis for trust in all forms of human relationships as examples of the different forms of relationships that are based in trust and honesty were reviewed.

C. The patient was asked to list the positive effects for others when he/she is honest and reliable.

11. List Dishonesty Consequences (11)

A. The patient was asked to list the positive effects for others when he/she is honest and reliable.

B. The patient was taught that pain and disappointment result when honesty and reliability are not given the highest priority in one's life.

12. Solicit a Commitment to Honesty (12)

A. The patient was asked to make a commitment to live a life based in honesty and reliability.

B. The patient was asked to sign a behavioral contract that focuses on keeping promises and being responsible to others.

C. The patient was asked to list five reasons why he/she should make a commitment to be honest and reliable.

13. Teach Empathy (13)

A. The patient was taught, through role playing and role reversal, the value of being empathetic to the needs, rights, and feelings of others.

B. The patient was asked to commit himself/herself to acting more sensitively to the rights and feelings of others.

14. Confront Disrespect (14)

A. The patient was confronted consistently and firmly when he/she exhibited an attitude of disrespect and rudeness toward the rights and feelings of others.

B. It was emphasized to the patient firmly and consistently that others have a right to boundaries to privacy and respect for their feelings and property.

15. Solicit Kind Actions (15)

A. The patient was required, in an attempt to get him/her to focus on the needs and feelings of others, to list three actions that would be performed as acts of kindness toward someone else.

B. The patient signed a contract in which he/she committed to performing three acts of service toward the community or others that would not result in direct benefit to himself/herself.

C. The patient's acts of kindness were reviewed, and the feelings associated with performing this assignment were processed.

16. Solicit an Apology (16)

A. The patient was asked to make a list of those people who deserve an apology because they were injured by the patient's insensitive, impulsive, aggressive, or dishonest behavior.

B. The patient was confronted when he/she attempted to project the blame for his/her aggressive or dishonest actions onto others.

17. Teach Acceptance of Responsibility (17)

A. The value of taking full responsibility for one's own behavior and then apologizing for the pain caused to others because of that behavior was reviewed and emphasized.

B. Role playing and modeling were used to teach how to apologize.

18. Review Elements of Apology (18)

A. The specific steps were laid out that would be necessary to begin to make amends to others who have been hurt by the patient's behavior.

B. The patient was asked to make a commitment to carry out those necessary steps that would make restitution for the hurt caused to others.

C. Behavioral rehearsal was used to teach how to make amends or give an apology to those who have been hurt by the patient's behavior.

D. The patient's implementation of apologizing to others was reviewed, and the feelings associated with this action were processed.

E. The patient was strongly reinforced for taking responsibility for causing pain to others and apologizing for this behavior.

19. Review Work Authority Conflicts (19)

A. The patient was asked to list the most important rules that should govern his/her behavior within the work setting.

B. The patient was assisted in developing a specific list of rules and duties related to the patient's employment behavior.

C. The patient reviewed the expectations regarding how he/she should respond to authority figures within the employment setting.

D. Role playing was used to teach respectful responses to directives from authority figures.

20. Reinforce Employment Attendance (20)

A. The patient's attendance at work and his/her respect for authority was reviewed and reinforced.

B. The patient was asked to keep a journal of work attendance and instances of acceptance of directives from authority figures.

C. The patient's work records and journal material were reviewed, and successful prosocial behavior was reinforced.

21. Teach Prosocial Work Behavior (21)

A. The patient was asked to list those negative behaviors that have led to conflicts within the work setting both with coworkers and authority figures.

B. The patient was assisted in developing prosocial responses toward resolving conflicts with coworkers and acceptance of directives from authority figures.

C. The patient has implemented more prosocial responses at work, and the positive results of this attitude were reviewed.

22. Confront Irresponsible Parenting (22)

A. The patient was asked to acknowledge and accept responsibility for a history of avoiding the obligations of parenthood.

B. The patient was confronted with a pattern of his/her behavior that demonstrates a lack of acceptance of responsibility for being a nurturant parent.

C. The patient was asked to list incidences from his/her past that are examples of avoidance of the responsibilities of parenting.

23. Reinforce Responsible Parenting (23)

A. The patient was asked to list specific behaviors that would indicate that he/she was taking on the responsibilities of being a reliable, responsible, and nurturant parent.

B. The patient was asked to list potential consequences to himself/herself and the children of avoiding the responsibilities of parenting.

24. Solicit a Commitment to Responsible Parenting (24)

A. The patient was assisted in developing a list of concrete steps that could be taken to demonstrate reliable, responsible parenting behavior.

B. The patient was asked to make a commitment toward implementation of specific steps that would demonstrate responsible parenting.

C. The patient has begun to implement specific steps toward demonstrating responsible parenting, and he/she was reinforced for this change in behavior.

D. The positive impact of the patient's implementation of positive parenting behavior was reviewed.

25. Confront Projection (25)

A. The patient was consistently confronted whenever he/she failed to take responsibility for his/her own actions and instead placed blame for them onto others.

B. As the patient's pattern of projecting blame for his/her actions onto others began to weaken, he/she was reinforced for taking personal responsibility.

C. The importance of taking responsibility for one's own behavior and the positive implications for this as to motivating change were reviewed.

26. Explore Reasons for Blaming (26)

A. The patient's history was explored with a focus on causes for the avoidance of acceptance of responsibility for behavior.

B. The patient's history of physical and emotional abuse was explored.

C. The patient's early history of lying was explored as to causes and consequences.

D. Parental modeling of projection of responsibility for their behavior was examined.

27. Reinforce Taking Personal Responsibility (27)

A. The patient was verbally reinforced in a strong and consistent manner when he/she took responsibility for his/her own behavior.

B. The patient was taught how others develop respect for someone who takes responsibility for his/her actions and admits to mistakes.

28. Explore Childhood Abuse and Neglect (28)

A. The patient described instances from his/her own childhood of emotional, verbal, and physical abuse.

B. The patient described feelings of hurt, depression, abandonment, and fear related to parental abuse or neglect.

C. The patient was rather matter-of-fact in his/her description and showed little affect while describing a history of violence within the family during his/her childhood.

D. The patient tended to minimize the negative impact of physical abuse that he/she suffered and, at times, even excused the behavior as something that he/she deserved.

29. Review Emotional Detachment (29)

A. The patient's pattern of emotional detachment from others was reviewed.

B. It was pointed out to the patient that his/her childhood history of abuse and neglect has led to a pattern of emotional detachment in current relationships.

30. Teach Forgiveness (30)

A. The patient was taught the value of forgiveness as a means of overcoming pain and hurt, rather than holding onto it and acting out the anger that results from it.

B. The patient was asked to list those parent figures from his/her childhood that have caused him/her pain and suffering.

C. The patient was assisted in developing a list of benefits of beginning a process of forgiveness toward those perpetrators of pain in his/her childhood.

31. Process Distrust (31)

A. The patient was asked to verbalize what he/she could be afraid of in placing trust in others.

B. The patient's fear of being taken advantage of, being disappointed, being abandoned, or being abused when trust is placed in another person were processed.

32. Encourage Trust (32)

A. The patient was assisted in identifying some personal thoughts and feelings that he/she could disclose to another person as a means of beginning the process of showing trust in others.

B. The patient was assisted in identifying one or two other people within his/her life that he/she could trust with personal information.

C. The patient was asked to commit to making a disclosure to a significant other that would demonstrate trust.

33. Process Trust Exercise (33)

A. The patient's feelings of anxiety regarding trusting someone were explored.

B. The patient's experience with placing trust in another person was reviewed, and the success was reinforced.

ANXIETY

PATIENT PRESENTATION

1. Excessive Worry (1)

A. The patient described symptoms of preoccupation with worry that something dire will happen.

B. The patient showed some recognition that his/her excessive worry is beyond the scope of rationality, but he/she feels unable to control it.

C. The patient described that he/she worries about issues related to family, personal safety, health, and employment, among other things.

D. The patient reported that his/her worry about life circumstances has diminished, and he/she is living with more of a sense of peace and confidence.

2. Motor Tension (2)

A. The patient described a history of restlessness, tiredness, muscle tension, and shaking.

B. The patient moved about in his/her chair frequently and sat stiffly.

C. The patient said that he/she is unable to relax and is always restless and stressed.

D. The patient reported that he/she has been successful at reducing levels of tension and increasing levels of relaxation.

3. Autonomic Hyperactivity (3)

A. The patient reported the presence of symptoms such as heart palpitations, dry mouth, tightness in the throat, and some shortness of breath.

B. The patient reported periods of nausea and some diarrhea when anxiety levels escalate.

C. The patient stated that occasional tension headaches are also occurring along with other anxiety-related symptoms.

D. Anxiety-related symptoms have diminished as the patient has learned new coping mechanisms.

4. Hypervigilance (4)

A. The patient related that he/she is constantly feeling on edge, that sleep is interrupted, and that concentration is difficult.

B. The patient reported being irritable and snappy in interaction with others as his/her patience is thin and he/she is worrying about everything.

C. The patient's family members report that he/she is difficult to get along with as his/her irritability is high.

D. The patient's level of tension has decreased, sleep has improved, and irritability has diminished as new anxiety-coping skills have been implemented.

---

* The numbers in parentheses correlate to the number of the Behavioral Definition statement in the companion chapter with the same title in *The Complete Adult Psychotherapy Treatment Planner,* second edition (Jongsma and Peterson) by John Wiley & Sons, 1999.

INTERVENTIONS IMPLEMENTED

1. Build Trust (1)

A. Unconditional positive regard and warm acceptance were used to increase rapport and build trust with the patient.

B. As the patient's trust level increased, he/she was able to tell his/her story of the experience of anxiety.

C. The patient described his/her attempts to resolve the anxiety problem.

D. The patient was quite open in describing triggers for anxiety and coping attempts.

2. Challenge Anxiety Bases (2)

A. The patient was asked to produce evidence of the anxiety and any logical basis for him/her to worry to such an extensive degree.

B. Challenging the patient's irrational basis for the anxiety has caused him/her to reexamine the anxiety problem.

C. The patient has begun to challenge himself/herself and to label his/her fear as unfounded.

3. List Life Conflicts (3)

A. The patient was asked to list his/her important past and present life conflicts that may contribute to his/her feelings of worry.

B. The patient's list of life conflicts that trigger anxiety were processed.

C. The patient has been able to clarify the causes for his/her worry and to put them into better perspective.

4. Identify Unresolved Conflicts (4)

A. The patient was assisted in becoming aware of unresolved life conflicts that contribute to his/her persistent fears.

B. The patient was assisted in clarifying his/her feelings of anxiety as they relate to unresolved life conflicts.

C. The patient was assisted in identifying steps that could be taken to begin resolving issues in his/her life that contribute to persistent fear and worry.

D. As the patient has worked toward resolving unresolved conflicts, his/her feelings of anxiety have diminished.

5. Assign *Ten Days to Self-Esteem!* (5)

A. The patient was asked to complete exercises in the anxiety section of the book *Ten Days to Self-Esteem!* (Burns).

B. The patient was able to identify cognitive distortions that generate anxiety after he/she worked on the anxiety exercise in *Ten Days to Self-Esteem!*.

C. The patient reported increased sensitivity to his/her own tendency to distort thoughts that precipitate anxiety.

---

* The numbers in parentheses correlate to the number of the Therapeutic Intervention statement in the companion chapter with the same title in *The Complete Adult Psychotherapy Treatment Planner,* second edition (Jongsma and Peterson) by John Wiley & Sons, 1999.

6. Medication Referral (6)

A. The patient was referred to a physician to evaluate him/her for psychotropic medication to reduce symptoms of anxiety.

B. The patient has completed an evaluation by the physician and has begun taking anti-anxiety medications.

C. The patient has resisted the referral to a physician and does not want to take any medication to reduce anxiety levels.

7. Monitor Medication Compliance (7)

A. The patient's compliance with the physician's prescription for psychotropic medication was monitored as to the medication's effectiveness and side effects.

B. The patient reported that the medication has been beneficial to him/her in reducing his/her experience of anxiety symptoms.

C. The patient reported that the medication does not seem to be helpful in reducing anxiety experiences.

D. The therapist conferred with the physician to discuss the patient's reaction to the psychotropic medication, and adjustments were made by the physician in the prescription.

8. Guided Imagery Training (8)

A. The patient was trained in the use of positive guided imagery that will induce relaxation as a coping mechanism to reduce anxiety symptoms.

B. The patient reported that using positive guided imagery has been effective in reducing the experience of anxiety.

C. The patient has not followed through with the implementation of guided imagery to reduce the experience of stress and anxiety.

9. Utilize Biofeedback (9)

A. EMG biofeedback techniques were used to facilitate the patient learning relaxation skills.

B. The patient reported that he/she has implemented his/her use of relaxation skills in daily life to reduce levels of muscle tension and the experience of anxiety.

C. The patient has not followed through on implementation of relaxation skills to reduce anxiety symptoms.

D. The patient reported that his/her level of anxiety has decreased since relaxation techniques were implemented.

10. Assign *Relaxation and Stress Reduction Workbook* (10)

A. The patient was assigned to read about one of the stress reduction techniques in the *Relaxation and Stress Reduction Workbook* (Davis, Eshelman, and McKay) and to then implement this chosen technique in daily life.

B. The patient has followed through with learning a new stress reduction technique from the *Relaxation and Stress Reduction Workbook* and is attempting to implement it on a daily basis.

C. The patient's implementation of the stress reduction technique has successfully reduced his/her experience of anxiety.

11. Teach Behavioral Coping Strategies (11)

A. The patient was taught behavioral coping strategies that are effective in reducing anxiety.

B. The patient was encouraged to increase his/her social involvement and to utilize physical exercise as a means of reducing stress.

C. The patient was encouraged to obtain consistent employment in order to reduce his/her preoccupation with anxiety-related symptoms.

D. As the patient has implemented behavioral coping strategies, his/her level of anxiety has successfully been reduced.

12. Confront Irrational Fears (12)

A. The patient's fears were examined closely, and he/she was assisted in identifying the irrational nature of his/her persistent worry.

B. As the patient has increased his/her awareness of the irrational nature of his/her excessive and persistent worries, a sense of peace and reassurance has been established.

C. Although the patient is able to label his/her fears as irrational, he/she continues to experience significant anxiety symptoms related to them.

13. Analyze Fears Logically (13)

A. The patient's fears were analyzed by examining the probability of his/her negative expectation becoming a reality, the consequences of the expectation if it occurred, his/her ability to control the outcome, the worst possible result if the expectation occurred, and his/her ability to cope if the expectation occurred.

B. The patient's ability to control the outcome of circumstances was examined, and the effectiveness of his/her worry on that outcome was examined also.

C. Cognitive therapy techniques have been effective at helping the patient understand his/her beliefs and distorted messages that produce worry and anxiety.

D. As the patient has increased his/her understanding of distorted, anxiety-producing cognitions, his/her anxiety level has diminished.

14. Explore Cognitive Messages (14)

A. The patient's cognitive, anxiety-mediating messages were identified.

B. The patient was assisted in developing positive, realistic, alternative thoughts that could mediate confidence, self-assurance, and relaxation.

C. As the patient has learned to implement positive self-talk, his/her anxiety level has diminished.

15. Develop Insight into Past Traumas (15)

A. The patient's past traumatic experiences that have become triggers for anxiety were examined.

B. The patient has developed insight into how past traumatic experiences have led to anxiety in present unrelated circumstances.

C. The patient's development of insight regarding past traumas has resulted in a reduction in the experience of anxiety.

16. Develop Positive Cognitions (16)

A. The patient was assisted in developing reality-based cognitive messages that will increase self-confidence in coping with irrational fears.

B. As the patient has learned positive self-talk and has implemented it in his/her daily life, anxiety has diminished.

C. The patient reported increased self-confidence since instituting positive self-talk.

D. The patient has found it difficult to implement positive self-talk, as he/she continues to be preoccupied with distorted, anxiety-mediating cognitive messages.

17. Teach Thought Stopping (17)

A. The patient was taught thought-stopping techniques that involve thinking of a stop sign and replacing negative thoughts with a pleasant scene.

B. The patient's implementation of the thought-stopping technique was monitored, and his/her success with this technique was reinforced.

C. The patient reported that the thought-stopping technique has been beneficial in reducing his/her preoccupation with anxiety-producing cognitions.

18. Assign "Cost-Benefit Analysis" (18)

A. The patient was asked to complete a "Cost-Benefit Analysis" as found in *Ten Days to Self-Esteem!* (Burns) in which he/she was asked to list the advantages and disadvantages of maintaining the anxiety.

B. Completing the "Cost-Benefit Analysis" exercise has been beneficial to the patient as he/she developed more insight into the impact of anxiety on his/her daily life.

C. The patient has not followed through on completing the "Cost-Benefit Analysis" of his/her anxiety and was encouraged to do so.

19. Assign *Friedman's Fables* (19)

A. *Friedman's Fables* (Friedman) was read within the session, and principles that pertain to anxiety reduction were processed with the patient.

B. The patient was able to verbalize some positive principles from the fables that reduce anxious thoughts.

C. The patient was not receptive to the fable exercise and could not identify any principles that he/she thought would be successful in helping him/her cope with anxiety.

20. Challenge Anxious Perspective (20)

A. The patient's persistent fears were challenged through the use of providing him/her with a more balanced, realistic perspective that was incompatible with anxiety-producing views.

B. The patient reported that his/her level of anxiety has diminished as he/she has implemented a more positive perspective on reality.

C. The patient has been successful at developing alternative views of reality that are more positive, and his/her anxiety has been reduced consistently with that change.

21. Utilize a Solution-Focused Approach (21)

A. The patient was assisted in identifying anxiety-coping skills that he/she has learned in the past and with which he/she has been successful at managing his/her anxiety.

B. The patient was assigned the task of consistently using successful coping mechanisms from the past to deal with present anxiety-related difficulties.

C. The patient reported success at reducing anxiety levels by using successful coping skills from the past.

D. The patient was unable to identify past successful coping mechanisms and believes that he/she has never successfully managed his/her anxiety.

22. Utilize Paradoxical Intervention (22)

A. A paradoxical intervention was developed with the patient in which he/she was encouraged to experience the anxiety at specific intervals each day for a defined length of time.

B. The patient has implemented the paradoxical intervention and reported that it was difficult for him/her to maintain the anxiety as he/she was eager to get on with other activities.

C. The patient has experienced, in general, a reduction of his/her anxiety as he/she has developed an insight into his/her ability to control it.

ATTENTION DEFICIT DISORDER (ADD)—ADULT

PATIENT PRESENTATION

1. ADD Childhood History (1)

A. The patient confirmed that his/her childhood history consisted of the following symptoms: behavioral problems at school, impulsivity, overexcitability, temper outbursts, and lack of concentration.

B. The patient had a diagnosed ADD condition in his/her childhood.

C. Although the patient's symptoms were not diagnosed as ADD, it can be concluded from the childhood symptoms that the ADD condition was present at that time.

2. Lack of Concentration (2)

A. The patient reported an inability to concentrate or pay attention to things of low interest, even though they may be important to his/her life.

B. The patient's lack of ability to concentrate has resulted in his/her missing out on the comprehension of important details.

C. The patient's ability to concentrate seems to be increasing as he/she reported increased attention skills.

3. Distractibility (3)

A. The patient reported that he/she is easily distracted, and his/her attention is drawn away from the task at hand.

B. The patient gave evidence of distractibility within today's session.

C. The patient's distractibility is diminishing, and his/her focused concentration is increasing.

4. Restless/Fidgety (4)

A. The patient reported that he/she cannot sit still for any length of time, but often feels restless and fidgety.

B. The patient gave evidence of being restless and fidgety within the session, often moving about in his/her chair.

C. The patient's ability to rest comfortably for a longer period of time has increased.

5. Impulsivity (5)

A. The patient reported a history of acting quickly without adequately thinking of the consequences, leading to negative results in his/her life.

B. The patient related incidences of making impulsive decisions that have resulted in harmful consequences for himself/herself and others.

C. The patient reported greater control over his/her impulses and is making more reasoned decisions.

---

* The numbers in parentheses correlate to the number of the Behavioral Definition statement in the companion chapter with the same title in *The Complete Adult Psychotherapy Treatment Planner,* second edition (Jongsma and Peterson) by John Wiley & Sons, 1999.

6. Rapid Mood Swings (6)

A. The patient reported that he/she has a history of rapid mood swings and general mood lability within short spans of time.

B. The patient reported that his/her mood can change several times throughout a day and that little frustrations can easily lead to anger or depression.

C. The patient's mood has begun to stabilize, and he/she is reporting less frequent mood swings.

D. The patient reported that he/she is not easily moved from a good mood to a bad mood in a short amount of time, as had been the case previously.

7. Disorganization (7)

A. The patient has a history of disorganization in many areas of his/her life.

B. The patient's disorganization is evident in areas related to home and work, leading him/her to be less efficient and less effective than he/she could be.

C. The patient has made significant progress in increasing his/her organization and is using that organization to become more efficient.

D. The patient uses lists and reminders to increase his/her organizational ability.

8. Lack of Project Completion (8)

A. The patient reported that he/she has started many projects and has a history of rarely finishing them.

B. Family members reported frustration at the patient's pattern of rarely finishing projects that he/she has begun.

C. The patient has shown progress in project completion and has moved to not begin a new project until the previous one is completed.

9. Low Frustration Tolerance (9)

A. The patient acknowledged that he/she is quite irritable and can become angry with only minor irritants.

B. The patient demonstrated within the session that he/she is quite irritable, becoming angry with only slight provocation.

C. The patient's family members indicate that he/she has an explosive temper, which has caused him/her to be out of control and abusive at times.

D. The patient reported that he/she has better control over his/her anger and has learned to increase his/her frustration tolerance.

10. Low Stress Tolerance (10)

A. The patient acknowledged that he/she has a low stress tolerance and is easily frustrated or upset.

B. The patient is making an effort to control his/her frustration and to remain calm in the face of stress.

C. The patient has demonstrated a calmer demeanor within the sessions and is not so easily upset.

D. The patient reported that several incidents have occurred recently that he/she has been able to accept easily, even though they were frustrating.

11. Low Self-Esteem (11)

A. The patient reported a history of feeling inadequate compared with others dating back to childhood.

B. The patient's low self-esteem was evident in his/her self-critical statements, lack of confidence in his/her abilities, and social withdrawal.

C. The patient is beginning to show evidence of improved self-esteem as he/she occasionally makes positive self-descriptive statements and has been willing to take some risk to get involved in new activities.

12. Addictive Behaviors (12)

A. The patient indicated that he/she has engaged in substance abuse on an impulsive basis and has used substances to cope with the frustration of distractibility and failure.

B. The patient acknowledged that substance abuse has not been beneficial and has led to negative consequences in his/her life.

C. The patient is committed to termination of substance abuse.

D. The patient has been successful at abstinence from substance abuse.

E. The patient has accepted a referral to substance abuse treatment to deal with his/her addictive behavior.

INTERVENTIONS IMPLEMENTED

1. Psychological Testing (1)

A. The patient was administered psychological testing in order to establish or rule out the presence of an ADD problem.

B. Psychological testing has established the presence of an ADD problem.

C. The psychological testing failed to confirm the presence of ADD.

2. Process Psychological Testing Results (2)

A. The psychological testing results were processed with the patient to assist him/her in understanding his/her condition and to answer any questions that he/she might have.

B. The patient understood the explanation of the psychological testing and has accepted the presence of an ADD problem.

C. The patient has denied the presence of ADD and refused to accept the confirming results of the psychological testing.

3. Medication Evaluation Referral (3)

A. The patient was referred to a physician for an evaluation for psychotropic medication to help in controlling the ADD symptoms.

B. The patient complied with the medication evaluation and has attended the appointment.

C. The patient refused to attend an evaluation appointment with the physician to be evaluated for psychotropic medication.

---

* The numbers in parentheses correlate to the number of the Therapeutic Intervention statement in the companion chapter with the same title in *The Complete Adult Psychotherapy Treatment Planner,* second edition (Jongsma and Peterson) by John Wiley & Sons, 1999.

4. Process Psychiatric Evaluation (4)

A. Results and recommendations of the psychiatric evaluation were processed with the patient, and all questions were answered.

B. As a result of the physician's evaluation, the patient was prescribed medication to assist in the control of ADD symptomatology.

5. Monitor Medication Compliance (5)

A. The patient's compliance with the medication prescription was monitored, and the medication's effectiveness on his/her level of functioning was evaluated.

B. The patient has been taking the medication consistently as prescribed and reported that the medication was effective in helping to control the ADD symptoms.

C. The patient has been taking the psychotropic medications as prescribed but reports that he/she has not noted any significant improvement in his/her ADD symptoms.

6. Confer with Physician (6)

A. Contact has been made with the physician who prescribed the patient's psychotropic medications to discuss the effectiveness and side effects of those medications.

B. The patient granted permission for release of information to be given to the prescribing physician for the psychotropic medications.

C. Because the medications have not yet been effective, the prescribing physician agreed to alter the prescription in an attempt to make the medication regimen more successful.

7. Conjoint Session to Give Evaluation Feedback (7)

A. A conjoint session was held with the patient and his/her significant others in order to present the results of the psychological and physician evaluations.

B. All questions regarding the evaluation results were processed.

C. The patient's family members were solicited for support regarding his/her compliance with treatment for his/her ADD symptoms.

D. The patient's family gave strong support to the patient regarding medical and psychological treatment for his/her ADD symptom.

8. Identify Medication Benefits (8)

A. The patient was asked to make a list of advantages and disadvantages regarding staying on the psychotropic medications for the treatment of his/her ADD symptomatology, even after much progress has been made in symptom control.

B. The patient was encouraged to stay on his/her medication even when his/her symptoms are diminished, in spite of temptations to terminate taking the medication.

C. The medication has proven to be beneficial in reducing the ADD symptom pattern.

9. Support Medication Compliance (9)

A. The patient was encouraged and supported in remaining on medications.

B. The patient was firmly confronted when he/she indicated an interest in terminating the medication use because the symptoms had improved.

C. The patient has agreed to continue medication use on a consistent basis.

10. Assign a List of Positive Medication Effects (10)

A. The patient was assigned to list the positive effects that have occurred for him/her since beginning to take the medication consistently.

B. The patient specifically indicated several symptoms that have reduced in intensity since beginning the medication.

C. The patient verbalized an understanding of the benefits of continuing with the pre-scribed psychotropic medications on a long-term basis.

11. Identify Difficult ADD Behaviors (11)

A. The patient was assisted in identifying the specific ADD behaviors that have caused him/her the most difficulty.

B. The patient listed such things as distractibility, lack of concentration, impulsivity, rest-lessness, and disorganization as the most difficult for him/her.

C. The patient was resistive to becoming specific about identifying ADD behaviors that cause him/her the most difficulty.

12. Review Evaluation Results (12)

A. The results of the psychological testing and physician's evaluation were reviewed again with the patient in order to affirm him/her in the choice of his/her most difficult, prob-lematic behaviors to address in counseling.

B. The patient selected those behaviors that were most difficult as focal points for treatment.

C. The patient has agreed to concentrate his/her efforts to change on these most difficult behavior arenas.

13. Family Rank Patient's Behaviors (13)

A. The patient was asked to request family members to complete a ranking of the three be-haviors that they perceive as those that interfere the most with the patient's daily func-tioning.

B. Family members have ranked the patient's behavior and have identified those three be-haviors that they perceive to be the most problematic for the patient.

C. The patient's family has refused to cooperate with ranking his/her behaviors and would not provide such a list for him/her.

D. The patient has failed to ask for the family's participation in his/her treatment and has not asked them to rank his/her problematic behaviors.

14. Teach Problem-Solving Skills (14)

A. The patient was taught problem-solving skills that involve identifying the problem, brain-storming solutions, evaluating options, implementing action, and evaluating results.

B. The patient verbalized an understanding of the problem-solving skill techniques.

C. Role playing was used to help the patient apply problem-solving techniques to daily problems in his/her life.

15. Assign Problem-Solving Homework (15)

A. The patient was assigned the homework of applying the problem-solving techniques pre-viously learned to specific, identified ADD behaviors.

B. The patient has followed through with the problem-solving homework, and the results of that effort were processed.

C. The patient reported success at implementing the problem-solving techniques, and he/she was reinforced for this success.

D. The patient has had difficulty applying problem-solving techniques, and he/she was redirected regarding implementation of these techniques.

16. Teach Self-Control Strategies (16)

A. The patient was taught the self-control strategy of "stop, listen, think, and act" to assist him/her in curbing impulsive behavior.

B. The patient was taught problem-solving self-talk as a means of reducing impulsivity.

C. Role playing was used to help the patient apply self-control strategies to daily life situations that are affected by his/her ADD symptoms.

D. The patient reported success at applying self-control strategies and indicated that his/her impulsivity has been diminished.

17. Teach Time-Limited Impulse Indulgence (17)

A. The patient was assigned to structure a specific time each week when he/she would indulge impulses that are not self-destructive, such as eating a favorite food, listening to favorite music, and so on.

B. The patient has followed through on establishing a time-limited period each week when harmless impulses are indulged.

18. Teach Time-Out Intervention (18)

A. The patient was taught to utilize a time-out intervention in which he/she removes himself/herself from a situation in order to calm down and consider behavioral alternatives as reactions to the situation.

B. The patient has implemented the time-out procedure and is controlling destructive impulses by considering alternative behaviors and their consequences.

19. Teach Relaxation Techniques (19)

A. The patient was taught various relaxation techniques including deep muscle relaxation, rhythmic breathing, meditation, and guided imagery to be used when stress levels increase.

B. The patient has implemented relaxation procedures to reduce tension and physical restlessness and reported that this technique is beneficial.

C. The patient has not followed through on implementation of relaxation techniques to reduce restlessness and tension and was encouraged to do so.

20. Develop Self-Reward System (20)

A. A self-administered reward system was designed for the patient to reinforce himself/herself for times when he/she exercises positive control over impulsivity, loss of temper, and attentiveness and other symptoms of his/her ADD.

B. The patient has implemented the self-reward system and has been reinforcing himself/herself for engaging positive alternatives to problem behaviors.

C. The implementation of the reward system has increased the frequency of positive alternative behaviors and decreased the frequency of problematic ADD behaviors.

21. Utilize Structured Reminders/Organizers (21)

A. The patient was encouraged to use such things as lists, sticky notes, files, and maintenance of daily routines in order to reduce forgetfulness and increase organization of his/her life.

B. The patient's implementation of structured reminders and organizers has been successful in reducing forgetfulness and helping him/her to complete necessary tasks.

22. Utilize Brainwave Biofeedback (22)

A. The patient was administered brainwave biofeedback to assist him/her in improving attention span, impulse control, and mood regulation.

B. The patient was successful at implementing the brainwave biofeedback technique within the session.

C. The patient has had difficulty regulating his/her brainwave using the biofeedback technique.

23. Transfer Biofeedback Skills (23)

A. The patient was encouraged to transfer the biofeedback training skills of relaxation and cognitive focusing to specific daily situations that were identified as particularly problematic because of the ADD symptoms.

B. The patient reported that since the use of brainwave biofeedback was initiated, he/she has had improved attention span and impulse control.

C. The patient reported that the brainwave biofeedback technique does not seem to improve his/her attention span, impulse control, or mood regulation.

24. Encourage Healthy Addictions (24)

A. The patient's tendency toward addictive behavior was directed at healthy alternatives such as exercise or volunteer community work.

B. The patient has followed through with becoming involved in an exercise routine on a daily basis and is also performing community service activities on a weekly basis.

C. The patient has not followed through on establishing healthy, alternative addictions.

25. Physical Fitness Trainer Referral (25)

A. After the patient obtained approval from his/her personal physician, he/she was referred to a physical fitness trainer to assist in the design of an aerobic exercise routine.

B. The patient has followed through with the referral to a physical fitness trainer and has begun to establish a daily aerobic exercise routine.

C. The patient reported that engaging in the physical fitness routine has helped to increase relaxation and reduce restlessness.

D. The patient has not followed through on establishing the daily exercise routine and was encouraged to do so.

26. List Negative ADD Consequences (26)

A. The patient was asked to make a list of the negative consequences that result from his/her problematic ADD behaviors.

B. The list of the negative consequences that result from ADD behaviors was processed to increase the patient's awareness of the impact of his/her behavior on himself/herself and others.

C. Coping strategies were reviewed that could be implemented as alternatives to the problematic ADD behaviors that produce negative consequences.

27. ADD Group Referral (27)

A. The patient was referred to group therapy for adults with ADD to help increase his/her understanding of ADD, boost self-esteem, and to receive feedback from others.

B. The patient has followed through on attendance at the ADD group therapy sessions and reported that they have been beneficial.

C. The patient has not followed through on consistent attendance at the ADD group therapy sessions and was encouraged to do so.

28. Teach Coach Technique (28)

A. The patient was taught the principles of a *coaching* technique, whereby he/she would pick a friend, colleague, or family member to help him/her get organized, stay focused on a task, and give encouraging support.

B. The patient was assisted in selecting a specific person from his/her social network that could serve as his/her coach.

29. Train the Coach in HOPE Technique (29)

A. The person selected by the patient to act as his/her coach was trained in the Help, Obligations, Plans, and Encouragement (HOPE) technique as described in the book *Driven to Distraction* (Hallowell and Raty).

B. The coach was trained in how to assist the patient with Help, Obligations, Plans, and Encouragement as part of the HOPE procedure.

C. The coach technique has been implemented, and the patient reported that it has been helpful in increasing his/her organization and task focus.

D. The patient and the coach have failed to implement the HOPE technique, and the patient was encouraged to initiate this procedure.

30. Teach Listening Skills (30)

A. Role playing and modeling were used to teach the patient how to listen to others and to accept their feedback regarding his/her behavior.

B. The patient reported that, on several occasions, he/she was able to use the new listening skills to accept direction and feedback from others.

C. The patient continued to report difficulties with listening as he/she becomes defensive whenever feedback or direction is given to him/her.

31. Assign Books on ADD (31)

A. The patient was referred to specific reading material designed to increase his/her knowledge about ADD.

B. The patient has followed through on reading the recommended books, and key concepts were processed within the session.

C. The patient has not followed through on reading the assigned material on ADD and was encouraged to do so.

32. Affirm a Positive Self-Image (32)

A. In a conjoint session, positive aspects of the patient's relationship with his/her significant other were pointed out, as well as affirming positive aspects of the patient's character.

B. The patient reported feelings of increased self-esteem as a result of affirming positive aspects of himself/herself and relationships with others.

C. The patient has made more positive affirming statements about himself/herself.

33. Significant Other Support Group Referral (33)

A. The patient's partner was referred to a support group for friends and family of people with ADD conditions.

B. The patient's partner was taught about the symptoms of ADD, its treatment, and prognosis.

C. The patient's partner refused to attend a support group.

D. The patient's partner has attended a support group and has reported an increased understanding of the ADD condition.

34. Communication Group Referral (34)

A. The patient and his/her partner were referred to a communication/relationship seminar to improve their conflict resolution and communication skills.

B. The patient and his/her partner followed through on the referral and have attended a communication/conflict resolution seminar and reported that they have benefited from the group instruction.

C. The patient and his/her partner have not followed through on the referral to a relationship seminar and were encouraged to do so.

35. List Relationship Expectations (35)

A. The patient and his/her partner were asked to list the expectations that each of them has for the relationship and for each other.

B. The relationship expectations of each partner were processed in a conjoint session with realistic expectations reinforced and unrealistic expectations discarded.

C. The patient reported that he/she feels that his/her relationship with his/her partner has improved and that both are more satisfied.

D. The patient's relationship with his/her partner continues to be conflictual and filled with poor communication.

36. Teach Communication Skills (36)

A. The patient and his/her partner were instructed in how to communicate effectively with each other.

B. The patient and his/her partner acknowledged conflicts between them and worked toward the resolution of these conflicts that have been a barrier to communication.

C. In a conjoint session, the patient and his/her partner were assisted in clarifying their thoughts and feelings, and communication between them was facilitated by teaching them listening skills.

D. The patient and his/her partner reported that their communication has improved significantly.

37. Assign Structured Communication Times (37)

A. The patient and his/her partner were assigned to schedule a specific time each day to spend together in communicating, expressing affection, recreating, or talking through problems.

B. The patient has followed through with establishing structured times for communication and reported that the relationship is benefiting from such an exercise.

C. The patient and his/her partner have not followed through with maintaining structured communication times, and their relationship continues to be conflictual.

38. Develop Conflict Signal System (38)

A. The patient and his/her partner were assisted in the development of a signal system as a means of indicating when conflict behaviors are beginning to escalate and communication has become destructive.

B. The patient reported that it has been helpful to implement the signal system to cause a time-out in interaction with his/her partner when conflicts between them escalate.

C. The patient and his/her partner have not adhered to the rules of the signal system, and communication between them continues to be problematic and destructive at times.

BORDERLINE PERSONALITY

PATIENT PRESENTATION

1. Emotional Reactivity (1)

A. The patient described a history of extreme emotional reactivity when minor stresses occur in his/her life.

B. The patient's emotional reactivity is usually quite short lived, as he/she returns to a calm state after demonstrating strong feelings of anger, anxiety, or depression.

C. The patient's emotional lability has been reduced, and he/she reported less frequent incidents of emotional reactivity.

2. Chaotic Interpersonal Relationships (2)

A. The patient has a pattern of intense, but chaotic, interpersonal relationships as he/she puts high expectations on others and is easily threatened that the relationship might be in jeopardy.

B. The patient has had many relationships that have ended because of the intensity and demands that he/she placed on the relationship.

C. The patient reported incidents that have occurred recently with friends, whereby he/she continued placing inappropriately intense demands on the relationship.

D. The patient has made progress in stabilizing his/her relationship with others by diminishing the degree of demands that he/she places on the relationship and reducing the dependency on it.

3. Identity Disturbance (3)

A. The patient has a history of being confused as to who he/she is and what his/her goals are in life.

B. The patient has become very intense about questioning his/her identity.

C. The patient has become more assured about his/her identity and is less reactive to this issue.

4. Impulsivity (4)

A. The patient described a history of engaging in impulsive behaviors that have the potential for producing harmful consequences for himself/herself.

B. The patient has engaged in impulsive behaviors that compromise his/her reputation with others.

C. The patient has established improved control over impulsivity and considers the consequences of his/her actions more deliberately before engaging in behavior.

---

* The numbers in parentheses correlate to the number of the Behavioral Definition statement in the companion chapter with the same title in *The Complete Adult Psychotherapy Treatment Planner,* second edition (Jongsma and Peterson) by John Wiley & Sons, 1999.

5. Suicidal/Self-Mutilating Behavior (5)

A. The patient reported a history of multiple suicidal gestures and/or threats.

B. The patient has engaged in self-mutilating behavior on several occasions.

C. The patient made a commitment to terminate suicidal gestures and threats.

D. The patient agreed to stop the pattern of self-mutilating behavior.

E. There have been no recent reports of occurrences of suicidal gestures, threats, or self-mutilating behavior.

6. Feelings of Emptiness (6)

A. The patient reported a chronic history of feeling empty and bored with life.

B. The patient's frequent complaints of feeling bored and that life had no meaning had alienated him/her from others.

C. The patient has not complained recently about feeling empty or bored, but appears to be more challenged and at peace with life.

7. Intense Anger Eruptions (7)

A. The patient frequently has eruptions of intense and inappropriate anger triggered by seemingly insignificant stressors.

B. The patient seems to live in a state of chronic anger and displeasure with others.

C. The patient's eruptions of intense and inappropriate anger have diminished in their frequency and intensity.

D. The patient reported that there have been no incidents of recent eruptions of anger.

8. Feels Others Are Unfair (8)

A. The patient made frequent complaints about the unfair treatment he/she believes that others have given him/her.

B. The patient frequently verbalized distrust of others and questions their motives.

C. The patient has demonstrated increased trust of others and has not complained about unfair treatment from them recently.

9. Black-or-White Thinking (9)

A. The patient demonstrated a pattern of analyzing issues in simple terms of right or wrong, black or white, trustworthy versus deceitful, without regard for extenuating circumstances before considering the complexity of the situations.

B. The patient's black-or-white thinking has caused him/her to be quite judgmental of others.

C. The patient finds it difficult to consider the complexity of situations, but prefers to think in simple terms of right versus wrong.

D. The patient has shown some progress in allowing for the complexity of some situations and extenuating circumstances, which might contribute to some other people's actions.

10. Abandonment Fears (10)

A. The patient described a history of becoming very anxious whenever there is any hint of abandonment present in an established relationship.

B. The patient's hypersensitivity to abandonment has caused him/her to place excessive demands of loyalty and proof of commitment on relationships.

C. The patient has begun to acknowledge his/her fear of abandonment as being excessive and irrational.

D. Conflicts within a relationship have been reported by the patient, but he/she has not automatically assumed that abandonment will be the result.

INTERVENTIONS IMPLEMENTED

1. Explore Trigger Situations (1)

A. The patient was asked to identify those situations that trigger feelings of fear, depression, and anger.

B. The patient has shown good insight into his/her ability to clearly identify the situations that stir intense feelings of fear, depression, and anger.

2. Assign a Feelings Journal (2)

A. The patient was assigned to record a daily journal of feelings, along with the circumstances that triggered those feelings.

B. The patient has completed a journaling of daily feelings and the stimulus situations that trigger those feelings, and this material was processed within the session.

C. Completing the exercise of journaling feelings on a daily basis has helped the patient identify those circumstances that trigger feelings of fear, depression, and anger.

3. Identify Distorted Thoughts (3)

A. The patient was assisted in identifying the distorted schemas and related automatic thoughts that mediate his/her anxiety response.

B. The patient has been accepting of the fact that he/she has held to distorted thoughts rather than realistic thoughts and that this distortion has increased his/her feelings of anger, depression, and anxiety.

4. Assign Journal of Self-Defeating Thoughts (4)

A. The patient was asked to keep a daily record of self-defeating thoughts, such as those of hopelessness, helplessness, worthlessness, and catastrophizing.

B. The patient has followed through on keeping a daily record of self-defeating thoughts, and this material was processed within the session.

C. The patient's dysfunctional thoughts were challenged for their inaccuracy, and each was replaced with a thought that is more positive, realistic, and self-enhancing.

5. Utilize Cognitive Restructuring (5)

A. The patient was trained in revising his/her core schema using cognitive restructuring techniques.

B. Dysfunctional, inaccurate thinking was challenged, and these thoughts were replaced with more positive, realistic thinking.

---

* The numbers in parentheses correlate to the number of the Therapeutic Intervention statement in the companion chapter with the same title in *The Complete Adult Psychotherapy Treatment Planner,* second edition (Jongsma and Peterson) by John Wiley & Sons, 1999.

6. Reinforce Positive Self-Talk (6)

A. The patient was reinforced for implementing positive, realistic self-talk that mediates a sense of peace.

B. The patient noted several instances from his/her daily life that reflected the implementation of positive self-talk, and these successful experiences were reinforced.

7. Assign Recording of Positive Self-Talk (7)

A. The patient was asked to record any and all instances of successful use of revised constructive cognitive patterns in his/her daily life.

B. The patient's record of successful use of constructive cognitive patterns was reviewed, processed, and reinforced.

C. The patient recalled several instances of using positive self-talk, and he/she noted the positive consequences of this technique in reducing his/her feelings of fear and anxiety and building a sense of calm.

8. List Negative Impulsivity Consequences (8)

A. The patient was assigned the task of listing the destructive consequences to himself/herself and others of his/her impulsive behavior.

B. The patient has listed and become aware of the negative consequences to himself/herself and others resulting from his/her impulsivity.

C. The patient has a lack of insight into the negative consequences that result from his/her impulsivity.

9. Teach Self-Control Strategies (9)

A. The patient was taught mediational and self-control strategies such as using "stop, look, listen, and think" to delay gratification and inhibit impulsivity.

B. Role playing, modeling, and behavior rehearsal were used to apply the self-control strategies to scenes from the patient's daily life.

10. Assign Implementation of Self-Control Strategies (10)

A. The patient was assigned to record instances of his/her successful implementation of using "stop, look, listen, and think" to control reactive impulses.

B. The patient reported implementing "stop, look, listen, and think" as an impulse control strategy on several successful instances.

C. The patient's impulsivity has been reduced as a result of using the self-control strategies.

11. Teach Cognitive Control (11)

A. The patient was taught cognitive methods thoughts, such as thought stopping, thought substitution, and reframing, as methods for gaining and improving control over impulsive actions.

B. The patient has implemented cognitive methods for impulse control and reported success and reducing impulsivity.

12. Teach Relaxation Techniques (12)

A. The patient was taught relaxation techniques, such as progressive deep muscle relaxation and self-hypnosis, to be used to reduce feelings of stress.

B. The patient was administered biofeedback to enhance relaxation skills.

C. The patient has developed his/her skill to relax.

13. Assign Recording Relaxation Usage (13)

A. The patient was asked to record instances of using relaxation techniques to cope with stress, rather than reacting with anger.

B. The patient was reinforced for sharing instances of successful implementation of relaxation in the face of stress.

C. The patient verbalized being pleased with himself/herself because he/she did not react with anger in the face of stress; instead, he/she utilized self-relaxation techniques.

14. Teach Assertiveness (14)

A. The patient was taught assertiveness skills through the use of role playing, modeling, and behavioral rehearsal.

B. The patient verbalized an understanding of the difference between assertiveness, aggressiveness, and passivity.

C. The patient was able to identify several areas in his/her life that could benefit from using assertiveness.

15. Assertiveness Group Referral (15)

A. The patient was referred to an assertiveness training group.

B. The patient has followed through with the referral to an assertiveness training group and has attended consistently.

C. The patient has not followed through with the referral to an assertiveness training group and has not attended the group consistently.

D. The patient reported that he/she believes that the assertiveness training group experience has been helpful in developing assertiveness skills in place of aggressive responses or passivity.

16. Review Assertiveness Implementation (16)

A. The patient's implementation of assertiveness skills was reviewed, and his/her feelings about the experience were processed.

B. The positive consequences of the patient's assertiveness implementation were emphasized and reinforced.

C. The patient reported difficulty in implementing assertiveness and was redirected.

17. Teach "I" Messages (17)

A. The patient was taught, through modeling, role playing, and behavioral rehearsal, to use "I" messages to communicate feelings directly.

B. The patient was taught to use "I" messages as an alternative to aggressive responding or possessiveness when he/she feels threatened.

18. Reinforce Use of "I" Messages (18)

A. The patient's implementation of the use of "I" messages to communicate feelings without aggression was reinforced.

B.   The patient recalled instances when he/she was able to implement the use of "I" messages rather than messages of aggression or possessiveness.

C.   The patient reported resistance to using "I" messages and was redirected in their use.

19. Explore Childhood Abuse/Abandonment (19)

A.   Experiences of childhood physical or emotional abuse, neglect, or abandonment were explored.

B.   As the patient identified instances of abuse and neglect, the feelings surrounding these experiences were processed.

C.   The patient's experiences with perceived abandonment were highlighted and related to his/her current fears of this experience occurring in the present.

D.   The patient identified instances of abuse and abandonment in his/her childhood, but denied any emotional impact of these experiences on himself/herself.

20. Confront Overcontrol of Others (20)

A.   The destructive effect of overcontrolling others when they pull back from relationships was pointed out to the patient.

B.   The patient was urged to separate the feelings of helplessness and desperation that originate in childhood experiences from current relationships in the present.

C.   The patient verbalized the effect that childhood experiences of abuse, neglect, and abandonment have had upon possessiveness in relationships and his/her sensitivity to a hint of loss of commitment in relationship to himself/herself.

D.   The patient refused to acknowledge the impact of childhood experiences of neglect and abuse as having any effect on current emotional reactivity.

21. Reinforce Anger Insight (21)

A.   The patient expressed insight into the effect of his/her childhood experiences of abuse and neglect on current urges to react with rage.

B.   The patient was reinforced for verbalizations of insight into his/her causes for frequent eruptions of intense, inappropriate anger or fear.

22. Teach Abandonment-Coping Strategies (22)

A.   The patient was taught various coping strategies such as using "stop, look, listen, and plan," relaxation and deep breathing techniques, expanded social network, and the use of "I" messages to deal with his/her intense fear of abandonment.

B.   The patient reported successfully implementing coping strategies to reduce his/her sensitivity to any hint of abandonment in relationships.

C.   The patient continued to show evidence of fear of abandonment, and this fear triggers intense emotional reactions.

23. Explore the Fear of Being Alone (23)

A.   The patient's fears associated with being alone were explored in detail.

B.   The patient acknowledged significant fear of being alone and recognized that it is tied to fears of abandonment based in childhood experiences.

24. Encourage Solitary Activities (24)

A. The patient was encouraged to break his/her pattern of avoiding being alone by initiating activities that are engaged in without a companion.

B. Activities that the patient could perform alone were identified and he/she was encouraged to initiate these activities.

C. The patient reported on successful initiation of enjoyable activities that were done alone and stated that he/she felt comfortable with this independence.

D. The patient resisted initiating solitary activities and continues to fear being alone.

25. Medication Evaluation Referral (25)

A. The patient was referred to a physician to be evaluated for psychotropic medications to stabilize his/her mood.

B. The patient has cooperated with a referral to a physician and has attended the evaluation for psychotropic medications.

C. The patient has refused to attend a physician evaluation for psychotropic medications.

26. Monitor Medication Compliance (26)

A. The patient's compliance with prescribed medications was monitored, and effectiveness of the medication on his/her level of functioning was noted.

B. The patient reported that the medication has been beneficial in stabilizing his/her mood.

C. The patient reported that the medication has not been beneficial in stabilizing his/her mood.

D. The patient reported side effects of the medication that he/she found intolerable.

27. Explore Self-Mutilating Behavior (27)

A. The patient's history and nature of self-mutilating behavior was explored thoroughly.

B. The patient recalled a pattern of self-mutilating behavior that has dated back several years.

C. The patient's self-mutilating behavior was reported to be associated with feelings of depression, fear, and anger, as well as a lack of self-identity.

28. Interpret Self-Mutilating Behavior (28)

A. The patient's self-mutilation was interpreted as an expression of the rage and helplessness that could not be expressed as a child victim of emotional abandonment and abuse.

B. The patient accepted the interpretation of his/her self-mutilation and more directly expressed his/her feelings of hurt and anger associated with childhood abuse experiences.

C. The patient rejected the interpretation of self-mutilating behavior as an expression of rage associated with childhood abandonment or neglect experiences.

29. Assess Suicidal Behavior (29)

A. The patient's history and current status regarding suicidal gestures was assessed.

B. The secondary gain associated with suicidal gestures was identified.

C. Triggers for suicidal thoughts were identified, and alternative responses to these trigger situations were proposed.

30. Elicit Nonsuicide Contract (30)

A. A promise was elicited from the patient that he/she will initiate contact with the therapist or an emergency helpline if the suicidal urge becomes strong and before any self-injurious behavior is enacted.

B. The patient promised to terminate self-mutilation behavior and to contact emergency personnel if urges for such behavior arise.

C. The patient has followed through on the non-self-harm contract by contacting emergency service personnel rather than enacting any suicidal gestures or self-mutilating behavior.

31. Emergency Helpline Referral (31)

A. The patient was provided with an emergency helpline telephone number that is available 24 hours a day.

B. The patient promised to utilize the emergency helpline telephone number rather than engaging in any self-harm behaviors.

32. Substitute "I" Messages for Self-Harm (32)

A. The patient was strongly encouraged to express feelings directly through using assertive "I" messages rather than indirectly through self-mutilating behavior.

B. The patient has implemented assertive "I" message communication, and his/her engagement in self-mutilating behavior has terminated.

33. Review Dichotomous Thinking (33)

A. The patient was assisted in examining his/her style of evaluating people, especially regarding his/her dichotomous thinking.

B. The patient was taught the risks of his/her judgmental style of evaluating people.

C. The patient was reminded of the harm that is caused to relationships as a result of his/her dichotomous thinking.

D. The patient accepted the observation that he/she must be sensitive to his/her pattern of black-or-white thinking.

34. Teach Negative Consequences of Judging (34)

A. The patient was assisted in understanding and identifying the negative consequences of judging people harshly and impulsively.

B. The patient listed the negative consequences that have resulted from his/her having judged people ridgedly and harshly.

C. The patient was resistant to seeing any negative consequences that result from his/her harsh judgments based in black-or-white thinking.

35. Challenge Dichotomous Thinking (35)

A. The patient was helped to understand how dichotomous thinking leads to feelings of interpersonal mistrust.

B. Attempts were made to help the patient see positive and negative traits in all people, as opposed to idealizing some and harshly condemning others.

C. The patient was able to identify positive and negative traits in several people within his/her social network.

36. List Others' Positive and Negative Traits (36)

A. Role reversal and modeling were used to help the patient recognize positive and negative qualities in other people within his/her social network.

B. The patient was able to verbalize the weaknesses or faults of those who had been judged to be perfect and the strengths or assets of those who had been judged to be worthless.

CHEMICAL DEPENDENCE

PATIENT PRESENTATION

1. Consistent Abuse of Alcohol (1)

A. The patient described a history of alcohol abuse on a frequent basis and, often, until intoxicated or passed out.

B. Family members confirmed a pattern of chronic alcohol abuse by the patient.

C. The patient acknowledged that his/her alcohol abuse began in adolescence and continued into adulthood.

D. The patient has committed himself/herself to a plan of abstinence from alcohol and participation in a recovery program.

E. The patient has maintained total abstinence, which is confirmed by his/her family.

2. Consistent Drug Abuse (1)

A. The patient described a history of mood-altering drug abuse on a frequent basis.

B. Family members confirmed a pattern of chronic drug abuse by the patient.

C. The patient acknowledged that his/her drug abuse began in adolescence and continued into adulthood.

D. The patient has committed himself/herself to a plan of abstinence from mood-altering drugs and participation in a recovery program.

E. The patient has maintained total abstinence, which is confirmed by his/her family.

3. Inability to Reduce Alcohol/Drug Abuse (2)

A. The patient acknowledged that he/she frequently has attempted to terminate or reduce his/her use of the mood-altering drug, but found that once use has begun, he/she has been unable to follow through.

B. The patient acknowledged that, in spite of negative consequences and a desire to reduce or terminate the mood-altering drug abuse, he/she has been unable to do so.

C. As the patient has participated in a total recovery program, he/she has been able to maintain abstinence from mood-altering drug use.

4. Negative Blood Effects (3)

A. The patient's blood work results reflect a pattern of heavy substance abuse in that his/her liver enzymes are elevated.

B. The patient's blood work results indicate that mood-altering drugs have been used.

C. As the patient has participated in the recovery program and has been able to maintain abstinence from mood-altering drugs, his/her blood work has shown improved status and has come back to within normal limits.

---

* The numbers in parentheses correlate to the number of the Behavioral Definition statement in the companion chapter with the same title in *The Complete Adult Psychotherapy Treatment Planner,* second edition (Jongsma and Peterson) by John Wiley & Sons, 1999.

5. Denial (4)

A. The patient presented with denial regarding the negative consequences of his/her substance abuse, in spite of direct feedback from others about its negative impact.

B. The patient's denial is beginning to break down as he/she is acknowledging that substance abuse has created problems in his/her life.

C. The patient now openly admits to the severe negative consequences in which substance abuse has resulted.

6. Amnesiac Blackouts (5)

A. The patient has experienced blackouts during alcohol abuse, which have resulted in memory loss for periods of time in which the patient was still functional.

B. The patient stated that his/her first blackout occurred at a young age and that he/she has experienced many of them over the years of his/her alcohol abuse.

C. The patient acknowledged only one or two incidents of amnesiac blackouts.

D. The patient has not had any recent experiences of blackouts, as he/she has been able to maintain sobriety.

7. Persistent Alcohol/Drug Abuse Despite Problems (6)

A. The patient has continued to abuse alcohol/drugs in spite of recurring physical, legal, vocational, social, or relationship problems that were directly caused by the substance use.

B. The patient has denied that the many problems in his/her life are directly caused by alcohol or drug abuse.

C. The patient acknowledged that alcohol or drug abuse has been the cause of multiple problems in his/her life and verbalized a strong desire to maintain a life free from using all mood-altering substances.

D. As the patient has maintained sobriety, some of the direct negative consequences of substance abuse have diminished.

E. The patient is now able to face resolution of significant problems in his/her life as he/she has begun to establish sobriety.

8. Increased Tolerance (7)

A. The patient described a pattern of increasing tolerance for the mood-altering substance as he/she needed to use more of it to obtain the desired affect.

B. The patient described the steady increase in the amount and frequency of the substance abuse as his/her tolerance for it increased.

9. Physical Withdrawal Symptoms (8)

A. The patient acknowledged that he/she has experienced physical withdrawal symptoms such as shaking, seizures, nausea, headaches, sweating, anxiety, and insomnia as he/she withdrew from the substance abuse.

B. The patient's physical symptoms of withdrawal have eased as he/she stabilized and maintained abstinence from the mood-altering substance.

C. There is no further evidence of physical withdrawal symptoms.

10. Suspension of Activities (9)

A. The patient has suspended his/her involvement in important social, recreational, and occupational activities, because they interfered with his/her substance abuse lifestyle.

B. The patient is beginning to recognize that all other aspects of his/her life became secondary to the primary object of obtaining and using the mood-altering substance.

C. The patient is resuming his/her responsibilities in the area of social, recreational, and occupational activities as he/she becomes established in a recovery lifestyle.

11. Excessive Time Investment (10)

A. The patient described an excessive investment of time and effort that he/she expended in order to obtain, use, or recover from using the mood-altering substance.

B. As the patient has stabilized in a recovery program, he/she has discovered large amounts of time to give to constructive activity.

12. Loss of Control (11)

A. The patient has frequently consumed greater amounts of the substance and used it for a longer period of time than he/she intended.

B. In spite of making promises to himself/herself and others to reduce the frequency of alcohol/drug abuse, the patient has been unable to fulfill those promises consistently.

C. The patient described many instances of telling himself/herself that he/she would only use a little bit of the drug or alcohol for a brief time but, instead, became consumed by the drug/alcohol and use was heavy.

13. Health Problems (12)

A. The patient acknowledged that he/she has been warned about the negative consequences of substance abuse by a physician.

B. The patient is suffering from poor health due to his/her substance abuse, but the substance abuse continued in spite of significant negative consequences.

C. The patient's physical health has stabilized, and some of the negative consequences have begun to reverse as he/she has maintained a life free from mood-altering substances.

INTERVENTIONS IMPLEMENTED

1. Gather Drug/Alcohol History (1)

A. The patient was asked to describe his/her alcohol/drug use in terms of the amount and pattern of use, symptoms of abuse, and negative life consequences that have resulted from chemical dependence.

B. The patient openly discussed his/her substance abuse history and gave complete data regarding its nature and extent.

C. The patient minimized his/her substance abuse and did not give reliable data regarding the nature and extent of his/her chemical dependence problem.

D. As therapy has progressed, the patient has become more open in acknowledging the extent and seriousness of his/her substance abuse problem.

---

* The numbers in parentheses correlate to the number of the Therapeutic Intervention statement in the companion chapter with the same title in *The Complete Adult Psychotherapy Treatment Planner,* second edition (Jongsma and Peterson) by John Wiley & Sons, 1999.

2. List Negative Consequences (2)

A. The patient was asked to make a list of the ways that substance abuse has negatively impacted his/her life.

B. The patient minimized the negative impact of substance abuse on his/her life.

C. The patient openly acknowledged the negative consequences of drug/alcohol abuse on his/her life.

3. Administer Alcohol Severity Index (3)

A. The Alcohol Severity Index test was administered to the patient.

B. The results of the Alcohol Severity Index, which indicated a significant substance abuse problem, were processed with the patient.

C. The results of the Alcohol Severity Index indicated that the patient's problem with chemical dependence is relatively minor.

4. Assign a Letter from Significant Others (4)

A. The patient was assigned to ask two or three significant others to write a letter to the therapist in which they identify how they perceive the patient's chemical dependence has negatively impacted his/her life.

B. The patient has followed through and asked people to write a letter describing the negative impact of substance abuse in his/her life.

C. The patient has not followed through on requesting a letter from significant others regarding negative consequences of substance abuse in his/her life, and he/she was redirected to do so.

D. The letters received from significant others indicated that the patient has had serious consequences in his/her life, and these results were processed with him/her.

5. Assign First Step Paper (5)

A. The patient was assigned to complete an Alcoholics Anonymous First Step paper and to share it with a group and the therapist.

B. The patient has completed a First Step paper and in it acknowledged that chemical dependence has dominated and controlled his/her life.

C. The patient has failed to complete a First Step paper and was redirected to do so.

6. Didactic Lecture Referral (6)

A. The patient was asked to attend didactic lectures related to chemical dependence and the process of recovery.

B. The patient was asked to identify in writing several key points attained from each didactic lecture.

C. Key points from didactic lectures that were noted by the patient were processed in individual sessions.

D. The patient has become more open in acknowledging and accepting his/her chemical dependence.

7. Reinforce Breakdown of Denial (7)

A. The patient was reinforced for any statement that reflected acceptance of his/her chemical dependence and acknowledgment of the destructive consequences that it has had on his/her life.

B. The patient has decreased his/her level of denial as evidenced by fewer statements that minimize the amount of his/her alcohol/drug abuse and its negative impact on his/her life.

8. Assign Readings on Disease Concept (8)

A. The patient was assigned to read material on the disease concept of alcoholism and to select several key ideas to discuss at a later session.

B. The patient has read the information provided on the disease concept of alcoholism, and key ideas gained from that reading were processed.

C. The patient has not followed through on reading the assigned material on alcoholism as a disease and was redirected to do so.

D. As a result of his/her reading about alcoholism, the patient has demonstrated an increased understanding of alcoholism and the process of recovery.

9. Assess Intellectual, Personality, and Cognitive Functioning (9)

A. The patient's intellectual, personality, and cognitive functioning were assessed by means of psychological testing.

B. The patient's intellectual, personality, and cognitive functioning were assessed by means of clinical interview.

C. The results of the psychological assessment were given to the patient, and the factors that may contribute to his/her chemical dependence were highlighted.

10. Assess Stress Factors (10)

A. Situational stress factors that may foster the patient's chemical dependence were explored.

B. Several stressors that exist within the patient's life were identified, and their contribution to the patient's attraction to substance abuse was noted.

C. The patient was assisted in developing steps to be taken to reduce the level of stress in his/her life so as to increase the probability of successful substance abuse recovery.

11. Explore Chemical Dependence in the Family (11)

A. The patient's immediate nuclear family was reviewed for any history of chemical dependence.

B. The patient identified parent figures and siblings who have a history of substance abuse.

C. The patient related incidents from his/her childhood in which he/she was exposed to repeated substance abuse by others within the family.

D. The patient has verbalized an understanding of how his/her family history and childhood experiences have contributed to his/her own substance abuse.

12. Explore Chemical Dependence in Extended Family (12)

A. The patient's extended family was explored for a chemical dependence history so as to relate this to a genetic vulnerability for the patient to also develop chemical dependence.

B. The patient did identify several members of his/her extended family who have a chemical dependence history, and he/she accepted the fact that he/she may be genetically vulnerable to chemical dependence because of this family history.

13. Physical Examination Referral (13)

A. The patient was referred for a thorough physical examination to determine any negative medical effects related to his/her chemical dependence.

B. The patient has followed through with obtaining a physical examination and was told that his/her chemical dependence has produced negative medical consequences.

C. The patient has obtained a physical examination from a physician and has been told that there are no significant medical effects of his/her chemical dependence.

D. The patient has not followed through with obtaining a physical examination and was again directed to do so.

14. List Positive Sobriety Effects (14)

A. The patient was asked to make a list of positive effects that maintaining sobriety could have on his/her life.

B. The patient has produced a list of positive sobriety effects, and this list was processed and reinforced.

C. The patient has not followed through with making a list of positive sobriety effects and was redirected to do so.

D. The patient was assisted in making a list of positive sobriety effects, and this list was processed and reinforced.

15. Review Negative Peer Influence (15)

A. A review of the patient's negative peers was performed, and the influence of these people on his/her substance abuse patterns was identified.

B. The patient accepted the interpretation that maintaining contact with substance-abusing friends would reduce the probability of successful recovery from his/her chemical dependence.

C. A plan was developed to help the patient initiate contact with sober people who could exert a positive influence on his/her own recovery.

D. The patient has begun to reach out socially to sober individuals in order to develop a social network that has a more positive influence on his/her recovery.

16. Identify Needed Life Changes (16)

A. The patient was assisted in identifying those life changes that will be necessary in order to maintain long-term sobriety.

B. The patient has identified necessary changes in his/her social life, vocational setting, living situation, recreational habits, and use of free time that will support recovery.

C. The patient has been resistive to making other changes in his/her life beyond the change of terminating the use of the mood-altering substance.

17. Plan Social and Recreational Activities (17)

A. A list of social and recreational activities that are free from association with substance abuse was developed.

B. The patient has agreed to begin involvement in new recreational and social activities that will replace substance abuse–related activities.

C. The patient has begun to make changes in his/her social and/or recreational activities and reported feeling good about this change.

D. The patient was very resistive to any changes in social and recreational activities that have previously been a strong part of his/her life.

18. Plan Project Completion (18)

A. The patient was assisted in developing a list of household- or work-related projects that could be accomplished in order to build his/her self-esteem, now that sobriety affords time and energy for such constructive activity.

B. The patient has begun to involve himself/herself in constructive projects that have affirmed his/her self-esteem.

C. The patient has not followed through with using his/her time constructively to accomplish household- or work-related projects.

19. Reinforce Making Amends (19)

A. The negative effects that the patient's substance abuse has had on family, friends, and work relationships were identified.

B. A plan for making amends to those who have been negatively affected by the patient's substance abuse was developed.

C. The patient reported on his/her implementation of a plan to make amends to those who have been hurt by his/her substance abuse.

D. The patient reported feeling good about the fact that he/she has begun to make amends to others who have been hurt by his/her substance abuse.

E. The patient has not followed through on making amends to others who have been negatively affected by his/her pattern of substance abuse.

20. Identify Sobriety's Positive Family Effects (20)

A. The patient was assisted in identifying the positive changes that will occur within family relationships as a result of his/her chemical dependence recovery.

B. The patient reported that his/her family is enjoying a reduction in stress and increased cooperation since his/her chemical dependence recovery began.

21. Evaluate Living Situation (21)

A. The patient's current living situation was reviewed as to whether it fosters a pattern of chemical dependence.

B. The patient agreed that his/her current living situation does encourage continuing substance abuse.

C. The patient could not see any reason why his/her current living situation would have a negative effect on his/her chemical dependence recovery.

22. List Negative Aspects of Living Situation (22)

A. The patient was assigned the task of listing all the negative influences that are inherent in the current living situation in terms of its impact on his/her chemical dependence recovery.

B. The patient has identified several reasons why his/her current living situation will exert a negative influence on his/her attempts at chemical dependence recovery.

C. The patient could not find any reason for identifying his/her current living situation as having the potential for negative influence on his/her chemical dependence recovery.

23. Change in Living Situation (23)

A. The patient was encouraged to develop a plan to find a more positive living situation that will foster his/her chemical dependence recovery.

B. The patient has found a new living situation, which is free from the negative influences that the current living situation brings to his/her chemical dependence recovery.

C. The patient is very resistive to moving from his/her current living situation.

24. Reinforce Change in Living Situation (24)

A. The patient's plan for moving to a new living situation was strongly reinforced.

B. The patient has made a move to a new living situation, which removes him/her from the strong negative influence on his/her attempts at substance abuse recovery.

C. Because substance abuse was so prevalent in the previous living situation, the patient has moved to a situation free of those influences, and this move has been strongly supported and reinforced.

25. Assign Good-Bye Letter to Drug (25)

A. The patient was assigned to write a good-bye letter to his/her drug of choice as a means of terminating his/her emotional and cognitive involvement with that drug.

B. The patient has followed through with writing the good-bye letter to his/her drug of choice, and the contents of it were processed.

C. The patient's feelings about writing a good-bye letter to the drug of choice were processed.

D. The patient reported that he/she felt some sense of relief at breaking emotional ties with his/her drug of choice.

E. The patient failed to follow through on the assigned good-bye letter to his/her drug of choice and was redirected to do so.

26. Develop Abstinence Contract (26)

A. The patient was asked to sign an abstinence contract in which he/she promises to avoid any and all contact with his/her drug of choice.

B. The patient has signed the abstinence contract, and the emotional impact of this action was processed.

C. Although the patient states that he/she would like to give up involvement with his/her drug of choice, he/she refused to sign an abstinence contract.

D. The patient indicated that he/she feels afraid of what his/her life will be like since there will be no contact with his/her drug of choice.

27. Develop Aftercare Plan (27)

A. The patient was assisted in developing an aftercare plan that will support the maintenance of long-term sobriety.

B. The patient has listed several components to an aftercare plan that will support his/her sobriety, such as family activities, counseling, self-help support groups, and sponsors.

C. The patient has not followed through on developing an aftercare plan and was redirected to do so.

28. Explore Positive Support System (28)

A. The patient was assisted in exploring within his/her own life the positive support system that will be available to him/her as he/she continues a life of sobriety.

B. The patient was able to identify several aspects of a positive support system available to him/her that will support recovery.

C. The patient is not able to identify significant aspects of a support system that are available to him/her that will support recovery.

D. The patient was helped to identify new sources of positive support for his/her recovery.

29. Assign AA/NA Member Contact (29)

A. The patient was assigned to meet with an Alcoholics Anonymous/Narcotics Anonymous (AA/NA) member who has been working the Twelve-Step program for several years in order to find out specifically how the program has helped him/her stay sober.

B. The patient has followed through on meeting with the AA/NA member and was encouraged about the role that AA/NA can play in maintaining sobriety.

C. The patient met with the AA/NA member but was not encouraged about the role of self-help groups in maintaining sobriety.

D. The patient has not followed through on meeting with an AA/NA member and was redirected to do so.

30. AA/NA Meetings Referral (30)

A. It was strongly recommended to the patient that he/she attend AA/NA meetings on a frequent and regular basis in order to obtain support for his/her sobriety.

B. The patient has followed through on consistent attendance at AA/NA meetings and reports that the meetings have been helpful.

C. The patient has not followed through on regular attendance at AA/NA meetings and was redirected to do so.

D. The patient has attended AA/NA meetings but reports that he/she does not find them helpful and is resistive to return to them.

31. Identify Relapse Triggers (31)

A. The patient was assisted in developing a list of situations that may trigger relapse into substance abuse.

B. Alternative ways of coping with situations that could trigger relapse were identified.

C. The patient has implemented positive coping strategies to deal with the identified triggers for relapse into substance abuse.

D. The patient has resisted identifying relapse triggers and is vulnerable to relapse because of this resistance.

32. Recommend Relapse Prevention Workbooks (32)

A. The patient was referred to books such as *Staying Sober: A Guide to Relapse Prevention* (Gorski and Miller) and *The Staying Sober Workbook* (Gorski) as material that would help develop strategies for constructively dealing with trigger situations.

B. The patient has obtained the recommended reading material on relapse prevention and stated that he/she has found the material helpful.

C. The patient has not followed through on obtaining the recommended reading material and was redirected to do so.

D. The patient has used the recommended reading material to identify potential relapse triggers and to help him/her develop strategies for constructively dealing with each trigger.

CHEMICAL DEPENDENCE—RELAPSE

PATIENT PRESENTATION

1. Relapse after Treatment (1)

A. The patient described having received treatment for substance abuse and then establishing sobriety for a length of time, followed by a return to mood-altering drug abuse.

B. The patient has been unable to maintain sobriety beyond a short time after being released from substance abuse treatment or another protective setting.

C. The patient reported that he/she was able to maintain sobriety for many months prior to relapsing.

D. The patient reported being able to maintain a life free from mood-altering drugs for more than two years after having received substance abuse treatment.

E. The patient reported that he/she feels confident that this latest establishment of a recovery plan will be successful.

2. Relapse with AA Attendance (2)

A. The patient has been attending AA meetings regularly, but was unable to maintain sobriety.

B. The patient has not made significant changes in his/her lifestyle, even though he/she attended AA meetings regularly, and this resulted in relapse.

C. The patient is now ready to make significant changes in his/her lifestyle along with attendance at AA to support chemical dependence recovery.

3. Relapse after Substantial Sobriety (3)

A. After having been free from mood-altering drugs for several years, the patient has relapsed.

B. The patient presented with low self-esteem and feelings of hopelessness and helplessness after reverting to substance abuse after a substantial period of sobriety.

C. The patient is confident that he/she can return to clean and sober living after having relapsed briefly following a period of substantial sobriety.

4. Chronic Sobriety/Relapse Pattern (4)

A. The patient has a history of several months' sobriety followed by a relapse and then reestablishing several months' sobriety followed by relapse.

B. The patient is discouraged about his/her relapse pattern after having established sobriety for several months on several different occasions.

C. The patient has become more confident of his/her efforts to maintain sobriety on a consistent basis, even though this would be different than his/her previous pattern.

---

* The numbers in parentheses correlate to the number of the Behavioral Definition statement in the companion chapter with the same title in *The Complete Adult Psychotherapy Treatment Planner,* second edition (Jongsma and Peterson) by John Wiley & Sons, 1999.

INTERVENTIONS IMPLEMENTED

1. Identify Relapse Triggers (1)

A. The patient was assisted in identifying specific behaviors, attitudes, and feelings that contributed to his/her last relapse.

B. The patient has specified the mistakes that he/she made in behavior, attitude, and emotional reactions that contributed to his/her relapse.

C. The patient acknowledged that he/she did not implement the coping behaviors necessary to maintain sobriety in the face of trigger situations.

D. The patient gave a clear, firm commitment to renew efforts toward developing a comprehensive recovery plan for sobriety.

2. Assess Ability to Detox (2)

A. The assessment of the patient concluded that he/she was able to detox and begin to establish sobriety.

B. The assessment of the patient found that he/she was not able to detox in an outpatient setting, but needed referral to a more intensive level of care in order to begin recovery and establish sobriety.

C. The patient was referred to a residential/hospital-based treatment program to begin recovery efforts.

3. Teach Structured Routine (3)

A. The importance of structure and routine in daily life were taught to the patient.

B. The patient was assisted in developing a daily routine for his/her life.

C. A balance of work, sleep, proper nutrition, exercise, social contact, recreation, spiritual support, and recovery support was established in the patient's structured life.

4. AA Attendance Referral (4)

A. The patient was urged to make consistent attendance at AA meetings a part of his/her routine structure.

B. The patient agreed to attend AA meetings on a consistent basis.

C. The patient has refused to commit to regular attendance at AA meetings.

D. The patient reported that he/she has been attending AA meetings on a frequent and regular basis every week.

5. Contact AA Sponsor (5)

A. The patient was encouraged to make contact with his/her sponsor as a critical step in reestablishing a recovery program.

B. The patient has made contact with his/her AA sponsor and has agreed to maintain consistent contact with him/her.

C. The patient is not satisfied with his/her AA sponsor and will ask another AA member to fulfill that role shortly.

* The numbers in parentheses correlate to the number of the Therapeutic Intervention statement in the companion chapter with the same title in *The Complete Adult Psychotherapy Treatment Planner,* second edition (Jongsma and Peterson) by John Wiley & Sons, 1999.

6. Assign Second AA/NA Sponsor (6)

A. The patient was assigned the task of finding a second AA/NA sponsor who has a different approach and style than the first sponsor.

B. The patient has made contact with a second sponsor and has agreed to meet with both sponsors at least weekly.

C. The patient reported that he/she is meeting with both the first and second sponsors on a weekly basis.

D. The patient has not followed through on establishing contact with a second sponsor and was redirected to do so.

7. Identify Negative Influences (7)

A. The patient was assisted in identifying the people and situations who exert a negative influence on his/her recovery and encourage relapse.

B. The patient listed several people and places that he/she needs to avoid because they too easily trigger relapse.

C. Specific ways to avoid contact with high-risk people and places were identified.

D. The patient reported that he/she is avoiding contact on a consistent basis with those people and places that are high risk for triggering relapse.

8. Assign Relapse Workbook (8)

A. The patient was assigned to complete a relapse workbook to process the results of that work in future sessions.

B. The patient followed through on completion of a relapse workbook, and the results of that assignment were processed.

C. The patient has not followed through on completing a relapse workbook and was redirected to do so.

D. Completion of the relapse workbook has helped the patient identify people and places that must be avoided to maintain recovery.

9. Assign Recovery Reading Material (9)

A. The patient was assigned reading material on chemical dependence recovery and asked to select relevant items for future discussion.

B. The patient has followed through on reading the assigned recovery material, and relevant content was processed.

C. The patient has not followed through on reading the assigned recovery material and was redirected to do so.

D. Reading the recovery material has helped the patient identify people and places that must be avoided to maintain recovery.

10. Explore Feelings about Relapse (10)

A. The patient was helped to identify and express his/her feelings that contributed to the relapse and the feelings resulting from the relapse.

B. The patient is becoming more skilled at identifying and expressing his/her feelings.

11. **Assign Material on Resentment (11)**

A. The patient was assigned to read *The Golden Book of Resentment* (Father John Doe) or *As Bill Sees It* (Bill Wilson) in order to better understand his/her feelings of resentment and how these feelings can contribute to relapse.

B. The patient has read the assigned material on resentment and identified several issues within his/her life that have precipitated feelings of resentment and contributed to relapse.

C. The patient's feelings of resentment were processed and alternative coping mechanisms were discussed to deal with these feelings rather than allowing them to contribute to relapse.

D. The patient has not followed through on reading the assigned material on resentment and was redirected to do so.

12. **Assign Talk with Successful AA/NA Members (12)**

A. The patient was assigned to interview successful AA/NA members who have maintained their sobriety for three or more years and to focus on what they have specifically done to accomplish this.

B. The patient has followed through with holding discussions with successful AA/NA members and reported important concepts learned from this discussion regarding maintaining his/her own sobriety.

C. The patient has not followed through on interviewing successful AA/NA members and was redirected to do so.

13. **Identify Sobriety Rewards (13)**

A. The patient was assisted in identifying the positive rewards that would accrue in his/her life from maintaining total abstinence.

B. The identification of positive consequences that can result from recovery has served to motivate the patient to strengthen his/her recovery plan.

14. **Assign "Cost-Benefit Analysis" (14)**

A. The patient was assigned to complete a "Cost-Benefit Analysis" regarding his/her relapse into substance abuse.

B. The patient has completed his/her "Cost-Benefit Analysis" regarding his/her return to substance abuse and was able to identify many negative consequences and few rewards from this incident.

C. The patient has failed to complete the "Cost-Benefit Analysis" and was instructed to do so.

15. **Physician Evaluation Referral (15)**

A. The patient was referred to a physician for an evaluation for Antabuse or antidepressant medication as aids to his/her recovery.

B. The patient has completed a medical assessment for Antabuse and/or antidepressant medication.

C. The patient has accepted a prescription for Antabuse and has begun its use.

D. The patient has accepted a prescription for antidepressant medication and has begun its use.

E. The patient has not followed through on the referral to a physician for a medication evaluation and was redirected to do so.

16. Acupuncture Referral (16)

A. The patient was referred to an acupuncturist for treatment on a regular basis in order to strengthen recovery from chemical dependence.

B. The patient has followed through with involvement with acupuncture treatment and reported that the urge to use mood-altering substances has been reduced.

C. The patient has not followed through on obtaining acupuncture treatment.

D. The patient reported that the acupuncture treatment that he/she obtained has not been helpful in reducing the urge for mood-altering substances.

17. Monitor Medication Compliance (17)

A. The patient was monitored for his/her compliance with the medication orders and other treatments.

B. The patient has shown compliance with his/her prescribed medications and other treatments.

C. The patient reported that the medication has been beneficial in terms of supporting his/her chemical dependence recovery and stabilizing his/her mood.

D. The patient has not been compliant with prescribed medications and was redirected to do so.

E. The patient reported that the medication has not been effective in reducing urges for mood-altering drugs.

18. Confer with Prescribing Provider (18)

A. The physician who has been providing prescribed medications for the patient was conferred with regarding the patient's reports of the effectiveness of the medication.

B. The physician has agreed to alter the prescribed medication since the patient reported a lack of benefit from the medication.

19. Identify Relapse Triggers (19)

A. The patient was assigned to develop a list of behaviors, attitudes, and feelings that may have contributed to his/her substance abuse relapse.

B. The patient has identified several behaviors, attitudes, and feelings that he/she believes contributed to his/her substance abuse relapse.

C. Coping mechanisms were identified to be applied to those behaviors, attitudes, and feelings that have contributed to the patient's relapse.

20. Assign an Autobiography (20)

A. The patient was assigned to write a focused autobiography dating from the first attempt to get sober until the present.

B. The patient has completed his/her focused autobiography, beginning with the first attempt to get sober and read it within the session prior to discussing triggers to relapse.

C. The patient has not followed through on writing a focused autobiography and was redirected to do so.

21. Assign a List of Significant Others' Observations (21)

A. The patient was asked to gather from significant others a list of his/her behaviors or attitudes prior to his/her relapse.

B. The patient has obtained the list of observations from significant others, and this list was processed to identify triggers to relapse.

C. Alternative coping behaviors were identified for those relapse triggers that were identified from the patient's significant others' list of observations.

D. The patient has failed to gather a list from significant others regarding observations of his/her behaviors and attitudes and was redirected to do so.

22. Develop a Symptom Line (22)

A. The patient was assisted in developing a symptom line that identified each relapse in terms of when it happened and what was occurring at the time of the relapse.

B. The symptom line helped the patient identify the specific behaviors, attitudes, and feelings that led up to his/her relapses.

C. Alternative, positive coping mechanisms were suggested for the patient's use to counteract those triggers that were identified from the symptom line.

23. Spiritual Leader Referral (23)

A. The patient was referred to his/her identified spiritual leader who has knowledge of substance abuse and recovery in order to support the patient through the completion of the fifth step.

B. The patient has followed through with meeting with his/her spiritual leader to complete his/her fifth step.

C. The patient has not followed through with meeting with his/her spiritual leader to complete his/her fifth step and was redirected to do so.

24. Assign Books on Recovery (24)

A. The patient was assigned to read *Many Roads, One Journey: Moving Beyond the 12 Steps* (Kasl-Davis) or *Stage II Recovery* (Larsen) to help him/her identify behavior patterns that will need to be changed to maintain sobriety.

B. The patient has followed through with the reading assignments and has identified behavior patterns that need to be changed to maintain sobriety.

C. The patient has not followed through with the reading assignments and was redirected to do so.

25. Teach Relaxation Methods (25)

A. The patient was taught various methods of relaxation, such as meditation and deep breathing, to assist him/her in reducing his/her negative reactions to stress.

B. The patient identified several situations in which stress reduction techniques might be beneficial to be implemented in his/her daily life.

C. The patient reported that implementation of the relaxation techniques has helped to reduce stress reactions in his/her daily life.

D. The patient has not followed through with applying the stress reduction techniques in his/her daily life and was redirected to do so.

26. Teach Coping Skills for Feelings (26)

A. The patient was taught ways to react to negative emotions in constructive ways rather than allowing them to be a trigger for relapse.

B. The patient has demonstrated the ability to tolerate uncomfortable emotions by implementing coping mechanisms, such as sharing feelings, engaging in diversion activities, and journaling.

27. Develop Trigger-Coping Strategies (27)

A. The patient was assisted in developing at least two coping strategies for each identified trigger to relapse.

B. The patient reported that implementation of the positive coping strategies has helped reduce his/her vulnerability to relapse.

28. Teach Assertiveness (28)

A. The patient was taught the principles of assertiveness in contrast to aggressiveness and passivity.

B. Role playing, behavioral rehearsal, and modeling were used to apply assertiveness techniques to situations from the patient's daily life.

C. The patient reported that he/she has implemented assertiveness to communicate feelings more directly and that this has been a rewarding experience.

D. The patient has difficulty in implementing assertiveness and was redirected to do so.

29. Explore Relationship Stressors (29)

A. Within a conjoint session, the stresses with significant others that exist within the patient's relapse were explored.

B. Conjoint sessions were used to assist the patient and significant others resolve conflicts within their relationship.

30. Educate the Family Regarding Relapse Triggers (30)

A. The patient's partner and significant others were taught how certain people, places, and things can function as relapse triggers for the patient.

B. Significant others were assisted in identifying ways in which they could be supportive of the patient's sobriety.

C. The patient's significant others were strongly encouraged to attend Al-Anon meetings on a regular basis to help support his/her recovery from substance abuse.

D. Significant others from the patient's family have been resistive to finding a way that they could be supportive of his/her recovery efforts.

31. Develop Sobriety Rituals (31)

A. The patient was assisted in identifying and encouraged to participate in rituals that will support and enhance sobriety.

B. The patient was encouraged to attend AA on a regular basis and to participate in the rituals within that self-help recovery group.

C. The patient has established a pattern of regular participation in AA and also meets on a regular basis with his/her sponsor at a set date and time.

D. The patient is resistive to participating in rituals that support recovery and was redirected to do so.

32. Utilize Solution-Focused Approach (32)

A. The patient was assisted in identifying specific things that he/she was doing to support sobriety when he/she was successful prior to relapse.

B. The patient was directed to implement those behaviors that were his/her chemical dependence supportive of sobriety but were unused just prior to relapse.

33. Read Fables (33)

A. Fables from *Stories for the 3rd Ear* (Wallar) were read with the patient in order to help him/her verbalize principles to live by that will support sobriety.

B. The patient clearly identified constructive principles to live by from the reading of the fables.

C. The patient resisted identifying any principles to live by from the reading of the fables.

34. Develop a Significant Other Relapse Contract (34)

A. The patient was assisted in completing a relapse contract with his/her significant others that identified previous relapse-associated behaviors, attitudes, and emotions.

B. The patient's significant others agreed to provide warnings to that patient if they noticed the previously identified behaviors, attitudes, and emotions that have triggered relapse.

C. The patient reported that significant others have been helpful in pointing out to him/her triggers for relapse.

D. Significant others have been resistive to play a supportive role in the patient's recovery plan.

35. Develop a Written Aftercare Plan (35)

A. The patient was assigned the task of developing a written aftercare plan that addresses specific relapse triggers along with positive coping behaviors.

B. The patient has followed through on developing a relapse prevention plan that identifies positive coping behaviors for each relapse trigger.

C. The patient has not followed through on writing out an aftercare plan for relapse triggers.

D. The patient reported that he/she has implemented his/her aftercare plan successfully and that relapse triggers have been coped with adaptively.

CHILDHOOD TRAUMAS

PATIENT PRESENTATION

1. Physical/Sexual/Emotional Abuse (1)

A. The patient reported that he/she had a history of physical, sexual, or emotional abuse.

B. The patient reported that painful memories of abusive childhood experiences are intrusive and unsettling.

C. The patient reported that nightmares and other disturbing thoughts related to childhood abuse interfere with his/her sleep.

D. The patient reported that his/her emotional reactions associated with the childhood abusive emotional experiences have been resolved.

E. The patient was able to discuss his/her childhood abusive experiences without being overwhelmed with negative emotions.

2. Neglect Experiences (2)

A. The patient reported a history of parents who were neglectful of his/her emotional and physical needs.

B. The patient's feelings of low self-esteem, lack of confidence, and vulnerability to depression are related to his/her childhood experiences of neglect.

C. The patient stated that his/her parents were involved with substance abuse and this led to neglect of their child-rearing responsibilities.

D. The parents' involvement in work and their own self-centered experiences led to neglect of the children.

E. The patient reported that his/her parents had limited intellectual capacity and failed to comprehend the full responsibilities of parenting.

3. Chaotic Childhood History (3)

A. The patient described his/her childhood history as chaotic, related to frequent moods, substitute caretakers, financial instability, multiple parental partners, and the in-and-out presence of stepsiblings.

B. The patient described growing up in an alcoholic household, which led to significant instability.

C. The patient described one of his/her parents as seriously mentally ill, resulting in multiple periods of hospitalization and instability at home.

D. The patient described his/her parents as irresponsible and antisocial, leading to many legal and interpersonal conflicts.

---

* The numbers in parentheses correlate to the number of the Behavioral Definition statement in the companion chapter with the same title in *The Complete Adult Psychotherapy Treatment Planner,* second edition (Jongsma and Peterson) by John Wiley & Sons, 1999.

4. Repressive Parents (4)

A. The patient described his/her parents as rigid, perfectionistic, and hypercritical, resulting in him/her consistently feeling inadequate.

B. The patient reported that his/her parents were threatening and demeaning, resulting in feelings of low self-esteem.

C. The patient reported that his/her parents were hyperreligious, resulting in rigid, high expectations of behavior and harsh discipline.

D. The patient described an emotionally repressive atmosphere at home during his/her childhood as a result of his/her parents' lack of nurturance, encouragement, and positive reinforcement.

5. Irrational Fears (5)

A. The patient's early life experiences have led to continuing irrational fears in the present.

B. As the patient has developed insight into conflicts related to his/her childhood, his/her irrational fears have begun to diminish.

C. The patient reported a greater sense of security and an absence of previously held irrational fears.

6. Suppressed Rage (5)

A. The patient reported that his/her early painful experiences have resulted in feelings of anger and unexpressed rage.

B. The patient has begun to express suppressed feelings of rage toward his/her parents for their treatment of him/her during childhood.

C. The patient's level of anger has diminished and he/she reported a greater sense of peace.

7. Depression and Low Self-Esteem (5)

A. The patient reported feelings of low self-esteem and depression related to painful experiences of childhood.

B. As the patient has shared his/her pain related to childhood experiences, the feelings of low self-esteem and depression have diminished.

C. The patient reported increased feelings of positive self-esteem and a lifting of depression.

8. Identity Conflicts/Anxious Insecurity (5)

A. The patient reported struggles with his/her identity and feelings of insecurity due to painful childhood experiences.

B. The patient reported a clearer sense of identity and more self-confidence as his/her painful childhood experiences were processed.

9. Dissociative Phenomena (6)

A. The patient reported the presence of dissociative phenomena during times of high stress as a result of childhood emotional pain.

B. The patient reported that his/her experiences of dissociative phenomena have terminated as he/she worked through the painful experiences of his/her childhood.

INTERVENTIONS IMPLEMENTED

1. Build Trust (1)

A. Consistent eye contact, active listening, unconditional positive regard, and warm acceptance were used to help build trust with the patient.

B. The patient began to express feelings more freely as rapport and the trust level increased.

C. The patient has continued to experience difficulty being open and direct in his/her expression of painful feelings.

2. Explore Childhood Experiences (2)

A. The patient's painful childhood experiences were explored.

B. The patient explained what it was like to grow up in the home environment, focusing on the abusive/neglectful experiences that he/she endured.

C. The patient has begun to open up about his/her childhood experiences, but still remains rather guarded.

D. The patient described, in detail, the facts and feelings associated with his/her painful childhood experiences.

3. Develop Family Symptom Line (3)

A. A genogram was developed for the patient's family, along with a list of symptoms and characteristics of each family member.

B. As the patient described what it was like to grow up in his/her home, he/she also described the dysfunction present within each family member that contributed to the chaotic atmosphere of abuse and neglect.

C. The patient was resistive to describing the dysfunction of each family member and became defensive out of a sense of loyalty to them.

D. The patient described his/her feelings toward each family member as they were experienced in the past and in the present.

4. Clarify Family Role (4)

A. The patient was assisted in clarifying his/her role within the family and the feelings associated with that role assignment.

B. The patient clearly understood the role that he/she played within the family and how that contributed to the dynamics of dysfunction.

C. The patient verbalized an understanding of how his/her role within the family as a child has had an impact on his/her current feelings toward self and others.

5. Encourage Feelings Expression (5)

A. The patient was supported and encouraged when he/she began to express feelings of rage, fear, and rejection relating to family abuse or neglect.

B. The patient has continued to clarify his/her understanding of feelings associated with major traumatic incidents in childhood.

---

* The numbers in parentheses correlate to the number of the Therapeutic Intervention statement in the companion chapter with the same title in *The Complete Adult Psychotherapy Treatment Planner,* second edition (Jongsma and Peterson) by John Wiley & Sons, 1999.

C. As the patient has clarified his/her feelings and shared them within the session, his/her feelings of emotional turmoil have diminished.

6. Assign Feelings Journal (6)

A. The patient was assigned to record his/her feelings in a journal that describes memories, behavior, and emotions tied to traumatic childhood experiences.

B. The patient has followed through on the journaling assignment and has developed an increased awareness of the impact that his/her childhood experiences have had on present feelings and behavior.

C. The patient identified how his/her experiences of childhood have influenced how he/she parents his/her own children today.

7. Assign Books on Childhood Trauma (7)

A. Reading materials relating to traumatic childhood experiences were recommended to the patient to assist him/her in developing insight.

B. The patient has followed through on reading the recommended childhood trauma material, and insights related to that reading were processed.

C. The patient has not followed through on reading the recommended material and was redirected to do so.

8. Explore Patient's Parenting (8)

A. The patient was assisted in comparing his/her own parenting behavior to that of parent figures of his/her childhood.

B. The patient expressed understanding of how his/her own parenting patterns have been influenced by the negative patterns of his/her own parents.

C. The patient was resistive to drawing any parallels between his/her own parenting style and that of his/her abusive and neglectful parents.

9. Explore Victim versus Survivor (9)

A. The patient was asked to consider the positive and negative consequences of considering himself/herself as a victim versus being a survivor of childhood trauma.

B. The patient verbalized an understanding of the advantages of perceiving himself/herself as a survivor of abuse and neglect rather than a victim.

C. The patient has continued to view himself/herself as a victim of painful childhood experiences and has not moved forward toward feeling empowered as a survivor.

10. Reinforce Survivor Self-Perception (10)

A. The patient was encouraged and reinforced to perceive himself/herself as a survivor rather than a victim of childhood abuse or neglect.

B. As the patient increased his/her statements that reflected a self-perception of survivorship rather than victimization, strong reinforcement was given.

C. The patient has continued to make statements of being a victim rather than statements of personal empowerment that reflect survivorship.

11. Assign Feelings Letter (11)

A. The patient was assigned the task of writing a letter to his/her parents regarding his/her feelings associated with the experience of childhood neglect or abuse.

B. The patient has followed through with writing a feelings letter to his/her parents regarding his/her childhood abuse/neglect.

C. The patient reported that writing the letter regarding his/her childhood abuse experiences has helped him/her decrease feelings of shame and affirm himself/herself as not being responsible for the abuse.

D. The patient has not followed through with writing the letter to his/her parents regarding the childhood abuse or neglect experiences and was redirected to do so.

12. Support Confrontation of Perpetrator (12)

A. A conjoint session was held where the patient confronted the perpetrator of his/her childhood abusive experiences.

B. The patient was supported in his/her confrontation of the perpetrator of abuse and neglect while responsibility for that neglect was placed clearly on the perpetrator.

C. The patient found it very difficult to be direct in his/her confrontation of the perpetrator of childhood abuse/neglect.

D. The perpetrator responded with defensive statements and denial in reaction to the patient's confrontation of him/her regarding childhood abuse and neglect.

E. Since the confrontation of the perpetrator, the patient has reported decreased feelings of shame and more clarity regarding not being responsible for the abuse that occurred to him/her.

13. Utilize Empty-Chair Exercise (13)

A. The patient was guided in an empty-chair exercise with the perpetrator of the abuse as the imagined person in the empty chair.

B. The patient was guided in an empty-chair exercise in which the nonperpetrating parent was imagined to be in the empty chair.

C. The patient expressed his/her feelings and clarified the impact that the childhood experiences of abuse had on him/her.

D. The patient affirmed himself/herself as not being responsible for the abuse and placed responsibility clearly on the perpetrator.

E. The patient confronted the nonperpetrating parent for not protecting him/her from the abusive experiences in childhood.

14. Reinforce Holding Perpetrator Responsible (14)

A. Any and all statements that the patient made that reflected placing blame on the perpetrators and nonprotective, nonnurturant adults for his/her painful childhood experiences were reinforced.

B. The patient was consistently reminded that he/she was not responsible for the abuse and neglect that occurred in his/her childhood but that it was the responsibility of his/her childhood parents or caretakers.

C. The patient continues to struggle with blaming himself/herself for the abusive experiences of his/her childhood.

15. Teach Share-Check Technique (15)

A. The patient was taught to build trust in relationships through the use of the share-check technique.

B. The patient reported that he/she has begun to share personal thoughts and feelings with others on a minimal basis in order to see if those feelings are dealt with respectfully and supportively.

C. The patient expressed difficulty with building trust and intimacy with others.

D. The patient expressed insight into his/her difficulty with building trust as related to childhood experiences of abuse and neglect.

16. Teach Trust in Others (16)

A. The patient was encouraged and taught the advantages of treating others as trustworthy while continuing to assess their character.

B. The patient reported that he/she is beginning to increase trust and interaction with others.

C. The patient continues to struggle with issues of trust and to be withdrawn in social relationships.

17. Teach Forgiveness Benefits (17)

A. The patient was taught the benefits of beginning the process of forgiving those adults who perpetrated abuse and neglect on him/her during childhood.

B. The patient has begun the process of forgiving the perpetrators of his/her childhood abuse and neglect.

C. As the patient has begun to forgive the perpetrators of his/her painful childhood experiences, he/she has also begun to release feelings of hurt and anger and put the issue in the past.

D. As the patient has begun forgiveness, he/she has been able to experience feelings of trust in others.

18. Recommend Forgiveness Books (18)

A. Reading books on forgiveness was recommended to the patient to increase his/her understanding of the process and benefits of forgiveness.

B. The patient has followed through with reading the recommended material on forgiveness, and key concepts were reviewed and processed.

C. The patient has not followed through on reading the recommended material on forgiveness and was redirected to do so.

D. Since the patient has read the forgiveness material, he/she has been able to identify the positive aspects for himself/herself of being able to forgive all those involved with the abuse.

19. Assign Forgiveness Letter (19)

A. The patient was assigned to write a letter of forgiveness to the perpetrator of the childhood hurt.

B. The patient has followed through with writing his/her forgiveness letter to the perpetrator of the childhood hurt and reported that he/she has experienced a sense of putting the issue in the past.

C. The patient reported that he/she has begun the process of forgiving the perpetrator of his/her childhood pain and others who may have been passive collaborators.

D. The patient has not followed through on writing the forgiveness letter to the perpetrator of his/her childhood pain and was redirected to do so.

20. Research Family Dysfunction (20)

A. The patient was assigned to ask his/her parents about their family backgrounds and develop insight into patterns of behavior and causes for his/her parents' dysfunction.

B. The patient has identified patterns of abuse, neglect, and abandonment within the parents' families of origin and within the extended family also.

C. The patient verbalized a recognition that his/her parents have followed a pattern that has been long established within the family of abuse and neglect of the children.

D. Recognizing that his/her parents were following an extended family pattern of abuse and neglect has helped the patient begin the process of forgiving them.

E. Recognition of the extended family pattern of abuse and neglect has alerted the patient to be vigilant against continuing this cycle of abuse and neglect within his/her own family.

21. Assess Substance Abuse (21)

A. A complete drug and alcohol history of the patient was gathered to assess whether substance abuse has been a means of coping with feelings regarding the childhood trauma.

B. Chemical dependence was found within the patient's behavior pattern and referral to substance abuse treatment was made.

C. The assessment of the patient's substance abuse determined that there is not a chemical dependence problem.

D. The patient acknowledged that he/she has abused substances as a means of coping with the pain resulting from childhood abuse and neglect.

22. Explore Dissociative Experiences (22)

A. The patient's history of experiencing dissociative phenomena to protect himself/herself from the pain of childhood abusive experiences was explored.

B. The patient was assisted in understanding the role of dissociation in protecting himself/herself from emotional pain.

C. The patient reported the experience of dissociative phenomena to such an extent that this problem was made a focus of treatment.

D. The patient denied that there was any significant and consistent pattern of dissociative experiences.

23. Assess Dissociation Severity (23)

A. The severity of the patient's dissociative phenomena was assessed.

B. Because the patient's dissociative phenomena were significantly severe, hospitalization was recommended to stabilize his/her condition.

C. The patient's dissociative phenomena were not found to be severe or persistent.

CHRONIC PAIN

PATIENT PRESENTATION

1. Chronic Pain Limits Activity (1)

A. The patient has experienced chronic pain beyond that which would be expected through the normal healing process and it significantly limits his/her physical activities.

B. The patient has not been able to discover ways to manage or decrease his/her pain effectively.

C. The patient reported that the pain management strategies have helped to reduce his/her preoccupation with chronic pain.

D. The patient has increased involvement in physical activities, as he/she has acquired the necessary pain management skills.

2. Generalized Pain (2)

A. The patient has complained of pain throughout his/her body and in many joints, muscles, and bones.

B. The patient's pain has interfered in his/her daily functioning.

C. The patient verbalized fewer complaints about generalized pain and is resuming some normal activities.

D. The patient stated that he/she has become significantly less preoccupied with his/her generalized pain and is functioning rather normally.

3. Pain Medication Use (3)

A. The patient reported that he/she has become heavily reliant on pain medication, but that in spite of this dependence, he/she experiences little pain relief.

B. The patient has increased his/her pain medication use beyond the prescription level in an attempt to obtain relief.

C. The patient has become dependent on the use of medication and may be physiologically addicted.

D. The patient has acknowledged his/her overuse of medication and has begun to reduce this dependency and utilize other pain management techniques.

E. The patient has terminated the use of pain medication that was offering little benefit and has found more adaptive ways to regulate pain.

4. Experiences Headaches (4)

A. The patient described a chronic history of headache pain that occurs almost daily.

B. The patient's headaches produce excruciating pain that interferes with daily functioning.

C. The patient reported a reduction in the frequency and severity of his/her headaches.

---

* The numbers in parentheses correlate to the number of the Behavioral Definition statement in the companion chapter with the same title in *The Complete Adult Psychotherapy Treatment Planner,* second edition (Jongsma and Peterson) by John Wiley & Sons, 1999.

D. Use of medical and behavioral techniques has virtually eliminated the experience of headaches for the patient.

5. Back Pain (5)

A. The patient complained of chronic back pain that extends into the neck.

B. The patient's back pain has interfered with his/her normal functioning at work and play.

C. The patient has adapted his/her entire life to accommodate his/her back pain.

D. The patient's complaints of back pain have been significantly reduced as he/she has found constructive ways to regulate and manage this pain.

6. Fibromyalgia Pain (5)

A. The patient has been diagnosed with fibromyalgia, a condition that results in generalized pain and fatigue.

B. The patient's entire life has been negatively affected by the fibromyalgia condition.

C. The patient is beginning to focus on positive aspects of his/her life and to regulate and manage the fibromyalgia pain.

D. The patient has returned to near normal functioning, in spite of the fibromyalgia condition.

7. Rheumatoid Arthritis (6)

A. The patient experiences intermittent severe pain related to the condition of rheumatoid arthritis.

B. The patient's rheumatoid arthritis condition has become increasingly severe, resulting in limitations in physical activity and debilitation of psychological functioning.

C. The patient is beginning to manage his/her pain more effectively and maximize daily functioning ability.

8. Irritable Bowel Syndrome (6)

A. The patient has been diagnosed with irritable bowel syndrome, which results in attacks of severe cramping and pain associated with diarrhea.

B. The patient's life has been significantly restricted because of the irritable bowel condition.

C. The patient has learned to regulate his/her irritable bowel condition and to maximize his/her daily functioning ability.

9. Decreased Activity (7)

A. The patient has significantly decreased or stopped activities related to work, household chores, socialization, exercise, and sexual pleasure because of pain.

B. The patient described considerable frustration and depression related to the termination of constructive activity because of his/her pain.

C. As the patient has learned to regulate his/her pain more effectively, he/she has increased normal activities.

D. The patient has returned to work and is performing household-related chores as pain management has become more effective.

E. The patient has increased his/her pleasurable activities related to socialization, exercise, and sexual interaction as effective pain management has been learned.

10. **Generalized Physical Symptoms (8)**

A. The patient complained of pain-related symptoms such as fatigue, insomnia, muscle tension, decreased concentration, and memory interference.

B. As the patient has learned pain management and regulation skills, there have been fewer complaints of generalized physical symptoms.

11. **Depression (9)**

A. The patient's experience of chronic pain has led to feelings of depression.

B. The patient expressed feelings of depression related to his/her inability to perform normal daily activities because of debilitating pain.

C. As the patient has learned pain management skills, his/her depression has decreased.

D. The patient reported an increase in self-esteem, interest in activities, increased energy, and enjoyment of socialization as his/her pain management has become more effective.

12. **Pessimistic Verbalizations (10)**

A. The patient made frequent pessimistic verbalizations about his/her inability to control the pain or live a normal life or be understood by others.

B. As the patient has learned pain management skills, he/she is making significantly fewer pessimistic statements about himself/herself and his/her future.

INTERVENTIONS IMPLEMENTED

1. **Gather Pain History (1)**

A. A history of the patient's experience of chronic pain and his/her associated medical conditions was gathered.

B. The patient described the nature of his/her pain and explained the causes for it.

C. The patient does not have a clear understanding of the causes for his/her pain or effective ways to manage it.

2. **Explore Pain's Negative Impact (2)**

A. The changes in the patient's social, vocational, familial, and intimacy life that have occurred in reaction to his/her pain were explored.

B. The patient clearly identified how the pain has made a negative impact on many types of daily activities.

C. The patient explained the serious debilitating effect that the pain has had on his/her role within the family.

3. **Explore Emotional Reaction (3)**

A. The patient's emotional reaction to his/her chronic pain was explored.

B. The patient verbalized the mood and attitude changes that have accompanied the experience of chronic pain.

C. The patient described feelings of depression, frustration, and irritability that have resulted from the way pain has interfered with his/her life.

* The numbers in parentheses correlate to the number of the Therapeutic Intervention statement in the companion chapter with the same title in *The Complete Adult Psychotherapy Treatment Planner,* second edition (Jongsma and Peterson) by John Wiley & Sons, 1999.

D. The patient acknowledged that he/she experiences periods of severe depression related to this significant pain and the negative changes that have occurred in his/her life because of it.

4. Physician Referral (4)

A. The patient was referred to a physician to undergo a thorough examination to rule out any undiagnosed condition and to receive recommendations for further treatment options.

B. The patient has followed through on the physician evaluation referral and has been informed of new treatment options.

C. The patient was encouraged by the prospect of new medical procedures that may offer hope in terms of pain relief.

D. The patient was discouraged to discover that no new medical procedures could offer hope of pain relief.

E. The patient has not followed through on obtaining a new evaluation by a physician and was encouraged to do so.

5. Discuss Pain Management/Rehabilitation Programs (5)

A. A discussion was held regarding available pain management alternatives and rehabilitation programs.

B. After considering the alternative programs available, the patient selected a pain management/rehabilitation program for himself/herself.

C. The patient was resistive to the notion of participating in a pain management program and did not believe it would be helpful.

6. Pain Management/Rehabilitation Referral (6)

A. All the necessary arrangements were made for the patient to begin treatment at the pain management/rehabilitation program.

B. The patient has agreed to follow through on the referral and attend the first appointment at the pain management/rehabilitation program.

C. The patient has refused to participate in the pain management/rehabilitation effort.

7. Request Confidentiality Releases (7)

A. Release-of-information forms were completed and signed by the patient that would allow regular contact with the pain management/rehabilitation staff.

B. Release-of-information forms were forwarded to pain management staff and they have agreed to provide regular progress reports.

8. Solicit Treatment Commitment (8)

A. The patient has agreed to cooperate with a full regimen of pain management treatment with specialists in this area.

B. The patient has refused to make a commitment to complete pain management treatment.

9. Medication Review Referral (9)

A. The patient was referred to a physician who specializes in chronic pain management in order to obtain a medication review.

B. The patient has followed through with attending an appointment with a physician who reviewed his/her medications.

C. The patient has begun taking the new medications prescribed by the physician to regulate the pain.

D. The patient has not followed through with a referral to a physician for a medication review and was redirected to do so.

10. Confer with Physician (10)

A. Contact was made with the patient's physician, who evaluated pain control medications.

B. The patient's physician was given a progress report regarding the patient's chronic pain management.

C. The patient's physician indicated that no further medication options were available to manage the patient's pain.

11. Teach Pain Ownership (11)

A. The patient was assisted in understanding the benefits of accepting his/her pain.

B. The patient was defensive in reaction to being told the advantages of accepting the chronic pain as his/her own.

C. The patient continued to work through his/her tendency to externalize the pain and reject ownership of it.

12. Reinforce Pain Ownership (12)

A. The patient was reinforced for statements that reflected ownership of his/her pain.

B. The patient continues to be resistive to making any statements of ownership of his/her pain.

C. The patient has made considerable progress and clearly takes ownership of his/her own pain as a problem that he/she must deal with.

13. Teach Key Pain Concepts (13)

A. The patient was educated regarding various aspects of pain such as rehabilitation versus biological healing, conservative versus aggressive medical interventions, acute versus chronic pain, benign versus nonbenign pain, cure versus management, and the role of exercise, medication, and self-regulation techniques.

B. The patient verbalized a good understanding of the key concepts of pain.

C. Comments made by the patient reflect an increasing understanding of the causes and treatment for his/her pain.

D. The patient continues to be confused by his/her pain and only talks of finding a way to end it.

14. Assign Pain-Related Literature (14)

A. Books were recommended for the patient to read to assist him/her in understanding the causes for, treatments of, and reactions to pain.

B. The patient has followed through on reading the recommended material, and key concepts gained from the reading were processed.

C. The patient has not followed through on reading the assigned material and was redirected to do so.

D. Reading the assigned material has helped the patient gain a deeper understanding of pain and how to constructively react to it and manage it.

15. Assign "Identifying Pain Triggers" (15)

A. The patient was assigned to read "Identifying Pain Triggers" from *Making Peace with Chronic Pain* (Hunter) and then make a list of his/her own pain triggers.

B. The patient has followed through on reading the pain trigger literature and has constructed a list of pain triggers for himself/herself.

C. The patient's list of pain triggers was clarified and processed.

D. Alternative behaviors that could be used as mechanisms for coping with pain triggers were discussed.

16. Assign Pain Journal (16)

A. The patient was asked to keep a pain journal in which he/she would record the time of day, where and what he/she was doing, the severity of the pain, and what was done to alleviate the pain.

B. The patient has followed through on completing the pain journal.

C. The patient reported that he/she has not kept a pain journal and was redirected to do so.

17. Process Pain Journal (17)

A. The material from the patient's pain journal was processed to assist him/her in developing insight into triggers for and the nature of his/her pain.

B. Interventions were discussed that could help the patient alleviate the frequency, duration, and severity of his/her pain.

18. Assign "Causes and Triggers" (18)

A. The patient was assigned to read "Causes and Triggers" in *Taking Control of Your Headaches* (Duckro, Richardson, and Marshall) to help him/her identify causes for and triggers of headache pain.

B. The patient has followed through on reading the assigned material on causes for and triggers of headache pain.

C. The patient has gained a greater understanding of the possible causes for his/her own headache pain.

D. The patient has not followed through on reading the assigned headache trigger material and was redirected to do so.

19. Teach the Dance of Pain (19)

A. The patient was taught to conceptualize his/her reaction to pain as if it were a dance.

B. The patient was assisted in identifying the particular steps of the dance of pain as it moved through his/her life.

C. The patient understood the concept of the dance of pain as applied to his/her life.

20. Challenge Dance Changes (20)

A. The patient was challenged to alter the steps of his/her present dance that is a reaction to his/her pain.

B. The patient was assisted in seeing possible alternative reactions that could change his/her dance of pain.

C. The patient has followed through on attempting to change his/her reactions to pain.

21. Assign Mind-Body Books (21)

A. Books on the concept of the connection between mind and body were recommended to the patient.

B. The patient has followed through on reading the mind-body literature that was recommended.

C. The patient has failed to follow through on the recommended reading on the concept of the mind-body connection and was redirected to do so.

22. Teach Mind-Body Connection (22)

A. The patient was taught the connection between his/her pain and mental states of stress, anger, tension, and depression.

B. The patient verbalized an understanding of how mental states of stress can exacerbate his/her physical pain.

C. The patient failed to see any connection between psychological states and physical pain.

23. Holistic Healing Referral (23)

A. The patient was referred to a holistic healing program that could help him/her establish the connection between stress management and pain management.

B. The patient accepted the referral to a holistic healing program that integrates mind and body treatment.

C. The patient was not open to a referral to a holistic referral healing program.

24. Teach Relaxation (24)

A. The patient was taught several different relaxation techniques to be used to reduce muscle tension and assist in pain management.

B. The patient demonstrated a good understanding of the relaxation techniques and committed himself/herself to implementing them.

C. The patient reported that implementation of the relaxation techniques has been helpful in reducing stress and the experience of pain.

D. The patient has not followed through on implementation of the relaxation techniques and was redirected to do so.

25. Assign Relaxation Tapes (25)

A. The patient was recommended to use audio- or videotapes to assist him/her in becoming more relaxed.

B. The patient reported that use of relaxation tapes has been beneficial in producing a relaxation state and reducing the experience of pain.

C. The patient has not followed through on the use of relaxation tapes and was redirected to do so.

D. The patient reported that the use of relaxation techniques has not been helpful in reducing the experience of pain.

26. Arrange for Biofeedback Training (26)

A. The patient was referred for biofeedback training in order to help him/her develop more precise relaxation skills.

B. The patient was administered biofeedback training in order to teach him/her more in-depth relaxation skills.

C. The biofeedback training sessions have been helpful in training the patient to relax more deeply.

D. The patient reported that his/her relaxation skills have been beneficial in managing chronic pain.

27. Assign *How to Meditate* (27)

A. It was recommended that the patient read *How to Meditate* (LeShan) in order to learn the principles of meditation that could be applied to pain management.

B. The patient has followed through on reading the meditation literature and has begun to implement the procedure into daily life.

C. The patient reported that implementation of the meditation procedure has helped him/her relax and manage his/her pain more effectively.

D. The patient has not followed through with reading the meditation literature and was redirected to do so.

28. Yoga Referral (28)

A. The patient was referred to a yoga class in order to assist him/her in developing meditation and relaxation skills.

B. The patient has followed through on attending the yoga class and has increased his/her ability to relax.

C. The use of yoga and relaxation techniques has helped the patient manage his/her pain.

D. The patient has not followed through with consistently attending the yoga class and was redirected to do so.

29. Teach Need for Exercise (29)

A. The patient was taught the importance of regular exercise as a benefit in pain management.

B. The patient has verbalized an understanding of the need for regular exercise in his/her life.

C. The patient has verbalized resistance to any kind of exercise regimen.

30. Exercise Program Referral (30)

A. The patient was referred for assistance in developing an individually tailored exercise program that is approved by the patient's personal physician.

B. The patient accepted the referral for the development of a physical exercise program and has committed to regular participation.

C. The patient refused to participate in an exercise program and would not accept a referral to such a program.

D. The patient postponed participation in the development of an exercise program and was encouraged to follow through.

31. Encourage Exercise Implementation (31)

A. The patient was encouraged to implement a daily exercise program into his/her life.

B. The patient reported on the implementation of exercise into his/her daily life and was reinforced for doing so.

C. The patient reported that he/she has not been consistent in maintaining exercise in his/her daily routine and was encouraged to do so.

D. The patient reported that implementation of exercise into his/her daily life has increased his/her sense of physical well-being and confidence in his/her body.

32. Assign *Managing Pain before It Manages You* (32)

A. Chapters 6 and 7 from the book *Managing Pain before It Manages You* (Caudill) were assigned to the patient to help him/her identify unhealthy attitudes regarding pain.

B. The patient has followed through with reading the assigned material on developing healthy attitudes about pain.

C. The patient verbalized an understanding of the need for healthy attitudes about pain, and specific healthy attitudes were identified.

D. The patient has not followed through with reading the material recommended on healthy pain attitudes and was redirected to do so.

33. Assign Dysfunctional Attitude Scale (33)

A. The patient was assigned to complete the Dysfunctional Attitude Scale (DAS) in the book *Managing Pain before It Manages You* (Caudill) in order to help him/her identify his/her dysfunctional attitudes about pain.

B. The patient has completed the Dysfunctional Attitude Scale, and his/her dysfunctional attitudes were identified and processed.

C. The patient acknowledged his/her tendency to develop dysfunctional attitudes about pain and the need to change this.

D. The patient was defensive about and resistive to identifying his/her dysfunctional attitudes about pain.

34. Assign Feedback from Others (34)

A. The patient was asked to gather feedback from significant others in his/her life regarding their perception of his/her negative attitudes about pain and life in general.

B. The patient has followed through with gathering feedback from others about his/her negative attitudes and was open to acknowledging these negative attitudes.

C. The patient was assisted in developing changes in negative attitudes that would be beneficial for enjoyment of life and management of his/her pain.

35. Develop Positive Attitudes (35)

A. The patient was confronted about his/her negative attitudes about pain.

B. The patient was assisted in developing more positive, constructive attitudes about his/her pain.

C. The patient was resistive to developing positive attitudes that would help him/her manage his/her pain and still enjoy life.

D. The patient reported that replacement of negative attitudes with those that are more positive about pain and life in general have increased his/her sense of peace and joy.

36. Reinforce Humor (36)

A. The patient was assisted in developing his/her sense of humor within his/her daily life.

B. The importance of humor in promoting healing was reviewed.

C. The patient was given suggestions about how to increase his/her enjoyment of humor through the use of tapes, books, jokes, or movies on a regular basis.

D. The patient reported that the increase in enjoyment of humor has contributed to less focus on pain and a perception of well-being.

37. Explore Alternative Medical Procedures (37)

A. Alternative medical procedures such as acupuncture, hypnosis, and therapeutic massage were discussed with the patient.

B. The patient was encouraged to explore alternative medical procedures for their beneficial effect on his/her management of pain.

C. The patient reported following through on the use of alternative medical procedures and has found some benefit in them.

D. The patient reported that the use of alternative medical procedures has not been beneficial to help him/her manage pain.

38. Dietician Referral (38)

A. The patient was referred to a dietician for a consultation about his/her eating and nutritional patterns.

B. The patient has followed through on attending an appointment with a dietician to consult about eating and nutritional patterns.

C. The patient has not followed through on the dietician referral and was redirected to do so.

39. Process Dietician Recommendations (39)

A. The results of the dietician consultation were processed.

B. The patient identified changes that he/she is beginning to implement regarding eating and nutritional patterns.

C. The patient reported that the changes in his/her diet have helped to promote health and fitness.

D. The patient has not followed through on implementing the changes recommended by the dietician and was redirected to do so.

40. Reinforce Pleasurable Activities (40)

A. The patient was assisted in creating a list of activities that give him/her pleasure.

B. The patient's list of pleasurable activities was processed and clarified.

C. A plan was developed for the patient to increase the frequency of implementation of the selected pleasurable activities.

D. Since implementation of the pleasurable activities, the patient has reported an increased sense of well-being.

E. The patient has not followed through on creating a list of or implementing pleasurable activities at an increased frequency.

41. Teach Assertiveness (41)

A. The patient was referred to an assertiveness training group to facilitate his/her learning assertiveness skills.

B. Role playing, modeling, and behavioral rehearsal were used to teach the patient assertiveness skills that he/she can implement in his/her daily life.

C. Scenarios were identified whereby the patient could implement assertiveness skills to help him/her in the management of his/her chronic pain.

D. The patient reported that he/she found opportunities to become more assertive and that this has resulted in improved pain management.

E. The patient has failed to implement assertiveness in his/her daily life and was encouraged to do so.

42. Assign "You Can Change the Way You Feel" (42)

A. The patient was encouraged to read the chapter "You Can Change the Way You Feel" from *The Feeling Good Handbook* (Burns) to help him/her identify cognitive distortions.

B. The patient has followed through with reading the assigned material on identifying cognitive distortions that impact his/her attitudes about pain and life in general.

C. The patient has not followed through with reading the assigned material on identifying cognitive distortions and was redirected to do so.

D. The patient reported that reading the assigned material has helped him/her identify negative self-talk that promotes helplessness, anger, and depression.

43. Explore Negative Self-Talk (43)

A. The patient was assisted in identifying his/her distorted automatic thoughts that promote depression, helplessness, and/or anger.

B. The patient has been successful in identifying his/her distorted automatic thoughts that promote depression, helplessness, and/or anger.

C. The patient reported instances in which he/she was able to spontaneously identify cognitive distortions in his/her daily life.

D. The patient was resistive to identifying his/her cognitive distortions.

44. Assign "You Feel the Way You Think" (44)

A. The patient was assigned the written exercise "You Feel the Way You Think" from *Ten Days to Self-Esteem!* (Burns) to help him/her identify the negative self-talk that he/she engages in that promotes helplessness, anger, and depression.

B. The patient has followed through with completing the written exercise on identifying negative self-talk.

C. The patient has not followed through with completing the exercise on identifying negative self-talk and was redirected to do so.

D. The patient reported that completing the exercise on identifying negative self-talk has been beneficial in helping him/her identify his/her patterns of distorted thinking.

45. Develop Positive Self-Talk (45)

A. The patient was assisted in replacing his/her negative distorted thoughts with more positive, reality-based thoughts that would help him/her manage his/her pain.

B. The patient's negative self-talk was replaced with positive, reality-based thoughts that would enhance his/her enjoyment of life and positive thoughts about the future.

C. The patient has more consistently verbalized positive self-talk that promotes empowerment, self-acceptance, and joy.

D. The patient is resistive to letting go of his/her negative, distorted automatic thoughts that promote depression, helplessness, and anger.

46. Utilize Transactional Analysis (46)

A. Using a Transactional Analysis approach, the patient was helped to become aware of "old tapes" about pain and his/her negative future and to replace these "old tapes" with more healthy self-talk messages.

B. The patient reported that replacing the "old tapes" with new messages has helped him/her become more positive about life.

47. Explore Life Stressors (47)

A. The patient was assisted in listing the daily stressors that he/she must cope with that contribute to his/her tension level.

B. The patient reported becoming more aware of the role of stress in his/her life and how it contributes to the exacerbation of his/her pain.

C. The patient has had difficulty identifying the role of stress exacerbating his/her chronic pain.

48. Teach Stress Awareness (48)

A. The patient was taught about the many types of internal, external, and interpersonal stresses that make an impact on him/her.

B. The patient verbalized an increased awareness of stress in his/her daily life and identified specific instances of it.

C. The patient was resistive to perceiving stress as contributing to his/her chronic pain management problems.

49. Teach Stress-Coping Techniques (49)

A. The patient was assisted in developing specific ways to cope effectively with the major stressors in his/her life.

B. The patient reported attempts at implementing new ways to react to the stressors in his/her life that will promote less tension.

C. Implementation of stress-coping techniques has helped the patient reduce the impact of stress on his/her physical health.

D. The patient has had difficulty implementing stress management techniques, and stress continues to have a serious negative impact on his/her health.

50. Develop Relapse Prevention Plan (50)

A. The patient was assisted in developing a written relapse prevention plan that had a special emphasis on pain- and stress-trigger identification, along with specific ways to adaptively react to these triggers.

B. The patient was resistive to developing a written relapse prevention plan and was encouraged to do so.

51. Monitor Relapse Prevention Plan (51)

A. The patient's relapse prevention plan was reviewed and monitored with the patient.

B. Changes and modifications were suggested for the patient's relapse prevention plan to help him/her become more effective at dealing with pain and stress triggers.

C. The patient has consistently implemented the relapse prevention plan and this has reduced his/her levels of pain and stress.

D. The patient has not consistently implemented the relapse prevention plan and was encouraged to do so.

52. Assign Sharing of Relapse Prevention Plan (52)

A. The patient was assigned to share his/her relapse prevention plan with those that are going to be a part of his/her support system.

B. The patient has shared his/her relapse prevention plan with significant others so that they might help with implementation, support, and feedback.

C. The patient's significant others have been supportive of the relapse prevention plan and this has helped the patient implement the plan.

D. The patient's significant others have not been supportive of his/her rehabilitation efforts and a family meeting was planned to try to increase their support.

COGNITIVE DEFICITS

PATIENT PRESENTATION

1. Concrete Thinking (1)

A. The patient presented with clear evidence of impaired abstract thinking and a tendency to think concretely.

B. The patient's concrete thinking continues to be problematic and cause difficulty for him/her in understanding important concepts in life.

C. The patient recognizes his/her tendency to think concretely and is taking steps to cope with this through reliance on others.

2. Lack of Insight (2)

A. The patient presented with a lack of insight into the consequences of his/her behavior or impaired judgment.

B. The patient has become slightly more aware of his/her impaired judgment and is stopping to consider the consequences of his/her behavior.

C. The patient has learned to solicit feedback from others regarding his/her plans for action rather than impulsively reacting.

3. Short-Term Memory Deficits (3)

A. The patient showed evidence of short-term memory deficits, although long-term memory remains intact.

B. The patient's short-term memory deficit has improved somewhat.

C. The patient has used coping techniques to adapt to his/her short-term memory deficit.

D. The patient continues to be inadequately aware of his/her short-term memory deficit.

4. Long-Term Memory Deficits (3)

A. The patient showed evidence of long-term memory deficits.

B. The patient's long-term memory has improved slightly.

C. The patient relied on others to provide historical review as a result of his/her long-term memory deficits.

5. Difficulty with Complex Directions (4)

A. The patient does not follow complex or sequential directions without becoming confused or forgetting some of the elements of the directions.

B. The patient is learning to break down complex or sequential directions into small steps.

C. The patient is using coping mechanisms to overcome his/her deficit in following complex or sequential directions.

D. The patient has a lack of insight into his/her inability to follow complex or sequential directions.

---

* The numbers in parentheses correlate to the number of the Behavioral Definition statement in the companion chapter with the same title in *The Complete Adult Psychotherapy Treatment Planner,* second edition (Jongsma and Peterson) by John Wiley & Sons, 1999.

6. Loss of Orientation (5)

A. The patient showed evidence of loss of orientation in terms of person, place, or time.

B. The patient is learning to rely more on external cues in order to become reoriented to person, place, or time.

C. The patient showed evidence of good orientation to person, place, and time.

7. Distractibility (6)

A. The patient showed evidence of high distractibility and low attention span.

B. The patient's distractibility causes problems in daily living, as he/she does not follow through with necessary tasks.

C. The patient was unable to perform instrumental activities of daily living on a consistent basis because of his/her distractibility.

8. Impulsivity (7)

A. The patient's impulsivity has led to behavior that violates social mores.

B. The patient has gradually attained more control over his/her impulses, resulting in more controlled behavior.

C. The patient's impulsivity has resulted in embarrassment to himself/herself and offense to others.

9. Speech/Language Impairment (8)

A. The patient's organic condition has resulted in significant speech and language problems.

B. The patient's speech and language problems have caused a serious impairment in communication.

C. The patient's speech and language problems are noticeable but he/she is still able to communicate in spite of the impairment.

D. The patient's speech and language impairment causes him/her significant frustration and depression.

E. The patient's speech and language impairment seems to be improving.

INTERVENTIONS IMPLEMENTED

1. Explore Neurological Impairment Signs (1)

A. The patient was assessed for signs and symptoms of his/her neurological impairment, including problems with memory, motor coordination, abstract thinking, speech and language, executive functions, orientation, impaired judgment, and attention.

B. The patient was aware of his/her neurological impairment and could describe the problematic symptoms.

C. The patient does not have insight or awareness regarding his/her neurological symptoms.

---

* The numbers in parentheses correlate to the number of the Therapeutic Intervention statement in the companion chapter with the same title in *The Complete Adult Psychotherapy Treatment Planner,* second edition (Jongsma and Peterson) by John Wiley & Sons, 1999.

2. Assess Cognitive Behavior (2)

A. The patient was observed and monitored in regard to signs and symptoms of his/her neurological deficit.

B. The patient's neurological deficits were noted with the session, but he/she seemed to be unaware of them.

C. The patient's neurological deficits were evident and he/she seemed to be aware of them.

3. Arrange Psychological Testing (3)

A. Psychological testing was discussed with the patient and arrangements were made for testing to be administered.

B. Psychological testing was ordered to determine the nature and degree of the patient's cognitive deficits.

C. The patient agreed to cooperate with psychological testing in order to determine the nature and degree of his/her cognitive deficits.

4. Administer Psychological Testing (4)

A. Psychological testing was administered to determine the nature, extent, and possible origin of the patient's cognitive deficits.

B. The psychological testing results indicate significant neurological impairment.

C. The psychological testing results do not confirm neurological deficits.

D. The patient cooperated with psychological testing.

E. The patient was not cooperative with psychological testing and it had to be canceled.

5. Neurologist Referral (5)

A. The patient was referred to a physician specializing in neurology to further assess his/her organic deficits and possible causes for those deficits.

B. The patient accepted and followed through with the referral to the neurologist.

C. The patient did not follow through with the neurological referral and was redirected to do so.

6. Discuss Assessment Results (6)

A. The results of the neurological assessment as well as the psychological testing were discussed with the patient.

B. Appropriate objectives for treatment were developed based on the test results.

C. The patient seemed to have a clear understanding of the results of the neurological testing.

D. The patient did not seem to understand the nature of his/her impairment as assessed through the neurological evaluations.

7. Explain Limitations (7)

A. The patient's limitations that result from his/her neurological impairment were explained.

B. The patient verbalized an understanding of his/her impairment that results from the brain injury.

C. The patient could not understand, nor accept, the cognitive limitations that result from his/her brain injury.

D. The patient agreed to work toward developing alternative coping mechanisms focused on his/her cognitive impairment.

8. Explore Feelings (8)

A. Feelings of anxiety and depression were explored as related to the patient's cognitive impairment.

B. The patient verbalized his/her feelings of grief and anxiety associated with acceptance of his/her cognitive impairment.

C. The patient showed no feelings related to his/her cognitive impairment due to his/her lack of insight and understanding of that impairment.

D. The patient denied feelings of grief or anxiety even though he/she was aware of the limitations that result from his/her cognitive impairment.

9. Assess Sequential Follow-Through (9)

A. Appropriate sequential tasks were assigned to the patient to assist in the assessment of his/her ability to follow through on such directions.

B. The patient showed evidence of confusion and inability to follow through on sequential tasking.

C. The patient showed good ability to follow sequential directions.

10. Assign Memory Enhancement Activities (10)

A. The patient was encouraged to implement memory enhancement activities such as utilization of crossword puzzles, playing card games, or watching TV game shows.

B. The patient was encouraged to use coping strategies, such as using lists, establishing routines, and labeling the environment, to adapt to his/her short-term memory loss.

C. The patient has implemented the memory-enhancing activities and reported some success at them.

D. The patient has implemented coping strategies for short-term memory loss and this has proven to be beneficial in enacting instrumental activities of daily living.

11. Develop Help-Seeking Guidelines (11)

A. The patient and significant others were assisted in developing guidelines for when it would be appropriate for the patient to seek assistance in performing daily living tasks because of his/her cognitive impairment.

B. The patient's significant others were encouraged to allow the patient a reasonable time to attempt to perform tasks before offering their assistance.

C. The patient reported that he/she is becoming more comfortable with seeking and accepting assistance from others.

12. Identify Resource People (12)

A. The patient was assisted in identifying qualified resource people who can provide regular supervision to him/her.

B. A schedule of supervision was developed with qualified supervisory people who can assist the patient in his/her daily living.

C. The patient was resistive to accepting monitoring and supervision from others, and these feelings were processed and resolved.

D. The patient has accepted the necessity for supervision by others and has committed to following through on developing such a plan.

13. Develop Supervisory Plan (13)

A. A supervision plan was written for those qualified persons who can provide assistance to the patient and monitor his/her daily living.

B. A written plan for daily supervisory contact has been developed and implemented.

C. The supervision plan has proven to be an adequate support system for the patient.

D. The supervision plan has not proven to be adequate and a more intense level of care has been recommended.

DEPENDENCY

PATIENT PRESENTATION

1. Lack of Self-Reliance (1)

A. The patient described a pattern of behavior that reflected consistent reliance on parents for economic and emotional support.

B. The patient acknowledged his/her emotional and economic dependence on parents but expressed fear of breaking that dependence.

C. The patient denied his/her dependence on parents, even though the facts confirm it.

D. The patient has begun to take steps to break his/her dependence on parents and move toward increased emancipation.

2. Sequential Intimate Relationships (2)

A. The patient described a history of many intimate relationships in sequence with little, if any, space between the ending of one and the start of the next.

B. The patient acknowledged a fear of being alone and a strong need of having a companion.

C. Acknowledging the unhealthy dependence that was present in previous relationships, the patient has begun to feel more comfortable with independence.

3. Fear of Being Alone (3)

A. The patient acknowledged strong feelings of panic, fear, and helplessness when faced with being alone, as a close relationship ends.

B. The patient is beginning to overcome feelings of fear associated with being alone and independent.

4. Easily Hurt by Criticism (4)

A. The patient acknowledged that he/she is hypersensitive to any hint of criticism from others.

B. The patient's lack of confidence in himself/herself is reflected in his/her sensitivity to criticism.

C. The patient showed more confidence in himself/herself as he/she related incidents of accepting criticism without feeling devastated.

D. The patient has made progress in overcoming his/her hypersensitivity to criticism.

5. Eager to Please (4)

A. The patient described a history of behaviors that are strongly influenced by a desire to please others.

B. A strong need for approval from others dominated the patient's motivation.

C. The patient has become more aware of his/her people-pleasing pattern and has begun to become more assertive and honest in his/her relationships with others.

* The numbers in parentheses correlate to the number of the Behavioral Definition statement in the companion chapter with the same title in *The Complete Adult Psychotherapy Treatment Planner,* second edition (Jongsma and Peterson) by John Wiley & Sons, 1999.

6. Need for Reassurance (5)

A. The patient has been unable to make decisions or initiate action without excessive reassurance from others.

B. The patient's dependency on others is reflected in his/her seeking out their approval before he/she can take any action.

C. The patient has shown the ability to make decisions on a small scale without seeking approval from others.

D. The patient has implemented problem-solving techniques to enhance his/her decision-making skills and increase his/her confidence in such decisions.

7. Fear of Abandonment (6)

A. The patient's fear of abandonment has dominated his/her life and influenced his/her interpersonal relationships.

B. With any hint of abandonment, the patient's anxiety escalates dramatically and his/her dependency needs come to the surface.

C. As the patient has become more aware of his/her fear of abandonment and processed this fear, he/she has become less dependent and less clingy in relationships.

8. Relationship-Based Self-Worth (7)

A. All the patient's feelings of self-worth, happiness, and fulfillment have been derived from relationships with others.

B. The patient lacks an inner sense of identity and self-worth that is independent from what others may think of him/her.

C. The patient has come to realize that his/her self-worth is not dependent on relationships with others but is inherent in his/her identity.

9. Tolerance for Physical Abuse (8)

A. The patient has a history of at least two relationships in which he/she was physically abused but continued in the relationship for some time.

B. The patient made excuses for the perpetrator of the physical abuse and blamed himself/herself for the abuse.

C. The patient acknowledged that his/her fear of being alone caused him/her to tolerate the physical abuse.

D. The patient has committed to a policy of zero tolerance for physical abuse as he/she has become more aware of his/her self-worth.

10. Fear of Rejection (9)

A. The patient has avoided disagreement with others consistently out of fear of being rejected.

B. The patient's fear of rejection is lessening and he/she is becoming somewhat more assertive.

C. The patient has begun to verbalize mild disagreement with others and has managed to cope with the insecurity surrounding that behavior.

D. The patient has become quite comfortable at expressing his/her thoughts and opinions without fear of rejection.

INTERVENTIONS IMPLEMENTED

1. Explore Dependency History (1)

A. The patient was asked to describe the style and pattern of his/her emotional dependence within emotional relationships.

B. The patient's history of emotional dependence beginning in the family of origin and extending into current relationships was explored.

C. The patient recognized his/her pattern of emotional dependence within relationships.

D. The patient was quite defensive and resistive to acceptance of the reality of his/her emotional and economic dependence on others.

2. Assign Books on Dependency (2)

A. It was recommended that the patient read specific literature on dependency.

B. The patient has followed through on reading the recommended literature on dependency, and key ideas from that reading were processed.

C. The patient has verbalized an increased awareness of his/her dependency patterns based on reading the recommended literature.

D. The patient has not followed through on reading the recommended literature and was redirected to do so.

3. Develop Family Genogram (3)

A. A family genogram was developed to increase the patient's awareness of patterns of dependence in relationships and how he/she is repeating them in the present relationship.

B. Seeing the persistent pattern of dependency throughout the generations of his/her family has helped the patient realize his/her need to break this pattern for himself/herself.

C. The patient verbalized observations of extended family members demonstrating their dependency.

4. Explore for Emotional Abandonment (4)

A. The family of origin was explored for experiences of emotional abandonment.

B. As the patient became aware of his/her emotional abandonment experiences, his/her fear of displeasing others became more clear.

C. The patient's insight into his/her experiences of emotional abandonment has reduced his/her motivation to continually strive to meet others' expectations.

5. Identify Fear of Disappointing Others (5)

A. The patient was assisted in identifying the basis for his/her fear of disappointing others.

B. The patient's need for nurturance, affirmation, and emotional support that was not met in his/her childhood was identified as the basis of fear in the present of disappointing others.

C. The patient's insight into the basis for his/her fear of disappointing others has reduced that people-pleasing behavior.

---

* The numbers in parentheses correlate to the number of the Therapeutic Intervention statement in the companion chapter with the same title in *The Complete Adult Psychotherapy Treatment Planner,* second edition (Jongsma and Peterson) by John Wiley & Sons, 1999.

6. Read "The Bridge" Fable (6)

A. The fable "The Bridge" in *Friedman's Fables* (Friedman) was read with the patient.

B. The patient reflected on the meaning of the fable and this was processed together.

C. The patient developed more insight into his/her practice of striving to meet other people's expectations.

7. Identify Social/Emotional Needs (7)

A. The patient was asked to list his/her social and emotional needs and a way that each of those needs could be constructively met.

B. The patient's list of social and emotional needs was processed, and adaptive ways to meet those needs were identified.

C. The patient has begun to implement more adaptive ways to meet his/her social and emotional needs.

8. List Steps toward Independence (8)

A. The patient was asked to list ways that he/she could start taking care of himself/herself.

B. Two or three steps toward independence were selected, and the patient committed to taking those steps.

C. The patient's attempts to begin emancipation and independence from others were processed and successes were reinforced.

D. The patient has increased his/her attempts to fulfill his/her own needs and these attempts were encouraged and reinforced.

9. Assign Assertiveness (9)

A. The patient was assigned the task of speaking his/her mind as freely and honestly as possible for one day.

B. The patient's experience at speaking his/her mind was processed, and successful enactment was reinforced.

C. The patient verbalized his/her fears associated with speaking his/her mind, and these fears were processed to be resolved.

D. The patient found it very difficult to speak up and has not followed through with the assignment to speak assertively.

10. Teach Assertiveness (10)

A. The patient was referred to an assertiveness training group that would educate and facilitate assertiveness skills.

B. Role playing, modeling, and behavioral rehearsal were used to train the patient in assertiveness skills.

C. The patient has demonstrated a clearer understanding of the difference between assertiveness, passivity, and aggressiveness.

11. Reinforce Assertiveness (11)

A. As the patient reported instances of implementing assertiveness, these experiences were supported and reinforced.

B. The patient's frequency of speaking up assertively has increased and he/she was supported for this change.

C. The patient continues to suppress his/her own thoughts and feelings, choosing to try to please others.

12. Assign Saying No (12)

A. The patient was given the assignment of trying to say no to others without excessive explanation, for a period of one week.

B. The patient's experience of refusing to comply with others' requests or agree with their positions was processed.

C. The patient experienced considerable anxiety at expressing any disagreement with others but was pleased with his/her ability to begin to do so.

13. Assign *When I Say No I Feel Guilty* (13)

A. The patient was assigned to read the book *When I Say No I Feel Guilty* (Smith) to increase his/her understanding of the dynamic of trying to please others.

B. The patient has followed through with reading the assigned book on saying no to others and has verbalized increased insight into his/her own behavior.

C. The patient has not followed through with reading the assertiveness book and was redirected to do so.

D. The patient has increased his/her practice of disagreeing with others and not complying with their requests so readily.

14. Explore Sensitivity to Criticism (14)

A. The patient's sensitivity to criticism was explored and new ways of receiving, processing, and responding to criticism were identified.

B. The patient verbalized a decreased sensitivity to criticism and has implemented new ways of responding to it.

C. The patient described instances of accepting criticism from others without feeling devastated or highly anxious.

15. Assign Receiving without Giving (15)

A. The patient was encouraged to allow others to do something for him/her and to receive this favor without feeling compelled to give back to this person.

B. The patient described instances of allowing others to give to him/her and the feelings associated with that experience.

C. The patient reported that he/she has felt less compelled to reciprocate to others when they do something for him/her.

D. The patient's pattern of giving to others and attempting to please them has diminished.

16. Identify Daily Independence Behaviors (16)

A. The patient was assisted in identifying ways that he/she could increase his/her level of independence in day-to-day life.

B. The patient was encouraged to implement steps toward independence in daily life.

C. The patient verbalized an increased sense of self-responsibility as he/she has taken steps toward becoming more independent.

17. Develop Boundaries (17)

A. The patient was assisted in developing new boundaries for not accepting responsibility for others' actions or feelings.

B. Role playing, modeling, and behavioral rehearsal were used to teach the patient to establish boundaries in his/her interaction with others that separate responsibility for actions and feelings.

C. The patient reported instances of interactions with others in which he/she has begun to set boundaries for not taking responsibility for other people's actions and feelings.

18. Explore Independence with Partner (18)

A. A conjoint session was held with the patient's partner in order to focus on ways to increase the patient's independence within the relationship.

B. Both the partner and the patient identified ways that the patient could practice more independent behaviors.

C. The patient reported that he/she has followed through with implementing independence behaviors within the relationship with the partner.

D. The patient finds it difficult to change the patterns of dependence within the relationship with the partner.

19. Journal Responsibility Boundaries (19)

A. The patient was asked to journal on a daily basis regarding boundaries for taking responsibility for himself/herself and not for others.

B. The journal of responsibility boundaries was reviewed and the patient became more aware of times when the boundaries were broken by himself/herself or others.

C. The patient verbalized an increased awareness of when he/she accepts responsibility for other people's behavior.

D. The patient verbalized an awareness of attempts by others to place responsibility for their behavior on him/her.

20. Assign *Boundaries: Where You End and I Begin* (20)

A. The patient was assigned to read *Boundaries: Where You End and I Begin* (Katherine) to increase his/her understanding of personal responsibility.

B. The patient has followed through with reading the assigned book on boundaries and verbalized increased understanding of this concept for himself/herself.

C. The patient described several instances of having to set boundaries within his/her daily life.

21. Assign *A Gift to Myself* (21)

A. The patient was assigned to read *A Gift to Myself* (Whitfield) with a specific focus on the chapter of setting boundaries and limits.

B. The patient was asked to complete a survey on personal boundaries that is found within the book *A Gift to Myself.*

C. The patient has followed through with reading the assigned book on boundaries and has completed the survey.

D. The patient has not followed through with reading the assigned book on boundaries and was redirected to do so.

E. Important concepts on boundaries that were learned from reading the assigned material were processed with the patient and applied to his/her personal life.

22. Reinforce Boundary Implementation (22)

A. As the patient described instances of clarifying boundaries with others, he/she was reinforced for doing so.

B. The patient described instances where he/she had failed to set boundaries, but was aware of it upon reflection.

C. The patient has significantly increased his/her frequency of setting boundaries with others and has become very aware of his/her need to do so.

23. Encourage Decision Making (23)

A. The patient's decision-making avoidance was confronted and specific areas in which decisions need to be made were identified.

B. The patient has committed to making independent decisions and following through on implementation of these.

C. The patient has increased the frequency of making decisions within a reasonable time and with some assurance and confidence in the process.

24. List Positive Attributes (24)

A. The patient was assisted in developing a list of his/her positive attributes and accomplishments.

B. The patient found it very difficult to identify positive attributes and accomplishments.

C. With encouragement, the patient has become more aware of his/her positive attributes and accomplishments and is able to identify them.

D. Listing positive attributes and accomplishments has built the patient's sense of identity and self-esteem.

25. Assign Personal Affirmation Time (25)

A. The patient was assigned to institute a ritual of beginning each day with 5 to 10 minutes of solitude, in which the focus is on personal affirmation.

B. The patient has followed through on the assignment of affirming himself/herself for several minutes per day and reported that his/her self-esteem has grown.

C. The patient was able to identify several positive things about himself/herself that have been the focus of his/her positive affirmation time each day.

D. The patient's feelings of anxiety and embarrassment about affirming himself/herself on a daily basis were processed and resolved.

26. Identify Distorted Thoughts (26)

A. The patient's distorted and negative automatic thoughts associated with being assertive, being alone, or not meeting others' needs were explored and identified.

B. The patient identified several distorted automatic thoughts that enter his/her mind whenever situations are encountered that require assertiveness, being alone, or not complying with others' requests.

27. Explore Fears of Independence (27)

A. The patient's feelings of fear associated with being more independent were explored.

B. The patient identified fears of abandonment and lack of self-confidence as fueling his/her fear of independence.

C. As the patient explored his/her fears of independence, they were tied with distorted automatic thoughts that precipitated such fears.

28. Develop Positive Self-Talk (28)

A. The patient was assisted in developing positive, reality-based messages for himself/herself that must replace the distorted negative self-talk.

B. The patient has implemented positive self-talk techniques and this practice has reduced feelings of fear and increased assertiveness and independence.

C. The patient has found it very difficult to replace the negative distorted messages with more positive, reality-based messages and was redirected to do so.

29. Al-Anon Referral (29)

A. It was recommended to the patient that he/she attend Al-Anon or another appropriate self-help group that would support breaking the dependency cycle with an alcoholic partner.

B. The patient has followed through with attending the self-help group of partners of alcoholics.

C. The patient reported an increased awareness of his/her need to break the dependency with his/her alcoholic partner.

30. Assign *The Verbally Abusive Relationship* (30)

A. It was recommended that the patient read *The Verbally Abusive Relationship* (Evans) in order to gain a better understanding of dependency within abusive relationships.

B. The patient has read the assigned material on abusive relationships and key ideas were processed and applied to his/her daily life.

C. The patient has not read the assigned material on abusive relationships and was encouraged to do so.

D. The patient reported that reading the assigned material on abusive relationships has increased his/her awareness of his/her own patterns of dependency and need to break from those patterns.

31. Safe House Referral (31)

A. The patient was referred to a safe house that would protect him/her from the physically abusive relationship existing within the home.

B. The patient has followed through on the referral to a safe house and has found protection from further abuse.

C. The patient verbalized fear of breaking away from his/her abusive partner and these fears were processed and resolved.

D. The patient has not followed through on the referral to a safe house and continues the dependency pattern within the abusive relationship.

32. **Domestic Violence Program Referral (32)**

A. The patient was referred to a program specifically focused on treating people involved with domestic violence.

B. The patient has followed through on attendance at the domestic violence treatment program and this attendance was encouraged and reinforced.

C. The patient has not followed through on the referral to the domestic violence treatment program and was encouraged to do so.

D. The patient reported that he/she was pleased with the domestic violence treatment program and has already learned important concepts for his/her life.

DEPRESSION

PATIENT PRESENTATION

1. Loss of Appetite (1)

A. The patient reported that he/she has not had a normal and consistent appetite.

B. The patient's loss of appetite has resulted in a significant weight loss associated with the depression.

C. As the depression has begun to lift, the patient's appetite has increased.

D. The patient reported that his/her appetite is at normal levels.

2. Depressed Affect (2)

A. The patient reported that he/she feels deeply sad and has periods of tearfulness on an almost daily basis.

B. The patient's depressed affect was clearly evident within the session as tears were shed on more than one occasion.

C. The patient reported that he/she has begun to feel less sad and can experience periods of joy.

D. The patient appeared to be more happy within the session and there is not evidence of tearfulness.

3. Lack of Activity Enjoyment (3)

A. The patient reported a diminished interest in or enjoyment of activities that were previously found pleasurable.

B. The patient has begun to involve himself/herself with activities that he/she previously found pleasurable.

C. The patient has returned to an active interest in and enjoyment of activities.

4. Psychomotor Agitation (4)

A. The patient demonstrated psychomotor agitation within the session.

B. The patient reported that with the onset of the depression, he/she has felt unable to relax or sit quietly.

C. The patient reported a significant decrease in psychomotor agitation and the ability to sit more quietly.

D. It was evident within the session that the patient has become more relaxed and less agitated.

5. Psychomotor Retardation (4)

A. The patient demonstrated evidence of psychomotor retardation within the session.

B. The patient moved and responded very slowly, showing a lack of energy and motivation.

---

* The numbers in parentheses correlate to the number of the Behavioral Definition statement in the companion chapter with the same title in *The Complete Adult Psychotherapy Treatment Planner,* second edition (Jongsma and Peterson) by John Wiley & Sons, 1999.

C. As the depression as lifted, the patient has responded more quickly and psychomotor retardation has diminished.

6. Sleeplessness/Hypersomnia (5)

A. The patient reported periods of inability to sleep and other periods of sleeping for many hours without the desire to get out of bed.
B. The patient's problem with sleep interference has diminished as the depression has lifted.
C. Medication has improved the patient's problems with sleep disturbance.

7. Lack of Energy (6)

A. The patient reported that he/she feels a very low level of energy compared to normal times in his/her life.
B. It was evident within the session that the patient has low levels of energy, as demonstrated by slowness of walking, minimal movement, lack of animation, and slow responses.
C. The patient's energy level has increased as the depression has lifted.
D. It was evident within the session that the patient is demonstrating normal levels of energy.

8. Lack of Concentration (7)

A. The patient reported that he/she is unable to maintain concentration and is easily distracted.
B. The patient reported that he/she is unable to read material with good comprehension because of being easily distracted.
C. The patient reported increased ability to concentrate as his/her depression has lifted.

9. Indecisiveness (7)

A. The patient reported a decrease in his/her ability to make decisions based on lack of confidence, low self-esteem, and low energy.
B. It was evident within the session that the patient does not have normal decision-making capabilities.
C. The patient reported an increased ability to make decisions as the depression is lifting.

10. Social Withdrawal (8)

A. The patient has withdrawn from social relationships that were important to him/her.
B. As the patient's depression has deepened, he/she has increasingly isolated himself/herself.
C. The patient has begun to reach out to social contacts as the depression has begun to lift.
D. The patient has resumed normal social interactions.

11. Suicidal Thoughts/Gestures (9)

A. The patient expressed that he/she is experiencing suicidal thoughts but has not taken any action on these thoughts.
B. The patient reported suicidal thoughts that have resulted in suicidal gestures.
C. Suicidal urges have been reported as diminished as the depression has lifted.
D. The patient denied any suicidal thoughts or gestures and is more hopeful about the future.

12. Feelings of Hopelessness/Worthlessness (10)

A. The patient has experienced feelings of hopelessness and worthlessness that began as the depression deepened.

B. The patient's feelings of hopelessness and worthlessness have diminished as the depression is beginning to lift.

C. The patient expressed feelings of hope for the future and affirmation of his/her own self-worth.

13. Inappropriate Guilt (10)

A. The patient described feelings of pervasive, irrational guilt.

B. Although the patient verbalized an understanding that his/her guilt was irrational, it continues to plague him/her.

C. The depth of irrational guilt has lifted as the depression has subsided.

D. The patient no longer expresses feelings of irrational guilt.

14. Low Self-Esteem (11)

A. The patient stated that he/she has a very negative perception of himself/herself.

B. The patient's low self-esteem was evident within the session as he/she made many self-disparaging remarks and maintained very little eye contact.

C. The patient's self-esteem has increased as he/she is beginning to affirm his/her self-worth.

D. The patient verbalized positive feelings toward himself/herself.

15. Unresolved Grief (12)

A. The patient has experienced losses about which he/she has been unable to resolve feelings of grief.

B. The patient's feelings of grief have turned to major depression as energy has diminished and sadness/hopelessness dominate his/her life.

C. The patient has begun to resolve the feelings of grief associated with the loss in his/her life.

D. The patient has verbalized feelings of hopefulness regarding the future and acceptance of the loss of the past.

16. Hallucinations/Delusions (13)

A. The patient has experienced mood-related hallucinations or delusions indicating that the depression has a psychotic component.

B. The patient's thought disorder has begun to diminish as the depression has been treated.

C. The patient reported no longer experiencing any thought disorder symptoms.

17. Recurrent Depression Pattern (14)

A. The patient reported a recurrent pattern of depressive episodes that have been treated with a variety of approaches.

B. The patient has a history of depression within the family that parallels his/her own experience of depression.

INTERVENTIONS IMPLEMENTED

1. Explore Depression Experiences (1)

A. The patient was asked to describe his/her experience of depression for the signs and symptoms that are present in his/her daily living.

B. The patient identified several signs and symptoms of depression such as depressed affect, low self-esteem, diminished interest, and lack of energy.

2. Identify Depression Causes (2)

A. The patient was asked to verbally identify the source of his/her depressed mood.

B. The patient listed several factors that he/she believes contribute to his/her feelings of hopelessness and sadness.

3. Clarify Depressed Feelings (3)

A. The patient was encouraged to share his/her feelings of depression in order to clarify them and gain insight into their causes.

B. The patient has continued to share his/her feelings of depression and has identified causes for them.

C. Distorted cognitive messages contribute to the patient's feelings of depression.

D. The patient demonstrated sad affect and tearfulness when describing his/her feelings.

4. Explore Childhood Pain (4)

A. Experiences from the patient's childhood that contribute to his/her current depressed state were explored.

B. The patient identified painful childhood experiences that have continued to foster feelings of low self-esteem, sadness, and sleep disturbance.

C. As the patient has described his/her childhood experiences within an understanding atmosphere, sad feelings surrounding those experiences have diminished.

5. Explore Suppressed Anger (5)

A. The patient was encouraged to share his/her feelings of anger regarding painful childhood experiences that contribute to his/her current depressed state.

B. As the patient described painful experiences from the past, feelings of anger, sadness, and suppressed rage were also expressed.

C. The patient reported that he/she has begun to feel less depressed as suppressed feelings of anger and hurt have been expressed.

6. Connect Anger with Depression (6)

A. The patient was taught the possible connection between previously unexpressed feelings of anger and helplessness and his/her current state of depression.

B. As the patient has gained insight into suppressed feelings from the past, his/her current feelings of depression have diminished.

* The numbers in parentheses correlate to the number of the Therapeutic Intervention statement in the companion chapter with the same title in *The Complete Adult Psychotherapy Treatment Planner,* second edition (Jongsma and Peterson) by John Wiley & Sons, 1999.

C. The patient verbalized an understanding of the relationship between his/her current depressed mood and the repression of anger, hurt, and sadness.

7. Physician/Medication Referral (7)

A. The patient was referred to a physician for a physical examination to rule out organic causes for depression.

B. A referral to a physician was made for the purpose of evaluating the patient for a prescription for psychotropic medication.

C. The patient has followed through on a referral to a physician and has been assessed for a prescription of psychotropic medication.

D. The patient has been prescribed antidepressant medication.

E. The patient has refused the prescription of psychotropic medication prescribed by the physician.

8. Monitor Medication Compliance (8)

A. As the patient has taken the antidepressant medication prescribed by his/her physician, the effectiveness and side effects of the medication were monitored.

B. The patient reported that the antidepressant medication has been beneficial in reducing sleep interference and in stabilizing mood.

C. The patient reported that the antidepressant medication has not been beneficial.

D. The patient has not consistently taken the prescribed antidepressant medication and was redirected to do so.

9. Psychological Testing (9)

A. Objective psychological testing was administered to the patient to assess the depth of his/her depression and monitor suicide potential.

B. The patient cooperated with the psychological testing and feedback about the results were given to him/her.

C. The psychological testing confirmed the presence of significant depression.

10. Explore Suicide Potential (10)

A. The patient's experience of suicidal urges and his/her history of suicidal behavior was explored.

B. The patient stated that he/she does experience suicidal urges but feels that they are clearly under his/her control and that there is no risk of engagement in suicidal behavior.

C. The patient identified suicidal urges as being present but contracted to contact others if the urges became strong.

D. Because the patient's suicidal urges were assessed to be very serious, immediate referral to a more intensive supervised level of care was made.

11. Identify Cognitive Distortions (11)

A. The patient was assisted in developing an awareness of his/her distorted cognitive messages that reinforce hopelessness and helplessness.

B. The patient identified several cognitive messages that occur on a regular basis and feed feelings of depression.

C. The patient recalled several instances of engaging in negative self-talk that precipitated feelings of helplessness, hopelessness, and depression.

12. Assign Dysfunctional Thinking Journal (12)

A. The patient was requested to keep a daily journal that lists each situation associated with depressed feelings and the dysfunctional thinking that triggered the depression.

B. The Socratic method was used to challenge the patient's dysfunctional thoughts and to replace them with positive, reality-based thoughts.

C. The patient reported instances of successful replacement of negative thoughts with more realistic positive thinking.

13. Reinforce Positive Self-Talk (13)

A. The patient was reinforced for any successful replacement of distorted negative thinking with positive, reality-based cognitive messages.

B. The patient reported that engaging in positive, reality-based thinking has enhanced his/her self-confidence and increased adaptive action.

14. Monitor Ongoing Suicide Potential (14)

A. The patient was asked to report any suicidal urges or increase in the strength of these urges.

B. The patient stated that suicidal urges are diminishing and that they are under his/her control.

C. The patient stated that he/she has no longer experienced thoughts of self-harm.

D. The patient stated that his/her suicide urges are strong and present a threat.

15. Hospitalization Referral (15)

A. Because the patient was judged to be harmful to himself/herself, a referral was made for immediate hospitalization.

B. The patient was resistive to hospitalization for treatment of his/her suicide potential, so a commitment procedure was utilized.

C. The patient cooperated with hospitalization to treat the serious suicidal urges.

16. Monitor Grooming/Hygiene (16)

A. The patient was encouraged to practice consistent grooming and hygiene.

B. The patient has taken more pride in his/her personal appearance as evidenced by improved grooming and hygiene practices.

C. The patient was reinforced for practicing improved grooming and hygiene behavior.

17. Assign Positive Affirmations (17)

A. The patient was assigned to write at least one positive affirmation statement on a daily basis regarding himself/herself and the future.

B. The patient has followed through on the assignment of writing positive affirmation statements and reported that he/she is feeling more positive about the future.

C. The patient was reinforced for making positive statements regarding himself/herself and his/her ability to cope with the stresses of life.

D. The patient has not followed through on the assignment of writing positive affirmation statements and was encouraged to do so.

18. Teach Normalization of Sadness (18)

A. The patient was taught about the variation in mood that is within the normal sphere.

B. The patient reported that he/she is developing an increased tolerance to mood swings and is not attributing them to significant depression.

C. The patient is verbalizing more hopeful and positive statements regarding the future and accepting some sadness as a normal variation and feeling.

19. Teach Behavioral Coping Strategies (19)

A. The patient was taught behavioral coping strategies such as physical exercise, increased social involvement, sharing of feelings, and increased assertiveness as ways to reduce feelings of depression.

B. The patient has implemented behavioral coping strategies to reduce feelings of depression and was reinforced for doing so.

C. The patient reported that the utilization of behavioral coping strategies has been successful at reducing feelings of depression.

D. The patient reported several instances in which behavioral coping strategies were helpful in reducing depressive feelings.

20. Assign Chemical Dependence Recovery Books (20)

A. Because the patient has a concomitant chemical dependence problem, he/she was referred to books that can help him/her overcome the dual problem with depression.

B. The patient has followed through with reading the alcohol-related depression material, and key concepts were processed.

C. The patient has not followed through with reading the recommended material on alcoholism and depression and was encouraged to do so.

21. Plan Recreational Activities (21)

A. The patient was encouraged to list those recreational activities that he/she has found pleasurable in the past.

B. A plan was developed to engage in specific recreational activities to increase socialization and reduce internal focus.

C. The patient reported that engaging in recreational activities was difficult but did seem rewarding.

D. The patient is regularly participating in social and recreational activities.

22. Reinforce Social Activity (22)

A. As the patient reported increased socialization and verbalization of his/her feelings, needs, and desires, he/she was reinforced and supported.

B. The patient is more regularly engaging in social activities and initiating communication of his/her needs and desires.

23. Explore Unresolved Grief (23)

A. The patient's history of losses that have triggered feelings of grief were explored.

B. The patient identified losses that have contributed to feelings of grief that have not been resolved.

C. The patient's unresolved feelings of grief are contributing to current feelings of depression and need special focus.

24. Recommend Depression Self-Help Books (24)

A. Several self-help books on the topic of coping with depression were recommended to the patient.

B. The patient has followed through with reading self-help books on depression and reported key ideas that were processed.

C. The patient has not followed through with reading the self-help books that were recommended and was encouraged to do so.

D. The patient reported that reading the self-help books on depression has been beneficial and identified several coping techniques that he/she has implemented as a result of the reading.

25. Teach Conflict Resolution Skills (25)

A. The patient was taught conflict resolution skills such as practicing empathy, active listening, respectful communication, assertiveness, and compromise.

B. Using role playing, modeling, and behavioral rehearsal, the patient was taught implementation of conflict resolution skills.

C. The patient reported implementation of conflict resolution skills in his/her daily life and was reinforced for this utilization.

D. The patient reported that resolving interpersonal conflicts has contributed to a lifting of his/her depression.

26. Address Interpersonal Conflict (26)

A. A conjoint session was held to assist the patient in resolving interpersonal conflicts with his/her partner.

B. The patient reported that there has been resolution of interpersonal conflicts with his/her partner and this has contributed to a lifting of his/her depression.

C. Ongoing conflicts with a partner have fostered feelings of depression and hopelessness.

27. Teach Assertiveness (27)

A. Role playing, modeling, and behavioral rehearsal were used to train the patient in assertiveness.

B. The patient was referred to an assertiveness training group for intense education about acquiring assertiveness skills.

C. The patient reported that he/she has become more assertive in expressing his/her needs, desires, and expectations.

D. The patient continues to have difficulties in being assertive, as lack of confidence, low self-esteem, and social withdrawal inhibit him/her.

28. Assign Mirror Exercise (28)

A. The patient was assigned to talk positively about himself/herself into a mirror once per day.

B. The patient has performed the assigned exercise of mirror talking and reported that he/she has found more acceptance of his/her positive qualities.

C. The patient has decreased the frequency of negative self-descriptive statements and increased the frequency of positive self-descriptive statements.

D. The patient has not followed through on the assigned mirror talking exercise and was redirected to do so.

29. Reinforce Positive Self-Descriptions (29)

A. The patient was supported and strongly reinforced when he/she made positive statements about himself/herself.

B. The frequency with which the patient makes positive self-descriptive statements has increased.

C. The patient continues to make self-disparaging statements and has been confronted about doing so.

30. Assign Dysfunctional Thinking Journal (12)

A. The patient was requested to keep a daily journal that lists each situation associated with depressed feelings and the dysfunctional thinking that triggered the depression.

B. The Socratic method was used to challenge the patient's dysfunctional thoughts and to replace them with positive, reality-based thoughts.

C. The patient reported instances of successful replacement of negative thoughts with more realistic positive thinking.

31. Reinforce Physical Exercise (31)

A. A plan for routine physical exercise was developed with the patient and a rationale for including this in his/her daily routine was made.

B. The patient agreed to make a commitment toward implementing daily exercise as a depression reduction technique.

C. The patient has performed routine daily exercise and he/she reports that it has been beneficial.

D. The patient has not followed through on maintaining a routine of physical exercise and was redirected to do so.

32. Recommend *Exercising Your Way to Better Mental Health* (32)

A. The patient was encouraged to read *Exercising Your Way to Better Mental Health* (Leith) to introduce him/her to the concept of combating stress, depression, and anxiety with exercise.

B. The patient has followed through with reading the recommended book on exercise and mental health and reported that it was beneficial.

C. The patient has not followed through with reading the recommended material on the effect of exercise on mental health and was encouraged to do so.

D. The patient has implemented a regular exercise regimen as a depression reduction technique and reported successful results.

DISSOCIATION

PATIENT PRESENTATION

1. Multiple Personalities (1)

A. The patient described instances of splitting into two or more distinct personalities that take full control of his/her behavior.

B. The patient showed evidence within the session of assuming the role of multiple personalities.

C. The dissociation into multiple personalities occurs more frequently as stress builds within the patient's life.

D. The patient reported more integration of his/her identity and less loss of control to multiple personalities.

E. The patient has had no recent incidences of the appearance of distinct personalities.

2. Amnesia Episodes (2)

A. The patient described episodes of a certain inability to remember important personal information.

B. The loss of personal information recall occurred after a traumatic stress was endured.

C. The patient reported instances of partial recall of personal information that had been forgotten.

D. Personal identity information is now recalled quite easily and normally.

3. Depersonalization Experiences (3)

A. The patient reports instances of feeling detached from or outside of his/her body, during which reality testing remains intact.

B. The depersonalization experiences occur primarily during times of high stress.

C. As the patient has learned coping mechanisms for his/her anxiety, the depersonalization experiences have diminished.

D. The patient reports no recent experiences of depersonalization.

4. Derealization Experiences (4)

A. The patient reported instances of feeling as if he/she were automated or in a dream.

B. The derealization experiences occur during times of high stress.

C. The patient reported decreasing frequency of derealization experiences.

D. No recent derealization experiences were reported by the patient.

5. Severe-Persistent Derealization (5)

A. The depersonalization experiences reported by the patient were severe and persistent enough to cause marked distress in his/her daily life.

---

* The numbers in parentheses correlate to the number of the Behavioral Definition statement in the companion chapter with the same title in *The Complete Adult Psychotherapy Treatment Planner,* second edition (Jongsma and Peterson) by John Wiley & Sons, 1999.

B. As the patient has overcome traumatic, painful experiences, the instances of depersonalization have diminished.

C. The patient reports being able to function normally without interference from depersonalization experiences.

INTERVENTIONS IMPLEMENTED

1. Build Trust (1)

A. Consistent eye contact, active listening, unconditional positive regard, and warm acceptance were used to help build trust with the patient.

B. The patient began to express feelings more freely as rapport and trust level increased.

C. The patient has continued to experience difficulty being open and direct in his/her expression of painful feelings.

2. Label and Explore Multiple Personalities (2)

A. The patient was asked to describe the various personalities that take control of him/her and the circumstances under which this occurs.

B. The patient was somewhat resistant to and anxious about describing the personality states out of fear that he/she would lose control.

C. The patient was reinforced and supported for exercising control over the core personality and giving executive functioning to that personality.

3. Medication Evaluation Referral (3)

A. The patient was referred for an evaluation for psychotropic medication.

B. The patient followed through with the referral to a physician for a psychotropic medication evaluation.

C. The physician prescribed psychotropic medication to help the patient decrease anxiety and increase mood stability.

D. The patient is resistant to accepting the medication through the physician.

4. Monitor Medication Compliance (4)

A. The patient is taking the prescribed medication at the times ordered by the physician.

B. The patient was monitored for consistent compliance with the physician's prescription for medication.

C. The patient reported that he/she is taking the medication on a consistent basis and that it is beneficial.

D. The patient reported that the medication does not seem to be helpful and has terminated taking it.

5. Explore Emotional Pain (5)

A. The patient's sources of emotional pain and feelings of fear, rejection, inadequacy, or abuse were explored.

* The numbers in parentheses correlate to the number of the Therapeutic Intervention statement in the companion chapter with the same title in *The Complete Adult Psychotherapy Treatment Planner,* second edition (Jongsma and Peterson) by John Wiley & Sons, 1999.

B. The patient identified severe emotional traumas that are unresolved and have triggered dissociative states.

C. The patient shows considerable affect when describing traumatic instances of abuse and rejection.

D. As the patient shared his/her traumatic experiences from the past, the emotional response has diminished.

6. Connect Emotional Conflict and Dissociation (6)

A. The patient was insistent about making an insightful connection between his/her dissociation disorder and the avoidance of facing unresolved emotional conflicts.

B. As the patient developed insight into the emotional conflicts that trigger his/her dissociative states, the frequency of that dissociation diminished.

7. Encourage Reality Focus (7)

A. As the patient stayed focused on reality, rather than escaping through dissociating, he/she was reinforced.

B. The integration of the patient's personality was supported by encouraging focus on the here-and-now, rather than on past unresolved issues.

C. As the patient was supported, encouraged, and reinforced for an integrated personality and for focusing on here-and-now issues, the frequency of dissociation diminished.

8. Reinforce Here-and-Now Focus (8)

A. The importance of a here-and-now focus on reality, rather than a preoccupation with traumas from the past, was repeatedly emphasized to the patient.

B. The patient was reinforced for an integrated reality focus, rather than the dissociation associated with stresses from the past.

9. Train in Relaxation Techniques (9)

A. The patient was taught several different relaxation techniques to be used to reduce muscle tension and assist in anxiety management.

B. The patient demonstrated a good understanding of the relaxation techniques and committed himself/herself to implementing them.

C. The patient reported that implementation of the relaxation techniques has been helpful in reducing stress and the experience of anxiety.

D. The patient has not followed through on implementation of the relaxation techniques and was redirected to do so.

10. Teach Calm Reaction to Symptoms (10)

A. The patient was taught a calm, matter-of-fact reaction to any brief dissociation phenomena so as not to accelerate anxiety symptoms and to stay focused on reality.

B. The patient reported that as he/she practiced acceptance of brief episodes of dissociation, the frequency and severity of the episodes has diminished.

11. Facilitated Family Session (11)

A. A conjoint session with significant others and the patient was held to assist the patient in regaining lost information.

B. The patient showed evidence of beginning to integrate previously lost information with facts that he/she is able to recall.

C. The patient's amnesia continues to be severe and problematic.

12. Neurologist Referral (12)

A. The patient was referred for a neurological examination to evaluate the possibility of any organic cause for memory loss experiences.

B. The patient has followed through with the referral to the neurologist and no organic causes were determined.

C. The patient has failed to follow through on a neurologist referral and was redirected to do so.

D. The neurological examination determined that there is some organic basis for the memory and further treatment will be needed.

13. Teach Patience (13)

A. The patient was encouraged to attempt to be patient in the face of the loss of recall of personal identity information through amnesia.

B. The patient was reinforced for remaining calm in the face of recall difficulties.

C. The patient continues to express frustration, anger, anxiety, and fear in the face of amnesia.

14. Utilize Memorabilia (14)

A. Photographs and other memorabilia were used to gently trigger the patient's memory recall.

B. The patient is beginning to recall personal identity information with the help of personal memorabilia.

C. The patient continues to experience severe amnesia.

EATING DISORDER

PATIENT PRESENTATION

1. Chronic Rapid Overeating (1)

A. The patient described a history of chronic, rapid consumption of large quantities of high-carbohydrate food.

B. The patient has engaged in binge eating on almost a daily basis.

C. The frequency of binge eating of nonnutritious foods has begun to diminish.

D. The patient reported that there have been no recent incidences of binge eating.

2. Self-Induced Vomiting (2)

A. The patient has engaged in self-induced vomiting out of a fear of gaining weight.

B. The patient's purging behavior using self-induced vomiting has occurred on almost a daily basis.

C. The patient has increased his/her control over the self-induced vomiting and the frequency of this behavior has decreased.

D. The patient reported no recent incidences of self-induced vomiting.

3. Weight Loss (3)

A. The patient's eating disorder has resulted in extreme weight loss and a refusal to consume enough calories to increase the weight to more normal levels.

B. The extreme weight loss has resulted in amenorrhea in the patient.

C. The patient's weight loss has plateaued and he/she is beginning to acknowledge the need for a gain in weight.

D. The patient has begun to gain weight gradually and endure the anxious feelings associated with that experience.

E. The patient is now at the lower end of normal in terms of his/her weight and has been able to maintain that.

4. Laxative Abuse (4)

A. The patient has a history of laxative abuse to purge his/her system of food intake.

B. The frequency of laxative abuse has begun to diminish.

C. The patient reported no recent incidences of laxative abuse as a purging behavior for food intake.

5. Limited Food Intake (4)

A. The patient has a history of very limited ingestion of food, resulting in weight loss.

B. Although the patient talked of eating three meals per day, a closer analysis indicated that the amount of food consumed was very limited.

---

* The numbers in parentheses correlate to the number of the Behavioral Definition statement in the companion chapter with the same title in *The Complete Adult Psychotherapy Treatment Planner*, second edition (Jongsma and Peterson) by John Wiley & Sons, 1999.

C. The patient has begun to increase his/her caloric intake as portions of food consumed have gradually increased.

D. The patient reported consuming a normal level of calories per day in the recent past.

6. Excessive Strenuous Exercise (4)

A. The patient has engaged in excessive strenuous exercise as a weight control measure.

B. In spite of the fact that the patient is extremely underweight and is eating too little, he/she continues to engage in excessive strenuous exercise to burn calories.

C. The excessive strenuous exercise is a ritual that is compulsively completed by the patient on a daily basis.

D. The patient has begun to control the frequency and amount of exercise that he/she engages in to burn calories.

E. The patient has terminated the excessive strenuous exercise routine and only engages in normal amounts of healthy exercise.

7. Body Image Preoccupation (5)

A. The patient has a history of persistent preoccupation with his/her body image and grossly inaccurately assesses himself/herself as overweight.

B. The patient is beginning to acknowledge that his/her body image is grossly inaccurate and that some weight gain is necessary.

C. As the patient has begun to gain some weight, his/her anxiety level has increased and the fear of obesity has returned.

D. The patient has been able to gain weight up to normal levels without a distorted fear of being overweight controlling him/her.

8. Irrational Fear of Becoming Overweight (6)

A. The patient has developed a predominating irrational fear of becoming overweight.

B. The patient's fear of becoming overweight has controlled his/her food intake to extreme levels.

C. The patient has used purging methods to overcontrol his/her weight.

D. The patient's fear of becoming overweight has diminished.

E. The patient has not reported any fear of becoming overweight recently.

9. Electrolyte Imbalance (7)

A. An electrolyte imbalance resulting from the patient's eating disorder is compromising his/her health.

B. The patient has accepted the fact that his/her eating disorder has resulted in a fluid and electrolyte imbalance.

C. The patient has agreed to terminate the binge eating/purging behavior that has resulted in the electrolyte imbalance.

D. The patient has agreed to increase his/her nutritious food intake and terminate purging behaviors in order to correct a fluid and electrolyte imbalance.

E. The patient's fluid and electrolyte imbalance has been corrected as he/she has increased food intake and terminated purging behavior.

10. Denial of Emaciation (8)

A. The patient strongly denies seeing himself/herself as emaciated even when severely under the recommended weight levels.

B. The patient's denial of being emaciated is beginning to waver.

C. The patient is no longer in denial about being emaciated and has begun to take steps toward increasing his/her weight through more normal caloric intake.

INTERVENTIONS IMPLEMENTED

1. Explore Dysfunctional Eating (1)

A. The patient was asked to describe his/her dysfunctional eating patterns.

B. The patient acknowledged that his/her eating patterns are dysfunctional in terms of the amount and type of food consumed.

C. The patient had difficulty acknowledging that his/her eating patterns are dysfunctional.

2. Evaluate Calorie Consumption (2)

A. The patient's calorie consumption was compared with an average adult rate of 1,500 calories per day in order to establish the reality of his/her pattern of under- or overeating.

B. The patient acknowledged that his/her calorie consumption was not within the normal limits.

C. The patient defended his/her calorie consumption being outside the normal limits.

3. Explore Vomiting Behavior (3)

A. The patient was asked to describe any self-induced vomiting to help control caloric intake.

B. The patient acknowledged engagement in vomiting behavior on a regular basis, after eating, in order to reduce caloric intake.

C. The patient defended his/her use of vomiting in order to control caloric intake because of his/her distorted belief that he/she would become overweight.

4. Explore Laxative Abuse (4)

A. The patient confirmed regular use of laxatives for the purpose of reducing body weight.

B. The patient minimized his/her use of laxatives to control body weight.

C. The patient reported no longer using laxatives to control body weight.

5. Assess Exercise (5)

A. The patient was asked to describe the frequency and vigorousness of his/her exercise regimen.

B. The patient acknowledged frequent use of vigorous exercise to control weight gain.

C. The patient made a commitment to reduce the amount and frequency of his/her exercise.

D. The patient reported a moderate and normal use of exercise.

---

* The numbers in parentheses correlate to the number of the Therapeutic Intervention statement in the companion chapter with the same title in *The Complete Adult Psychotherapy Treatment Planner,* second edition (Jongsma and Peterson) by John Wiley & Sons, 1999.

6. Monitor Vomiting, Exercise, and Laxative Usage (6)

A. The patient's use of purging techniques and strenuous exercise was monitored.

B. The patient reported a decreased use of purging and exercise to control weight.

C. The patient denied any recent engagement in vomiting, strenuous exercise, or laxative use.

7. Explore Body Image (7)

A. The patient's perception of his/her body image/size and the frequency and intensity of his/her thinking about it was explored.

B. The patient acknowledged a persistent preoccupation with body image/size.

C. The patient's preoccupation with body image/size has diminished.

D. The patient's perception of his/her body image/size has become more realistic and less distorted.

8. Physical Examination Referral (8)

A. The patient was referred to a physician for a complete physical examination.

B. The patient followed through on a referral to a physician for an exam and reported that negative consequences from the eating disorder were discovered.

C. The patient's physical examination ruled out any serious negative consequences as a result of the eating disorder.

D. The patient reported that he/she has developed an electrolyte imbalance that resulted from the eating disorder.

9. Physician Consultation (9)

A. The patient's physician has been contacted about the patient's medical condition and nutritional habits.

B. The patient's physician confirmed that the patient's eating disorder has resulted in serious negative consequences.

10. Dentist Referral (10)

A. The patient was referred to a dentist for a complete dental examination.

B. The dental examination results indicate that the patient has experienced negative consequences from vomiting and poor nutrition.

C. The dental examination results indicated that there are no negative consequences from the eating disorder.

11. Assess for Psychotropic Medication (11)

A. The patient's need for psychotropic medication was assessed.

B. It was determined that the patient would benefit from psychotropic medication.

C. A need for psychotropic medication was not found and thus no referral was made.

12. Physician Medication Referral (12)

A. The patient was referred to a physician to be evaluated for psychotropic medication.

B. The patient cooperated with the physician referral and psychotropic medication has been prescribed.

C. The patient has failed to follow through on the physician referral and was encouraged to do so.

13. Monitor Medication (13)

A. The effectiveness of psychotropic medication and its side effects were monitored.

B. The patient reported that the medication has been effective in stabilizing mood.

C. The patient reported that the psychotropic medication has not been effective or helpful.

D. The patient has not taken the medication on a consistent basis and was encouraged to do so.

14. Psychological Testing (14)

A. Psychological testing was ordered to assess the patient's current emotional functioning and to aid in any differential diagnosis of coexisting conditions.

B. The patient cooperated with the psychological testing recommendation.

C. The patient resisted and refused to cooperate with the psychological testing.

15. Psychological Testing Feedback (15)

A. The patient was given feedback on the results of the psychological testing.

B. The psychological testing results indicated that the patient is struggling with some emotional conflicts.

C. The psychological testing results indicate the lack of any emotional conflicts or personality disturbance outside of the normal ranges.

16. Hospitalization Referral (16)

A. Since the patient's weight loss has been severe and his/her physical health is jeopardized, the patient was referred for hospitalization.

B. The patient cooperated with admission into treatment and acknowledged that his/her fragile medical condition necessitated such treatment.

C. The patient refused hospitalization that was recommended.

D. Because the patient's condition was so fragile and he/she was thought to be harmful to himself/herself, a commitment to hospitalization has been pursued.

17. Establish Minimum Calorie Intake (17)

A. The patient was assisted in developing a minimum daily caloric intake.

B. The patient committed to eating meals at regular intervals and consuming at least the minimum daily calories necessary to gain weight.

C. The patient has refused to make a commitment to consuming a minimum daily amount of calories.

18. Assist in Meal Planning (18)

A. Specific menus for meals were developed for each of the three meals per day.

B. The patient has agreed to follow through on eating the planned foods from the menu.

C. The patient reported following through on eating the meals that had been planned earlier.

D. The patient reported that he/she has not followed through on eating the planned menu items.

19. Monitor Weight (19)

A. A plan was made to monitor the patient's weight on a regular basis.

B. The patient was weighed and the results reflected a modest gain.

C. The patient was weighed and the results reflected no weight gain.

D. The patient was weighed and the results reflected a weight loss.

20. Establish Weight Goals (20)

A. The body mass index was used to establish healthy weight goals for the patient.

B. The patient has made gradual progress toward maintaining healthy weight goals.

C. The patient has not made any progress toward the healthy weight goals established.

21. Assign Eating Journal (21)

A. The patient was asked to keep a journal of food intake, as well as his/her thoughts and feelings at the time of eating and after eating.

B. The patient has followed through on keeping a journal, and the results of that journaling were processed.

C. The patient has not followed through on keeping a journal of food consumption and was encouraged to do so.

22. Process Journal Information (22)

A. The information from the patient's daily journal of food consumed, as well as his/her associated thoughts and feelings, were processed.

B. The patient discovered through the journaling process that he/she has been eating very little food and his/her thoughts and feelings about the eating behavior are distorted.

C. The journaling activity has helped the patient realize and accept that he/she has not been eating enough nutritious foods.

23. Monitor Electrolyte Balance (23)

A. The patient was encouraged to maintain regular contact with his/her physician in order to monitor electrolyte balance levels.

B. The patient has resisted maintaining regular contact with his/her physician and was encouraged to do so.

C. The patient's latest monitoring of his/her electrolyte levels indicates that he/she has attained and maintained balanced fluids and electrolytes.

24. Assign Thoughts and Feelings Journal (24)

A. The patient was assigned to keep a journal of daily thoughts and feelings associated with his/her eating behavior.

B. The patient has followed through with the assignment of journaling thoughts and feelings associated with his/her eating behavior.

C. The patient has not followed through with journaling thoughts and feelings regarding his/her eating behavior and was encouraged to do so.

25. Identify Negative Cognitive Messages (25)

A. The patient was assisted in identifying the negative cognitive messages that mediate his/her avoidance of food intake.

B. The patient was able to identify his/her irrational beliefs and distorted self-talk that are associated with eating normal amounts of food.

C. The patient regularly engages in catastrophizing or exaggerating when he/she thinks about caloric intake and weight gain.

26. Teach Realistic Self-Talk (26)

A. The patient was trained in using realistic cognitive messages regarding food intake and body size.

B. The patient reported that he/she has begun to verbalize to himself/herself positive, healthy, rational messages associated with eating and body size.

C. The patient has not consistently implemented the use of realistic cognitive self-talk and was encouraged to do so.

27. Reinforce Positive Self-Talk (27)

A. The patient was reinforced for implementation of realistic positive self-talk regarding food intake and body size.

B. The patient reported an increased frequency of positive self-talk regarding food intake and body size.

28. Teach Realistic Body Appraisal (28)

A. The patient was confronted about his/her unrealistic assessment of his/her body image.

B. The patient was assigned exercises that would reinforce a healthy, realistic body appraisal, such as positive self-talk in front of a mirror or shopping for clothes that flatter his/her appearance.

C. The patient has verbalized an increased awareness of his/her unrealistic assessment of his/her body image.

D. The patient has begun to make more positive statements about his/her body and acceptance of normal body size.

29. Confront Body Image Perfectionism (29)

A. The patient's irrational perfectionism and body image expectations were confronted.

B. The patient was assisted in developing reasonable acceptance of his/her body with normal and typical flaws.

C. The patient has begun to verbalize positive, reality-based self-talk regarding weight status and body size.

30. Explore Sexuality Fears (30)

A. The patient's fears regarding sexual development and sexual impulses were explored.

B. The patient verbalized an understanding of how his/her fear of sexual development could influence severe weight loss.

C. The patient's fears regarding sexual development were processed and his/her sexual impulses were normalized.

D. The patient expressed diminished fears regarding sexual development and increased acceptance of his/her sexual impulses.

31. Resolve Sexual Impulse Fears (31)

A. The patient's fear of losing control of his/her sexual impulses was explored.

B. The relationship between the patient's fear of his/her sexual impulses and his/her eating disorder to keep himself/herself unattractively thin or fat was explored.

C. The patient has developed insight into the relationship between fears regarding sexuality and his/her eating disorder.

32. Normalize Sexual Impulses (32)

A. The patient was reinforced for his/her acceptance of sexual impulses and a desire for normal sexual intimacy.

B. The patient verbalized acceptance of his/her sexual impulses and a desire for intimacy.

33. Explore Perfectionism (33)

A. The patient's fear of failure and the role of perfectionism in the search for avoidance of failure were explored.

B. The patient identified the relationship between the fear of failure, a drive for perfectionism, and the roots of low self-esteem.

C. The patient verbalized increased acceptance of himself/herself in spite of typical and normal failure experiences.

34. Reinforce Positive Qualities (34)

A. The patient was assisted in identifying his/her positive qualities and successes.

B. The patient reported a reduction in his/her fear of failure and an increase in a positive sense of self.

C. The patient verbalized acceptance of shortcomings and normal failures as a part of the human condition.

35. Reinforce Acceptance of Imperfection (35)

A. The patient was taught the importance of acceptance of himself/herself and others as human and subject to failure and shortcomings.

B. The patient's spiritual belief system was utilized to support self-acceptance.

C. The patient reported that he/she has made progress in accepting himself/herself with shortcomings and imperfections.

36. Explore Passive-Aggressive Control (36)

A. The role of passive-aggressive control in rebelling against authority figures as it applies to the patient's eating disorder was explored.

B. The patient acknowledged that he/she does engage in passive-aggressive behavior that is a rebellion against authority figures, especially in the area of food consumption.

C. The patient was encouraged to more directly address his/her conflicts with authority figures in order to avoid the contribution of passive-aggressive behavior to the eating disorder.

D. The patient reported that he/she has begun to address his/her conflicts with the authority figures in his/her life.

37. Explore Fear of Loss of Weight Control (37)

A. The patient's fears regarding loss of control over eating or his/her weight were explored.

B. Fears surrounding loss of control over eating or weight were processed and reported to be diminished.

38. Explore Independence Fears (38)

A. The patient acknowledged separation anxiety and emancipation anxiety.

B. The basis for the patient's fears related to independence and emancipation were explored and resolved.

C. The patient has begun to express more confidence in himself/herself regarding independence and emancipation.

39. Facilitate Family Emancipation (39)

A. A family therapy session was held that focused on issues of separation, dependency, and emancipation.

B. The patient acknowledged his/her fears regarding separation and emancipation.

C. Family members were encouraged to reinforce the patient's attempts at independence and emancipation, rather than reinforcing dependence behaviors.

D. Family members reported that the patient is taking steps toward independence.

40. Reinforce Independence (40)

A. The patient was encouraged to make a declaration of independence from his/her family and to take responsibility for his/her own behavior.

B. The patient disclosed to family members his/her feelings of ambivalence regarding their control in his/her dependency.

C. The patient has made a statement of independence to his/her family members and has begun to show evidence of that independence.

41. Teach Assertiveness (41)

A. The patient was taught elements of assertiveness and how it is distinguished from passivity and aggressiveness.

B. The patient was referred to an assertiveness training class.

C. Role playing, behavioral rehearsal, and modeling were used to teach the patient assertiveness that would apply to his/her daily life situations.

D. The patient acknowledged his/her fears in regard to assertiveness, and these fears were processed.

42. Reinforce Assertiveness (42)

A. The patient reported success in implementation of assertiveness behaviors, and these successes were reinforced.

B. The patient reported on not following through with practicing assertiveness and was encouraged to do so.

43. Facilitate Assertiveness in Family (43)

A. A family therapy session focused on each member owning his/her own feelings, clarifying messages, and identifying control conflicts.

B. The patient was reinforced for assertively expressing his/her needs and emotions within family sessions.

C. The family was assisted in developing age-appropriate boundaries for all members.

D. The patient reported that there is a decreased level of stress within the family as he/she has been more direct in expressing thoughts and feelings.

44. Explore Emotional Struggles (44)

A. The patient's emotional struggles that are camouflaged by the eating disorder were explored.

B. The patient verbalized feelings of low self-esteem, depression, loneliness, anger, and a need for nurture that underlie the eating disorder.

C. As the patient has begun to address the underlying emotional conflicts, his/her eating disorder has come under better control.

45. Identify Self-Worth (45)

A. The patient was assisted in identifying the basis for his/her self-worth, separate from body image.

B. The patient's talents, successes, positive traits, importance to others, and intrinsic spiritual value were reviewed and reinforced.

C. The patient acknowledged a benefit from developing a positive identity that is based on character traits, relationships, and intrinsic value.

D. The patient has verbalized statements of positive self-esteem more frequently.

46. Assign *Body Traps* (46)

A. The patient was encouraged to read the book *Body Traps* (Rodin) in order to better understand his/her tendency toward distorting body image.

B. The patient has followed through on reading the body image book, and key ideas from the book were processed.

C. The patient has not followed through on reading the body image book and was encouraged to do so.

D. The patient made statements about a positive identity that was not based on weight and appearance, but on intrinsic values.

47. Connect Emotions to Eating Behavior (47)

A. The patient was taught the connection between his/her suppressed emotions, interpersonal conflict, and his/her dysfunctional eating behavior.

B. The patient verbalized an understanding of the connection between his/her suppressed emotional conflicts and unhealthy food usage.

C. The development of insight has helped the patient to resolve his/her eating problems.

48. Connect Dieting to Binge Eating (48)

A. The patient was taught the relationship between binge eating and a lack of regular mealtimes or deprivation from specific foods through dieting.

B. The patient has terminated his/her pattern of a too-restrictive diet and it has resulted in less binge eating.

49. Recommend Books on Binge Eating (49)

A. The patient was encouraged to read books on binge eating, such as *Overcoming Binge Eating* (Fairburn), to increase his/her awareness of the components of eating disorders.

B. The patient has followed through on reading the materials about binge eating and it has increased his/her understanding of eating disorders.

C. The patient has not followed through on reading the materials about binge eating and has been encouraged to do so.

50. Teach Detachment to Family Members (50)

A. A conjoint session was held in which family members were encouraged to detach themselves from taking responsibility for the patient's eating behavior without showing hostility or indifference.

B. Family members verbalized the commitment to placing full responsibility for nutritious eating on the patient alone.

51. Recommend *Surviving an Eating Disorder* to Family (51)

A. Family and friends of the patient were encouraged to read *Surviving an Eating Disorder* (Siegel, Brisman, and Weinshel), in order to help them detach themselves from the patient's eating disorder.

B. Family members have followed through on reading the assigned eating disorder material and key concepts were processed within a conjoint session.

C. Family members have not followed through on reading material about eating disorders and they were encouraged to do so.

52. Dietician Referral (52)

A. The patient was referred to a dietician to become more educated about healthy eating patterns and nutritional meals.

B. The patient has followed through on attending an appointment with the dietician and verbalized concepts that were learned through that appointment.

C. The patient has not followed through on attending a dietician appointment and was encouraged to do so.

53. Reinforce Personal Responsibility (53)

A. The patient was reinforced for all statements that indicated that he/she was taking responsibility for normal food intake.

B. The patient's success at weight gain was reinforced.

C. The patient has verbalized personal responsibility for adequate nutrition and has reported gradually increasing his/her weight without supervision from others.

D. The patient continues to try to hook others into taking responsibility for changing his/her eating habits.

54. Set Goal of No Laxative Use (54)

A. A goal of termination of inappropriate use of laxatives was established.

B. The patient reported success at termination of inappropriate laxative use.

C. The patient stated that there has been no recent inappropriate laxative use.

55. Set Goal to Terminate Vomiting (55)

A. A goal of termination of self-induced vomiting was established.

B. The patient reported that he/she has been successful at significantly reducing the frequency of self-induced vomiting.

C. The patient reported the termination of self-induced vomiting, with no recent incidences occurring.

56. Set Goal to Terminate Food Hoarding (56)

A. A goal to terminate food hoarding was established.

B. The patient reported that he/she has successfully terminated food-hoarding behavior.

57. Set Goal to Limit Exercise (57)

A. The patient established a goal of very limited exercise that is not strenuous or vigorous.

B. The patient reported success at setting reasonable limits on his/her physical exercise.

C. The patient reported that he/she has not engaged in any strenuous exercise to control weight gain.

58. Set Weight Gain Goal (58)

A. The patient established a goal of gaining two pounds per week until the total weight gain goal that was established through use of the body mass index was attained.

B. The patient has successfully gained weight at a rate of two pounds per week.

C. The patient has not met his/her goal of a weight gain of two pounds per week and was redirected toward an attempt to meet that.

59. Make Meal Plans (59)

A. The patient's meeting with the nutritionist was processed and concrete plans were established for meals and calorie consumption.

B. The patient reported significantly improving his/her dietary habits.

60. Support Group Referral (60)

A. The patient was referred to a support group for people with eating disorders.

B. The patient has followed through on the referral to a support group for people with eating disorders and reported having benefited from the meeting.

C. The patient has not followed through on attendance at a support group for those with eating disorders and was encouraged to do so.

D. Attendance at the support group for people with eating disorders has helped the patient maintain his/her gains in weight and healthy eating.

EDUCATIONAL DEFICITS

PATIENT PRESENTATION

1. No High School Diploma or GED (1)

A. The patient dropped out of high school before graduation and has not pursued a GED.

B. The patient indicated an interest in completing the requirements for a GED.

C. The patient has enrolled in classes to obtain his/her GED.

D. The patient has enrolled in classes to obtain credit for completion of his/her high school diploma.

2. Needs Vocational Training (2)

A. The patient possesses no marketable employment skills and is in need of vocational training.

B. The patient indicated a strong interest in obtaining vocational training.

C. The patient has taken the steps necessary to obtain vocational training.

D. The patient is involved in a vocational training program.

3. Functional Illiteracy (3)

A. The patient has virtually no reading or spelling skills.

B. The patient has indicated an interest in availing himself/herself of opportunities for learning to read.

C. The patient has enrolled in classes to learn to read.

4. Feelings of Shame/Embarrassment (3)

A. The patient verbalized strong feelings of shame and embarrassment in regard to his/her reading ability.

B. The patient's feelings of shame and embarrassment associated with his/her lack of reading ability have caused him/her to deny this deficit and fake it.

C. As the patient has taken steps toward reading skills, his/her feelings of shame and embarrassment have diminished.

5. Difficulties in Learning (4)

A. Although the patient has shown evidence of motivation to learn, he/she has a long history of failure or near failure in academic situations.

B. The patient's intellectual deficits have contributed to a history of failure in the academic arena.

C. The patient's learning disability has contributed to a lifelong history of struggle in any learning situation.

---

* The numbers in parentheses correlate to the number of the Behavioral Definition statement in the companion chapter with the same title in *The Complete Adult Psychotherapy Treatment Planner,* second edition (Jongsma and Peterson) by John Wiley & Sons, 1999.

INTERVENTIONS IMPLEMENTED

1. Explore Education Termination Causes (1)

A. The patient's attitude toward education was assessed and other factors that contributed to the termination of his/her education were explored.

B. The patient identified his/her negative attitude toward education as being based in failure experiences related to his/her learning disability.

C. The patient identified a negative attitude toward education that was fostered by family values and a lack of parental encouragement.

D. The patient blamed association with a negative peer group for his/her failure to persevere in the academic setting.

2. Teach Education Need (2)

A. The patient was confronted with his/her need for further education.

B. The patient acknowledged his/her need for further education and agreed to take steps to pursue it.

C. The patient denied the need for further education and indicated a lack of interest in pursuing it.

3. List Negative Consequences (3)

A. The patient was assisted in listing the negative consequences that have occurred because of his/her lack of a high school diploma or GED.

B. The patient identified the lack of vocational opportunities that were available to him/her because of his/her educational deficits.

C. The patient complained of the low-paying jobs that were available to him/her because of his/her lack of academic credentials.

4. Support Academic Advancement (4)

A. The patient was encouraged to obtain further academic training.

B. As the patient indicated an interest in further academic training, he/she was reinforced and guided toward possible resources to pursue.

5. Reinforce Educational/Vocational Training (5)

A. The advantages of pursuing educational/vocational training were pointed out to the patient.

B. The patient acknowledged that there would be social, monetary, and self-esteem advantages if he/she would pursue educational/vocational training.

6. Gather Educational History (6)

A. The patient's history of educational experiences was documented.

B. The patient was asked to describe the educational and vocational levels of achievement obtained by his/her family members.

---

* The numbers in parentheses correlate to the number of the Behavioral Definition statement in the companion chapter with the same title in *The Complete Adult Psychotherapy Treatment Planner,* second edition (Jongsma and Peterson) by John Wiley & Sons, 1999.

C. The patient described learning difficulties that were encountered in specific subject areas in the academic arenas.

D. The patient acknowledged that his/her lack of achievement in education follows a pattern of similar outcomes on the part of many extended family members.

7. Psychoeducational Testing (7)

A. The patient was referred to an educational learning specialist for testing in regard to his/her learning style, cognitive strengths, and possible learning disabilities.

B. The patient has followed through on referral for educational testing.

C. The patient has not followed through on the referral for educational testing and was encouraged to do so.

8. Perform ADD Assessment (8)

A. A psychological assessment was performed to determine whether the patient suffers from Attention Deficit Disorder (ADD).

B. The psychological assessment results indicate the presence of Attention Deficit Disorder.

C. The psychological assessment results did not confirm the presence of Attention Deficit Disorder that contributed to his/her educational problems.

9. ADD Medication Referral (9)

A. The patient was referred to a physician for a medication evaluation to treat his/her ADD.

B. The patient followed through with the referral to a physician for a medication evaluation and is taking the prescribed medication to treat his/her ADD.

C. The patient followed through with the medication evaluation and no medication was prescribed for his/her ADD.

D. The patient was prescribed medication for his/her ADD condition but has refused to consistently take this medication.

10. Monitor Medication Effects (10)

A. The patient is taking his/her medication as prescribed and has reported that it has been effective in reducing his/her ADD problems.

B. The patient stated that the medication to treat ADD has not been effective in reducing his/her attention deficit problems.

C. The patient has not taken his/her medication consistently and was encouraged to do so.

11. Encourage Recommendation Implementation (11)

A. The patient was encouraged to implement the recommendations of the educational, psychological, and medical evaluations.

B. The patient has agreed to implement the recommendations resulting from the evaluations and has taken steps to do so.

C. The patient has not followed through on implementing the recommendations of the evaluations and was encouraged to do so.

12. Support Educational Progress (12)

A. The patient was given encouragement and verbal affirmation as he/she described steps that are being taken to increase his/her educational levels.

B. The patient verbalized more positive attitudes about education and expressed pleasure with his/her educational achievement.

C. The patient expressed fears and anxiety associated with entering a learning situation.

13. Develop Fear-Coping Strategies (13)

A. The patient was taught behavioral and cognitive coping strategies to help him/her reduce anxiety related to learning situations.

B. The patient reported successful implementation of behavioral and cognitive coping strategies for reducing anxiety and fear in learning situations.

C. The patient verbalized decreased anxiety and negativity associated with learning situations.

14. List Negative Learning Experiences (14)

A. The patient was asked to list the negative messages he/she has received in learning situations from teachers, parents, peers, and others.

B. The patient expressed the emotional pain, frustration, and reduced confidence that resulted from the critical messages he/she has experienced in learning situations.

C. The patient's negative experiences surrounding learning situations and the painful emotions associated with these experiences were processed.

15. Explore Shame/Embarrassment (15)

A. Feelings of shame and embarrassment were expressed by the patient regarding his/her reading ability, educational achievement, and vocational skill.

B. The patient has begun to express fuller statements regarding his/her learning ability.

C. The patent was taught self-worth based on intrinsic value rather than achievement.

16. Teach Positive Self-Talk (16)

A. The patient's negative appraisal of himself/herself was reframed in terms of his/her potential to succeed and in terms of past noneducational accomplishments.

B. The patient has begun to verbalize positive self-descriptive statements and confidence in his/her ability to succeed educationally.

17. Identify Academic Strengths (17)

A. The patient was assisted in realistically evaluating and identifying his/her academic strengths.

B. Based on his/her academic strengths, the patient has developed an educational/vocational plan.

18. Assess Reading Deficits (18)

A. The patient's reading recognition and comprehension ability were assessed.

B. It was determined that the patient has very little reading ability and would benefit from educational assistance in this area.

C. The patient appears to have some basic reading skills and could benefit from further training.

19. Reading Education Referral (19)

A. The patient was referred to an educational resource that will help him/her obtain reading skills.

B. The patient has followed through on the referral to an educational resource to learn reading skills and reported some initial success in this area.

C. The patient has failed to follow through on pursuing education in the reading area and was encouraged to do so.

20. Provide Community Resource Information (20)

A. The patient was provided with information regarding community resources available for adult education specifically in the areas of high school completion, GED certification, and vocational skill training.

B. The patient was open to accepting information about educational training resources and agreed to obtain further information from these resources.

C. The patient was resistant to pursuing further information regarding educational and vocational training.

21. Assign Educational/Vocational Training Contact (21)

A. The patient was assigned to make preliminary contact with vocational/educational training agencies and report back regarding the experience.

B. The patient has made preliminary contact with educational/vocational agencies and the results of that contact were discussed.

C. The patient has not followed through on making contact with vocational/educational resources and was encouraged to do so.

22. Elicit Educational Commitment (22)

A. An attempt was made to elicit a commitment from the patient to pursue further academic/vocational training.

B. The patient stated a commitment to obtain further academic/vocational training.

C. The patient refused to verbalize a commitment to obtain further academic/vocational training.

23. Support Educational/Vocational Participation (23)

A. The patient was asked to describe his/her experience of attendance at educational/vocational training classes.

B. The patient stated that he/she has attended classes on a consistent basis in order to obtain further vocational/educational training.

C. The patient's consistent participation in educational/vocational training was strongly supported and reinforced.

D. The patient indicated that he/she has not been consistent in his/her participation in the educational/vocational training and was redirected to do so.

FAMILY CONFLICT

PATIENT PRESENTATION

1. Frequent Conflict with Parents/Siblings (1)

A. The patient described an atmosphere of frequent conflict with parents and siblings.

B. The patient projects blame onto others for his/her conflict with family members.

C. The patient is beginning to accept responsibility for his/her role in the family conflict and to attempt to find resolution.

D. The patient reported increased harmony and support between family members.

2. Lack of Contact (2)

A. The patient stated that his/her family members have little or nothing to do with each other, and, therefore, they are not seen as a positive influence or source of support.

B. The patient has taken the initiative to try to increase the degree of family members' involvement with each other.

C. The patient indicated that he/she is more a part of a family unit, now that the family members see each other more and interact together.

3. Dependence/Independence Conflict (3)

A. The patient describes ongoing conflict with his/her parents, which is characterized by the parents fostering the patient's dependence and the patient feeling that the parents are overly controlling.

B. The parents are attempting to nurture the patient's independence, and the patient is taking some steps toward emancipation.

C. The degree of conflict with parents has decreased significantly, and the patient is exercising reasonable independence.

4. Residence with Parents (4)

A. The patient has lived with his/her parents consistently since childhood.

B. The patient has made periodic attempts at emancipation and living independently but has always returned to live with his/her parents.

C. Plans have been made for the patient to emancipate to independent living.

D. The patient has successfully emancipated from his/her parents and is living independently from their constant emotional and economic support.

5. Alienation from Parents (5)

A. The patient has sustained long periods of noncommunication from his/her parents and describes himself/herself as the "black sheep."

B. Overtures have been made to bridge the gap between the patient and his/her parents and to build a supportive relationship.

---

* The numbers in parentheses correlate to the number of the Behavioral Definition statement in the companion chapter with the same title in *The Complete Adult Psychotherapy Treatment Planner,* second edition (Jongsma and Peterson) by John Wiley & Sons, 1999.

C. The patient is now in regular contact with his/her parents and feels as if he/she is an accepted member of the family.

6. Stepfamily Conflict (6)

A. Since the marriage of the two previously married partners, there has been conflict between the members of this reconstituted family.

B. Stepsiblings and stepparents have increased their understanding of and communication with each other.

C. The blended family unit has become more functional and bonded to one another.

INTERVENTIONS IMPLEMENTED

1. Reinforce Independent Thought (1)

A. The patient was encouraged to express his/her thoughts and feelings and was reinforced for having an independent perspective from other family members.

B. The patient's pattern of dependence interfered with his/her ability to openly and honestly describe his/her thoughts and feelings.

C. The patient has become more open in describing his/her thoughts and feelings and has described a sense of autonomy from other family members.

2. Explore Family Conflict (2)

A. Family members were asked to describe the nature, frequency, and intensity of their conflict with one another.

B. The causes for family conflict were explored from the perspective of each family member.

C. The patient outlined the nature of the family conflicts and his/her perspective on the causes for them.

3. Facilitate Family Communication (3)

A. A family therapy session was conducted to facilitate healthy communication, conflict resolution, and the emancipation process.

B. The family showed evidence of controlled reciprocal and respectful communication of their thoughts and feelings with each other.

4. Create a Family Genogram (4)

A. A family therapy session was conducted in which a genogram was developed that was complete with denoting family members, patterns of interaction, rules, and secrets.

B. The dysfunctional communication patterns between family members within the nuclear and extended family units was highlighted.

C. Family members acknowledged the lack of healthy communication that permeates the extended family.

---

* The numbers in parentheses correlate to the number of the Behavioral Definition statement in the companion chapter with the same title in *The Complete Adult Psychotherapy Treatment Planner,* second edition (Jongsma and Peterson) by John Wiley & Sons, 1999.

5. Facilitate Expression of Feelings (5)

A. Each family member was supported and encouraged to express his/her concerns, fears, and expectations regarding the family.

B. An increased oneness within the family unit was demonstrated through each family member sharing his/her thoughts and feelings.

C. The family members' resistance to openness communication was evident, and attempts were made to process and resolve this resistance.

6. Confront Responsibility Avoidance (6)

A. The patient was confronted when he/she was not taking responsibility for his/her own thoughts, feelings, and behavior and contribution to the family conflict.

B. The patient was reinforced for owning responsibility for his/her role in the family conflict.

C. The patient acknowledged an increased insight into his/her contribution to the family conflict.

7. Making Peace with Your Parents (7)

A. The patient was asked to read the book, *Making Peace with Your Parents* (Bloomfield and Felder), to increase his/her understanding of the dynamics of family conflict.

B. The patient has followed through on reading the book on family conflict, and key concepts of the book were identified for application in the patient's family situation.

C. The patient has not followed through on reading the book and was encouraged to do so.

D. The patient's reading of the book on family conflict has helped him/her understand dynamics within the family system.

8. Teach the Role of Resistance (8)

A. All family members were taught that resistance to change in the style of relating to one another can be expected to be high and that change would require concerted effort on the part of all family members.

B. Family members verbalized an increased awareness of how the family system has reinforced and will continue to reinforce the status quo in terms of patterns of communication and conflict resolution.

C. As family members have acknowledged their resistance to change, they have also become more open to and motivated for change.

9. Identify Dependence (9)

A. The patient was asked to make a list of the ways that he/she is dependent on his/her parents.

B. The patient has identified facets that reinforce his/her dependence on the family.

C. The patient showed denial and minimization as he/she was asked to honestly acknowledge ways that he/she is dependent on the parents.

10. Develop Dependence Reduction Plan (10)

A. A plan was developed to reduce the patient's dependence on his/her parents and each of those arenas where he/she has acknowledged a dependent pattern.

B. The patient has begun to implement a plan to reduce his/her pattern of dependence on his/her parents.

C. The patient was reinforced for all planful steps that were implemented toward becoming more independent and autonomous.

11. Family Experiential Weekend Referral (11)

A. The family was referred for participation in an experiential weekend retreat at a center for family education.

B. The family has followed through on participation in an experiential weekend and reported that it did build a sense of family unity and confidence in working together.

C. The patient has not followed through on accepting the referral for participation in the family weekend and was encouraged to do so.

12. Assign Parenting Books (12)

A. The parents were assigned to read books on effective parenting, and specific recommendations were made.

B. The parents have followed through with reading books on parenting, and key concepts were processed to encourage the implementation of healthy changes.

C. The parents have not followed through on reading books on parenting and were encouraged to do so.

13. List of Family Activities (13)

A. The patient was assisted in developing a list of positive family activities in which he/she and the family could engage to promote harmony.

B. Selected family activities that promote harmony were placed in the family schedule.

C. The family members have increased the number of positive family interactions in the implementation of planned family activities.

14. Identify Chemical Dependence Triggers (14)

A. The patient was assisted in identifying how family conflict has operated as a trigger for chemical dependence relapse.

B. The patient identified a pattern of escaping into substance abuse as a means of avoiding the feelings associated with family conflict.

C. The patient acknowledged using family conflict as an excuse for substance abuse.

15. Assign Family Substance Abuse Books (15)

A. The patient was asked to read books on the role of family dynamics in chemical dependence.

B. The patient has followed through on reading books on family substance abuse patterns, and key issues from this reading were processed.

C. The patient has not followed through on reading the books on family issues in substance abuse and was encouraged to do so.

16. Chemical Dependence Treatment Referral (16)

A. The patient was confronted with his/her need for chemical dependence treatment and a referral was made.

B. The patient acknowledged that his/her chemical dependence has played a significant role in precipitating family conflict.

C. The patient has acknowledged his/her chemical dependence and has accepted a referral for treatment.

D. The patient has denied a need for treatment for his/her chemical dependence and has rejected a referral.

17. Parenting Class Referral (17)

A. The parents were referred to a class to help them expand their understanding of children and to build skills in disciplining negative behavior and reinforcing positive behavior.

B. The parents have accepted a referral to a parenting class and have reported that they have found it to be beneficial.

C. Key concepts learned from the parenting class were reviewed and applied to the specific family situations.

D. The parents have not followed through on attending a parenting class and were encouraged to do so.

18. Tough-Love Group Referral (18)

A. The parents were referred to a tough-love group to help them learn to set boundaries firmly.

B. The parents have followed through on attending a tough-love group and have found meaningful support to help them deal with their own parenting situation.

C. The parents have not followed through on attending a tough-love group and were encouraged to do so.

19. Train Parents in the Barclay Method (19)

A. The parents were trained in the Barclay Method of understanding and managing defiant and oppositional behavior on the part of children.

B. The parents have responded favorably to being taught the principles of the Barclay Method and have begun to implement them in their parenting at home.

C. Both parents have reported that their involvement in the parenting process has increased and that they have become more effective in dealing with their children.

D. The parents reported that they have been supportive of each other in the parenting process and that this has produced more effective limit setting on the children.

20. Read Fables (20)

A. Within a family therapy session, selections from *Freedman's Fables* (Freedman) were read to help the family understand the dynamics of their interaction.

B. The family responded favorably to the fable exercise, and members were able to identify their role within the family dynamics.

21. Assign *Siblings Without Rivalry* (21)

A. The parents were assigned to read the book *Siblings Without Rivalry* (Faber and Mazlish) to help them understand the dynamics of sibling rivalry.

B. The parents have followed through on reading the book about sibling rivalry, and key concepts were processed.

C. Specific ways were identified for the parents to implement parenting techniques to reduce the degree of sibling rivalry.

D. The parents reported that the degree of sibling rivalry has diminished as they have implemented new parenting techniques.

E. The parents have not followed through on reading the assigned book and were encouraged to do so.

22. Teach Parenting Techniques (22)

A. The parents were taught effective parenting techniques and were referred to specific literature to educate them further in these concepts.

B. The parents have begun to implement more effective parenting techniques for their young children and were reinforced for doing so.

C. The parents described problematic interactions with the children as they have tried to implement new techniques, and these problems were processed and resolved.

D. The parents have shown considerable resistance to making changes in their parenting technique.

23. Confront Continuation of Dependence Pattern (23)

A. The patient's pattern of emotional and economic dependence on his/her parents was confronted.

B. The patient acknowledged that he/she has avoided taking on consistent employment responsibilities that would allow for independent living.

24. Teach Conflict Resolution (24)

A. Role playing, modeling, and behavioral rehearsal were used to teach the patient ways to resolve conflict effectively with his/her parents.

B. The patient was taught assertiveness skills and respectful communication using eye messages to help reduce conflict effectively.

C. The patient reported an increase in resolving conflicts with parents by talking calmly and assertively rather than aggressively and defensively.

25. Increase Family Structure (25)

A. The parents were assisted in developing rituals such as establishing dinnertimes, bedtime routines, and weekly family activities so as to increase structure and promote bonding within the family.

B. The parents have followed through on increasing the amount of structure within the family by implementing routine family activities.

C. The parents have been resistive to increasing the degree of family structure and were encouraged to do so.

26. Assist Developmental Structure (26)

A. The parents were assisted in increasing the degree of structure and setting firm limits.

B. Parents have implemented a family meeting that will promote communication and bonding within the family unit.

C. The parents have followed through on increasing the amount of structure and boundary setting.

27. Assign Family Drawings (27)

A. Each family member was assigned to bring to a family session a self-produced drawing of themselves in relationship to the family.

B. Each family member's drawing of their relationship to the family was reviewed and processed.

28. Assign a Family Collage (28)

A. The family was assigned to make a collage out of pictures cut from magazines.

B. The family collage that was created by the family members was processed.

C. The family members were assisted in developing a "coat of arms" that will signify the new, blended family unit.

29. Assign a Family Activity Plan (29)

A. Within a family session, the family was assigned the task of selecting and planning an activity in which all members could participate.

B. The family members described their participation in the planned family activity, and such bonding experiences were reinforced.

30. Create a Revised Genogram (30)

A. Family members were assisted in developing a revised genogram that depicted how new, healthy relationships are being developed.

B. Family members reported an increased sense of bonding and a desire for more connectedness with each other.

31. Assign *Changing Families* (31)

A. The parents were assigned to read the book *Changing Families* (Fassler, Lash, and Ives) with the family at home.

B. The parents have followed through on reading the book and reported the positive impact that this experience had on the family dynamics.

C. The parent have not followed through on reading the book on changing families and were encouraged to do so.

32. Explore Emancipation Fears (32)

A. The patient's fears regarding emancipation were explored and highlighted.

B. The patient's fears regarding emancipation were processed toward resolution.

C. The patient reported an increased desire for emancipation and a reduced fear of implementing a plan of emancipation.

D. The patient reported an increased level of independent functioning that will support emancipation.

33. Develop Emancipation Plan (33)

A. The patient was assisted in developing a specific plan of emancipation from his/her parents in a healthy and responsible way.

B. The patient stated his/her goal of emancipation and has shared his/her plan of emancipation with his/her parents.

C. The patient has begun to implement a plan for emancipation and was reinforced for doing so.

D. The patient has continued to resist emancipation, and his/her resistance was processed.

FEMALE SEXUAL DYSFUNCTION

PATIENT PRESENTATION

1. Lack of Sexual Desire (1)

A. Patient describes a consistently very low desire for or pleasurable anticipation of sexual activity.

B. The patient's interest in sexual contact is gradually increasing.

C. Patient verbalized an increased desire for sexual contact, which is a return to previously established levels.

2. Avoidance of Sexual Contact (2)

A. The patient reported a strong avoidance of and repulsion for any and all sexual contact with her respectful partner.

B. The patient's repulsion for sexual contact has begun to diminish.

C. The patient no longer has a strong avoidance of sexual contact and, in fact, has expressed pleasure with such contact.

3. Lack of Physiological Sex Response (3)

A. The patient has experienced a recurrent lack of the usual physiological response of sexual excitement and arousal.

B. Instead of indicating an interest in sexual contact, the patient's physiological response to excitement is not present.

C. The patient is gradually regaining the usual physiological response of sexual excitement and arousal.

D. The patient reported that sexual contact resulted in a satisfactory level of physiological response of sexual excitement.

4. Lack of Subjective Enjoyment (4)

A. The patient reported a consistent lack of a subjective sense of enjoyment and pleasure during sexual activity.

B. The patient reported an increased sense of pleasure and enjoyment during recent sexual contact.

C. The patient reported a satisfactory level of enjoyment and pleasure during recent sexual activity.

5. Delay in/Absence of Reaching Orgasm (5)

A. The patient reported a persistent delay in or absence of reaching orgasm after achieving arousal and in spite of sensitive sexual pleasuring by a caring partner.

B. The patient reported an improvement in time to reach orgasm during sexual contact.

* The numbers in parentheses correlate to the number of the Behavioral Definition statement in the companion chapter with the same title in *The Complete Adult Psychotherapy Treatment Planner,* second edition (Jongsma and Peterson) by John Wiley & Sons, 1999.

C. The patient reported a satisfactory response time to reaching orgasm during sexual contact.

6. Genital Pain (6)

A. The patient reported persistent genital pain before, during, or after sexual intercourse.

B. The patient's genital pain associated with sexual intercourse has diminished.

C. The patient reported no experience of genital pain before, during, or after sexual intercourse.

7. Vaginismus (7)

A. The patient reported a consistent or recurring involuntary spasm of the vagina that prohibits penetration for sexual intercourse.

B. The patient reported experiencing minimal vaginal penetration during sexual contact without the experience of pain.

C. The patient reported normal vaginal penetration during sexual intercourse without any experience of involuntary contraction or pain.

INTERVENTIONS IMPLEMENTED

1. Assess Relationship (1)

A. The patient was asked to share her thoughts and feelings regarding her relationship with her sexual partner.

B. The patient described a lack of harmony and fulfillment within the relationship with her partner.

C. The patient outlined several areas of significant conflict that exist in the relationship with her partner.

2. Conjoint Sessions (2)

A. Conjoint sessions were held between the patient and her partner that focused on conflict resolution, expression of feelings, and sex education.

B. Both partners shared their thoughts and feelings regarding their perception of the relationship.

C. Both partners identified what each perceived as significant problems within their relationship that influenced their sexual activity.

3. Explore Family-of-Origin Sexual Attitudes (3)

A. The patient was asked to describe her perception of sexual attitudes that she learned from her family of origin.

B. The patient outlined what she saw as causes for her sexual inhibition and feelings of guilt, fear, and repulsion associated with sexual activity.

---

* The numbers in parentheses correlate to the number of the Behavioral Definition statement in the companion chapter with the same title in *The Complete Adult Psychotherapy Treatment Planner,* second edition (Jongsma and Peterson) by John Wiley & Sons, 1999.

4. Gather Sexual History (4)

A. A detailed sexual history was gathered that examined current sexual functioning as well as childhood and adolescent experiences, level and sources of sexual knowledge, typical sexual practices, medical history, and use of mood-altering substances.

B. The patient provided detailed sexual history material regarding those things that she perceives had influence over her sexual attitudes, feelings, and behavior.

5. Explore Origin of Negative Sexual Attitudes (5)

A. The patient described her history of experiences within her family of origin that caused her to develop a negative attitude regarding sexuality.

B. The patient outlined the family-of-origin experiences in which the subject of sexuality was taboo.

C. The patient described learning negative sexual attitudes from her mother, who shared her distaste for sexual interaction.

6. Explore Religious Training/Sexual Attitudes (6)

A. The role of religious training and reinforcing feelings of guilt and shame surrounding sexual behavior and thoughts was explored with the patient.

B. The patient verbalized an understanding of how her religious training negatively influenced her sexual thoughts, feelings, and behavior.

7. Explore Sexual Abuse (7)

A. The patient's history was explored for sexual traumas or abuse.

B. The patient identified a history of sexual abuse as a child and acknowledged how this abuse has had a negative impact on sexual feelings and thoughts.

8. Process Sexual Trauma (8)

A. The patient's feelings surrounding an emotional trauma in the sexual arena were processed.

B. The patient verbalized a resolution of feelings regarding her sexual trauma.

C. The patient's childhood sexual abuse experiences have been resolved to the point that they no longer exercise a strong negative impact over current sexual attitudes, behavior, and feelings.

9. Teach Insight into the Past (9)

A. The patient was helped to develop insight into the role of past negative sexual experiences in creating current adult dysfunction.

B. The patient verbalized an understanding of the role of past negative sexual experiences and the development of dysfunctional sexual attitudes and responses in the present.

C. The patient made a commitment to put the negative attitudes and experiences in the past and to make a behavioral effort to become free from those influences.

10. Explore Sex Role Models (10)

A. The patient's sex role models who influenced her during her childhood or adolescence were explored.

B. The patient verbalized an understanding of the connection between the lack of positive sexual role models in childhood and her current adult sexual dysfunction.

11. Explore Automatic Thoughts (11)

A. The patient's automotive thoughts that trigger negative emotions before, during, and after sexual activity were explored.

B. The patient identified several negative cognitive messages that trigger feelings of fear, shame, anger, and grief during sexual activity.

12. Teach Healthy Self-Talk (12)

A. The patient was taught healthy alternative thoughts that will mediate pleasure, relaxation, and disinhibition during sexual activity.

B. The patient has begun to implement positive and healthy self-talk and reported that she is experiencing more relaxed feelings of pleasure during sexual activity.

13. Model Open Sexual Communication (13)

A. The patient was taught, through modeling, to talk freely and respectfully regarding sexual body parts, feelings, and behavior.

B. The patient is beginning to speak more freely and openly regarding her sexual feelings and behavior as well as using anatomically correct labels for sexual body parts.

C. The patient has continued to show strong inhibition regarding talking openly and freely regarding sexual material.

14. Assign Sexuality Books (14)

A. The patient was assigned books on human sexuality that provide accurate sexual information and outline sexual exercises that disinhibit and reinforce sexual sensate focus.

B. The patient has followed through on reading the assigned books on human sexuality and has found them informative and healthy in reducing her inhibition in the sexual arena.

C. The patient has not followed through on reading the books on human sexuality and was encouraged to do so.

D. As a result of reading books on human sexuality, the patient has verbalized more positive and healthy attitudes regarding her sexual feelings and behavior.

15. Reinforce Open/Positive Sexual Communication (15)

A. The patient was reinforced for talking freely, knowledgeably, and positively regarding sexual thoughts, feelings, and behavior.

B. The patient has demonstrated healthy and accurate knowledge of sexuality by freely verbalizing adequate information of sexual functioning using appropriate terms for sexually related body parts.

C. The patient continues to experience strong inhibition regarding talking openly and knowledgeably regarding her experience of human sexuality.

16. Assess Biochemical Causes for Dysfunction (16)

A. The role that substance abuse, diabetes, hypertension, or thyroid disease may have on the patient's sexual functioning was identified and assessed.

B. The patient identified a pattern of substance abuse that could have a very negative effect on sexual functioning.

C. The patient identified a medical condition that may have an impact on sexual functioning, and she was referred to a physician for further evaluation.

17. Review Medications (17)

A. The patient's use of medication was reviewed as to the possible negative side effects on sexual functioning.

B. The patient was referred to her physician for a more comprehensive review of the impact on sexual functioning that the medication she is taking may have.

C. The patient acknowledged that medication side effects may be a powerful contributing factor to her sexual problems.

18. Physician Evaluation Referral (18)

A. The patient was referred to a physician for a complete physical to rule out any organic basis for her sexual dysfunction.

B. The patient has cooperated with a referral to a physical and has submitted to an examination to rule out any organic basis for her sexual dysfunction.

C. The patient's physical did identify medical conditions and or medications that may have a harmful effect on her sexual functioning.

D. An evaluation by a physician found no organic basis for the patient's sexual dysfunction.

19. Medication Referral (19)

A. The patient was referred to a physician to evaluate whether a prescription of medication may help her overcome her sexual arousal disorder.

B. The physician has prescribed medication in an attempt to increase the patient's sexual arousal.

C. The patient reported that the medication prescribed by the physician to enhance sexual arousal has had a positive impact.

D. The patient reported that the medication prescribed by the physician to increase sexual arousal has not had any noticeable impact.

20. Assess Depression (20)

A. The patient's symptoms of depression were assessed for their frequency and severity.

B. The patient reported experiencing several key symptoms of depression and that depression of sexual desire coincided with the onset of the depression.

C. The patient reported that her feelings of depression began long after the depression of sexual desire and performance.

D. As the patient's depression has lifted, her sexual desire and performance have improved significantly.

21. Antidepressant Medication Referral (21)

A. The patient was referred for an evaluation for antidepressant medication.

B. As the patient has consistently taken her antidepressant medication, she reported an improvement in mood and increase in sexual desire.

C. Consistently taking antidepressant medication has not improved the patient's sexual dysfunction.

22. Explore Failed Relationships (22)

A. The patient's fears surrounding intimate relationships were explored along with her history of previously failed relationships.

B. The patient acknowledged that fear of intimacy was related to a history of painful, previously failed relationships.

C. As the patient has resolved some of her fears regarding intimate relationships, sexual dysfunction problems have dissipated.

23. Explore a Secret, Sexual Affair (23)

A. The patient identified a secret, sexual affair that has contributed to her sexual dysfunction with her partner.

B. The patient acknowledged her need to terminate one of her intimate relationships in order to focus emotional investment into the other intimate relationship.

C. The patient acknowledged that keeping a secret affair from her current partner has interfered with her ability to be sexually intimate.

24. Explore a Lesbian Interest (24)

A. The patient identified lesbian sexual urges that have predominated any heterosexual interests.

B. The patient acknowledged that her lesbian attraction is a major factor in her sexual dysfunction with her partner.

C. The patient has agreed to share her lesbian interest with her male partner and to discuss termination of their relationship.

25. Assign Sexual Awareness Exercises (25)

A. The patient was assigned body exploration and sexual awareness exercises to reduce her inhibition and to desensitize her to sexual aversion.

B. The patient has followed through on body exploration and sexual awareness exercises and reports a reduction in sexual inhibitions.

C. The patient has not followed through on implementing the body exploration and sexual awareness exercises and was encouraged to do so.

26. Assign Sexual-Pleasuring Exercises (26)

A. The patient was assigned graduated steps of sexual-pleasuring exercises with her partner to reduce performance anxiety and focus on experiencing bodily arousal sensations.

B. The patient has followed through on practicing sensate focus exercises both alone and with her partner.

C. The patient shared her feelings associated with her sexual-pleasuring exercises and reports an increased satisfaction with the sexual activity.

D. The patient has not followed through on performing the graduated steps of sexual-pleasuring exercises and was encouraged to do so.

27. Reinforce Disinhibition (27)

A. The patient was given encouragement for less inhibited, less constricted sexual behavior with her partner.

B. The patient was assigned body-pleasuring exercises that would focus on decreasing inhibition and increasing the freedom of sexual behavior with her partner.

C. The patient has followed through on completing the body-pleasuring exercises and has reported an increased feeling of freedom to express herself sexually.

E. The patient has not followed through on the body-pleasuring exercises with her partner and was encouraged to do so.

28. Assign a Sexuality Journal (28)

A. The patient was encouraged to keep a journal of sexual thoughts and feelings to increase her awareness and acceptance of them as a normal occurrence.

B. The patient has followed through on keeping a journal of sexual thoughts and feelings, and the material was processed as the patient was reinforced for this normal experience.

C. The patient has failed to follow through on journaling her sexual thoughts and feelings, and her resistance to doing so was processed to resolution.

29. Encourage Sexual Fantasies (29)

A. The patient was encouraged to indulge herself in normal sexual fantasies that could mediate and enhance sexual desire.

B. The patient reported success at becoming aware of and indulging in sexual fantasies that have increased sexual desire.

C. The patient reported resistance to indulging sexual fantasies because feelings of guilt, embarrassment, and shame predominated.

30. Encourage Sexual Experimentation (30)

A. The patient was encouraged to experiment with coital positions and environmental settings for sexual play that could increase her feeling of security, arousal, and satisfaction.

B. The patient has implemented changes in coital positions and environmental settings for sexual play and reported increased feelings of security, arousal, and satisfaction.

C. The patient has been resistant to making changes in the pattern of sexual activity with her partner and was encouraged to do so.

31. Encourage Sexual Assertiveness (31)

A. The patient was encouraged to be more assertive in expressing her feelings of sexuality and sexual play with her partner.

B. The patient reported that she has engaged in more assertive behaviors that have allowed her to share her sexual needs, feelings, and desires with her partner.

C. The patient reported behaving in a more sensuous way and expressing pleasure more freely in sexual contact.

32. Explore Extrarelational Stressors (32)

A. Stressors that may interfere with the strength of sexual desire or performance were explored.

B. The patient identified stressors in the areas of work, social relationships, family responsibilities, and other areas that drain energy away from sexual desire.

C. The patient was assisted in developing coping strategies to reduce the degree of stress that interferes with sexual interest or performance.

D. The patient reported that sexual arousal and performance have increased as the degree of stress with other areas of life has been reduced.

33. Explore Fears of Sexual Inadequacy (33)

A. The patient's fear of inadequacy as a sexual partner was explored.

B. As the patient acknowledged her fears of inadequacy regarding sexual performance and body image, a connection to avoidance of sexual activity with her partner was made.

C. An attempt was made to reduce the patient's fears of sexual inadequacy and to give her feelings of positive self-image associated with sexuality.

D. As the patient has developed a more positive self-image and increased her feelings of self-esteem, her interest in sexual activity has increased.

34. Explore Feelings of Threat (34)

A. The patient's feelings of threat, brought on by the perception of her partner as being sexually aggressive, were explored.

B. The patient has communicated her feelings of threat to her partner, which were based on a perception of her partner being too sexually aggressive or too critical of her.

C. As the patient has been freer to communicate her feelings of threat to her partner, sexual satisfaction has increased.

35. Encourage Positive Body Image (35)

A. The patient was asked to list assets of her body that she feels positively about.

B. The patient was encouraged to be less critical about her body image.

C. As the patient has become less self-critical regarding her body, she has begun to develop greater freedom of sexual expression.

36. Explore Feelings about Body Image (36)

A. The patient's feelings regarding body image were explored with a focus on identifying causes for her negativism.

B. The patient was confronted for being too self-critical and expecting perfection of herself.

C. The patient was encouraged to be more self-accepting of a body with normal flaws.

D. As the patient has become more accepting of her body and verbalized a more positive body image, she has become more sexually active.

37. Reinforce Sexual Desire (37)

A. The patient's expressions of desire for, and pleasure with, sexual activity were strongly reinforced.

B. As the patient has made progress in resolving sexual dysfunction issues, she has reported an increased desire for, and pleasure with, sexual activity.

C. The patient was encouraged to express her renewed desire for, and pleasure with, sexual activity to her partner.

38. Assign Vaginal Relaxation Exercises (38)

A. The patient was encouraged to use masturbation and a vaginal dilator, penetration devices to reinforce relaxation and success surrounding vaginal penetration.

B. The patient reported that the implementation of masturbation and vaginal penetration exercises has increased her feelings of confidence surrounding sexual penetration.

C. The patient reported experiencing sexual penetration from her partner without pain or involuntary spasm of the vagina.

39. Assign Sexual Partner Participation (39)

A. The patient's sexual partner was directed in sexual exercises that allow for the patient to control the level of genital stimulation and vaginal penetration.

B. As the patient has had complete control over vaginal penetration and stimulation, she has been able to experience penetration without pain.

FINANCIAL STRESS

PATIENT PRESENTATION

1. Excessive Indebtedness (1)

A. The patient described severe indebtedness and overdue bills that exceed his/her ability to meet the monthly payments.

B. The patient has developed a plan to reduce his/her indebtedness through increasing income and making systematic payments.

C. The patient has begun to reduce the level of indebtedness and is making systematic payments.

D. The patient has significantly reduced his/her indebtedness.

2. Unemployment (2)

A. The patient has become unemployed and has no source of income.

B. The patient has developed a plan to obtain emergency financial relief through community services.

C. The patient has developed a plan to immediately seek employment.

D. The patient has become employed again, and income has been restored.

3. Employment Change (3)

A. The patient's employment change has resulted in a reduction in income.

B. The patient has adjusted his/her budget for living to accommodate the reduction in income.

4. Spousal Monetary Conflict (4)

A. The patient described a pattern of conflict with his/her spouse over money management and the definition of necessary expenditures and savings goals.

B. The patient and his/her spouse have begun to talk constructively about spending and savings guidelines.

C. Agreement has been reached between the spouses regarding a budget and savings goals.

5. Hopelessness (5)

A. The patient described a feeling of hopelessness and low self-esteem associated with the lack of sufficient income to cover the cost of living.

B. As financial arrangements have been adjusted, the patient's mood has improved.

C. The patient has developed a sense of hope for the future as financial assistance has been attained and the cost of living is covered.

6. Poor Money Management Skills (6)

A. The patient has a long-term lack of discipline in money management that has led to excessive indebtedness.

---

* The numbers in parentheses correlate to the number of the Behavioral Definition statement in the companion chapter with the same title in *The Complete Adult Psychotherapy Treatment Planner,* second edition (Jongsma and Peterson) by John Wiley & Sons, 1999.

B. The patient has filed for bankruptcy to protect himself/herself from creditors.

C. The patient has never established a budget with spending guidelines and savings goals that would allow for prompt payment of bills.

D. The patient has developed a budget and has begun to live within it, making timely payment of bills.

7. Uncontrollable Financial Crisis (7)

A. Due to a crisis beyond the patient's control, his/her income is not sufficient to cover the monthly expenses.

B. The patient's bills have become past-due, and he/she is in need of financial assistance.

C. The patient has obtained financial assistance, and the pressure has been relieved from monthly obligations.

8. Loss of Housing Threat (8)

A. Because of an inability to meet monthly mortgage payments, the patient is under a threat of losing his/her shelter.

B. The patient has obtained relief in terms of extended payments to allow him/her to keep his/her housing.

C. The patient has caught up on monthly mortgage/rental payments, allowing him/her to remain in his/her housing.

9. Impulsive Spending (9)

A. The patient described a pattern of his/her impulsive spending that does not consider the eventual financial consequences of such action.

B. The patient was in defensive denial regarding his/her pattern of impulsive spending.

C. The patient acknowledged his/her impulsive spending and has begun to develop a plan to help cope with this problem.

D. The patient has established a pattern of delay of any purchase until the financial consequences of the purchase can be planned for and met.

INTERVENTIONS IMPLEMENTED

1. Build Trust (1)

A. Consistent eye contact, active listening, unconditional positive regard, and warm acceptance were used to help build trust with the patient.

B. The patient began to express feelings more freely as rapport and trust level increased.

C. The patient has continued to experience difficulty being open and direct in his/her expression of painful feelings.

2. Explore the Financial Situation (2)

A. The patient's current financial situation was explored in detail.

B. The patient described the details of his/her financial crisis, including his/her level of indebtedness and other monthly obligations.

---

* The numbers in parentheses correlate to the number of the Behavioral Definition statement in the companion chapter with the same title in *The Complete Adult Psychotherapy Treatment Planner,* second edition (Jongsma and Peterson) by John Wiley & Sons, 1999.

C. The patient described the past-due bills that have mounted and created a financial crisis.

D. The patient described his/her change of employment status that has reduced his/her level of income.

3. List Financial Obligations (3)

A. The patient was assisted in compiling a complete list of his/her financial obligations.

B. The patient has a pattern of minimization and denial in the area of acknowledging financial obligations.

4. Identify the Causes for the Financial Crisis (4)

A. The patient was assisted in identifying and clarifying the causes for the current financial crisis.

B. The patient was helped to reconstruct the history of his/her financial problems in an attempt to isolate the sources and causes of the excessive indebtedness.

C. The patient was confronted when excuses were made for the financial problems that continued a pattern of avoidance of taking responsibility.

5. Explore Hopelessness (5)

A. The patient's feelings of hopelessness and helplessness that are associated with the financial crisis were explored.

B. The patient verbalized feelings of depression and shame related to his/her current financial status.

C. The patient was encouraged to consider alternative actions that could be taken to begin to cope with the financial crisis.

6. Assess Despondency (6)

A. The depth of the patient's despondency over the financial crisis was assessed.

B. The patient's despondency was so serious that suicide precautions were taken until a sense of hope can be restored.

C. Although the patient is discouraged about his/her financial situation, his/her despondency was not so severe as to cause concern for his/her life.

7. Assess Suicide Potential (7)

A. The patient was directly assessed for any suicidal urges that have been experienced.

B. The patient denied any suicidal urges.

C. Because the patient described serious suicidal urges, steps were taken to ensure his/her safety.

8. Develop Spending Priorities (8)

A. The patient was assigned the task of listing the priorities that he/she believes should give direction to how money is spent.

B. The patient's list of priorities regarding how money is spent was processed and clarified.

C. The patient has agreed that an established set of priorities should govern his/her spending and has committed himself/herself to implementing that control.

D. The patient has demonstrated that his/her priorities have control over spending.

9. Explore the Family-of-Origin Financial Patterns (9)

A. The patient's family-of-origin patterns of earnings, saving, and spending money were identified.

B. The patient acknowledged that the financial patterns that he/she learned from his/her family of origin have influenced his/her own money management decisions.

C. The patient has allowed reasonable priorities to control financial decision making rather than following mismanagement patterns learned from his/her family of origin.

10. Identify Steps to Immediate Financial Relief (10)

A. The patient was assisted in reviewing possibilities for immediate financial relief such as filing for bankruptcy, applying for welfare, and/or obtaining credit counseling.

B. The patient has selected and pursued steps toward immediate financial relief to deal with expenses that exceed his/her income.

11. Community Assistance Referral (11)

A. The patient was referred to church and community resources that can provide welfare assistance and support.

B. The patient has met with community agency personnel to apply for immediate welfare assistance.

C. The patient's feelings related to applying to welfare assistance were processed.

12. Develop a Financial Plan (12)

A. The patient was directed to write a budget and long-range savings and investment plan.

B. The patient was referred to a professional financial planner.

13. Review Budget (13)

A. The patient's budget was reviewed as to its completeness and reasonableness.

B. The patient has written a budget that balances income with expenses.

C. The patient has implemented a budget, and spending has been strictly controlled by it.

14. Credit Counseling Referral (14)

A. The patient was referred to a nonprofit credit counseling service for the development of a budgetary plan of debt repayment.

B. The patient has accepted the referral to a credit counseling service and has attended planning meetings.

C. The patient has resisted a referral to a credit counseling service and was encouraged to follow through with the attendance at such meetings.

15. Encourage Credit Counseling (15)

A. The patient was strongly encouraged to continue following through with credit counseling sessions and to strictly adhere to the budgetary guidelines established.

B. The patient was reinforced for following through with credit counseling and implementing a strict repayment plan.

16. Attorney Referral (16)

A. The patient was referred to an attorney to discuss the feasibility and implications of filing for bankruptcy.

B. The patient has met with an attorney and has decided to file for bankruptcy.

C. The patient has met with an attorney and has decided to not file for bankruptcy.

17. Explore the Emotional Vulnerability to Spending (17)

A. The patient was assessed as to feelings of low self-esteem, need to impress others, loneliness, or depression that may accelerate unnecessary and unwanted spending.

B. The patient identified negative emotional states that he/she attempts to cope with through unnecessary spending.

18. Assess Mood Swings (18)

A. The patient was assessed for characteristics of bipolar disorder that could contribute to careless spending due to an impaired mania-related judgment.

B. The patient acknowledged impulsive spending as a part of a general pattern of impulsivity that is based on mood swings.

C. The patient was referred for a psychiatric evaluation to consider the possibility of medication to control mood swings.

19. Screen for Substance Abuse (19)

A. The patient's pattern of other drug usage was evaluated as to any possible contribution to his/her financial crisis.

B. The patient described a pattern of substance abuse that definitely contributes to the financial crisis.

C. The patient denied any substance abuse problem.

D. The patient was referred for substance abuse treatment.

20. Explore Family Substance Abuse (20)

A. Substance abuse by family members other than the patient was assessed.

B. The patient acknowledged a problem of substance abuse with other family members that contributes to the financial stress.

C. The patient denied any substance abuse problems by other family members that could contribute to the financial stress.

D. Arrangements were made for an intervention to confront the substance abuse by family members.

21. Plan a Job Search (21)

A. The patient was assisted in formulating a job search plan.

B. The patient has begun to implement a job search plan in order to raise his/her level of income.

C. The patient has been active in applying for employment and was reinforced for doing so.

D. The patient has been successful in obtaining employment that will raise his/her income and reduce financial stress.

22. Reinforce Conjoint Financial Planning (22)

A. A conjoint session was held to develop a mutually agreed-upon financial plan.

B. Both partners have committed themselves to a financial plan and have reinforced each other for implementing it consistently.

23. Reinforce Cooperative Financial Management (23)

A. The patient was reinforced for making changes in financial management that reflect compromise, reasonable planning, and respectful cooperation with his/her partner.

B. The patient has set financial goals and made budgetary decisions with his/her partner that allow for equal input and balanced control over financial matters.

24. Assign Financial Recordkeeping (24)

A. The patient was assisted in developing a plan of weekly and monthly recordkeeping that reflects income and payments made.

B. The patient has consistently kept weekly and monthly records of financial income and expenses and was reinforced for doing so.

25. Reinforce Debt Resolution (25)

A. The patient has reported successful resolution of debt and was strongly supported for this disciplined behavior.

B. The patient expressed a sense of pride and accomplishment at resolution of some of his/her debt.

26. Role-Play Resisting Spending Urges (26)

A. Role playing and modeling were used to teach the patient to resist spending beyond reasonable limits.

B. The patient was taught positive self-talk that compliments himself/herself for being disciplined over urges to spend.

27. Role-Play Resistance to External Pressure (27)

A. Role playing and behavioral rehearsal were used to help the patient develop coping mechanisms for external pressure to spend beyond what he/she can afford.

B. The patient identified pressure from family members and friends to spend beyond what he/she can afford.

C. The patient reported success at being graciously assertive in refusing pressure from others to spend money.

28. Reinforce Successful Resistance (28)

A. The patient has reported the use of cognitive and behavioral strategies to control the impulse to make unnecessary and unaffordable purchases and was reinforced for this constructive action.

B. The patient reported resisting the urge to overspend and was reinforced for this discipline.

29. Teach Cognitive Strategies (29)

A. The patient was taught to resist impulsive spending by implementing self-talk that asks questions regarding the necessity of the purchase and the affordability of the expense.

B. The patient reported success at reducing the impulse to spend as he/she has used cognitive checking methods.

30. Teach Purchase Delay (30)

A. The patient was taught the importance of delaying an impulse to make a purchase to allow time for reflection regarding the affordability and consequences of the expense.

B. The patient has successfully implemented the delay of impulses to spend, and this delay has resulted in a reduction of unnecessary purchases.

GRIEF/LOSS UNRESOLVED

PATIENT PRESENTATION

1. Preoccupation with Loss (1)

A. The patient's thoughts have been dominated by the loss experienced and he/she has not been able to maintain normal concentration on other tasks.

B. The patient reported a reduction in preoccupation with the experience of loss and slightly improved concentration.

C. The patient's concentration has improved significantly and his/her thoughts are no longer dominated by the loss experience.

2. Tearful Spells (1)

A. The patient reported waves of depression and grief that result in tearfulness on a frequent basis.

B. The patient's tearful spells have diminished somewhat in frequency.

C. The patient reported better control over his/her emotions and no incidence of spontaneous tearful spells.

3. Confusion about the Future (1)

A. The patient reported being confused about what the future of his/her life would be like after the traumatic loss.

B. The patient is beginning to talk about his/her future with slightly more certainty and is making short-term plans.

C. The patient has developed a future perspective and has made long-term plans.

4. Serial Losses (2)

A. The cumulative effect of several sequential losses in the patient's life has been depression and discouragement.

B. The patient has begun to be more hopeful about his/her future as he/she struggles to resolve the experience of loss.

C. The patient has returned to a more normal hopeful outlook on his/her life.

5. Emotional Lability (3)

A. The patient experiences a strong grief reaction whenever the losses are discussed.

B. The patient's emotional reactions to the discussion of the loss are more controlled.

C. The patient is able to discuss his/her losses without losing control of his/her emotions.

6. Depression Symptoms (4)

A. The patient described a lack of appetite and sleep disturbance as well as other depression signs that have occurred since the experience of the loss.

---

* The numbers in parentheses correlate to the number of the Behavioral Definition statement in the companion chapter with the same title in *The Complete Adult Psychotherapy Treatment Planner,* second edition (Jongsma and Peterson) by John Wiley & Sons, 1999.

B. The patient's depression symptoms have diminished as he/she has begun to resolve the feelings of grief.

C. The patient's depression symptoms have lifted.

7. Feelings of Guilt (5)

A. The patient verbalized guilt over believing that he/she had not done enough for the lost significant other.

B. The patient verbalized an unreasonable belief of having contributed to the death of the significant other.

C. The patient's feelings of guilt have diminished.

D. The patient reported that he/she no longer experiences guilt related to the loss.

8. Grief Avoidance (6)

A. The patient has shown a pattern of avoidance of talking about the loss except on a very superficial level.

B. The patient's feelings of grief are coming more to the surface as he/she faces the loss issue more directly.

C. The patient is able to talk about the loss directly without being overwhelmed by feelings of grief.

9. Support Network Loss (7)

A. Because of a geographic move, the patient has lost a positive support network that was in place at his/her previous place of residence.

B. The patient is beginning to take steps to develop a positive support network.

C. The patient reported success at reaching out to new friends within this new community.

INTERVENTIONS IMPLEMENTED

1. Build Trust (1)

A. Consistent eye contact, active listening, unconditional positive regard, and warm acceptance were used to help build trust with the patient.

B. The patient began to express feelings more freely as rapport and trust level increased.

C. The patient has continued to experience difficulty being open and direct in his/her expression of painful feelings.

2. Explore Losses (2)

A. The patient was asked to elaborate autobiographically on the circumstances, feelings, and effects of the loss or losses in his/her life.

B. The patient identified the losses that have been experienced in his/her life and shared the feelings of pain and grief associated with these losses.

C. The patient talked about the losses experienced, but the feelings associated with those losses were not shared.

---

* The numbers in parentheses correlate to the number of the Behavioral Definition statement in the companion chapter with the same title in *The Complete Adult Psychotherapy Treatment Planner,* second edition (Jongsma and Peterson) by John Wiley & Sons, 1999.

3. Assign Exploring Others' Grief (3)

A. The patient was encouraged to talk to others who have experienced loss in their lives as to how they reacted to those losses and how they coped with them.

B. The patient has followed through on the assigned task of speaking to others about their grief and he/she has learned new coping mechanisms.

C. The patient has not followed through on talking to others about their experience with grief and was encouraged to do so.

4. Teach Grief Stages (4)

A. The patient was educated regarding the stages of the grieving process.

B. The patient verbalized an increased understanding of the steps of the grieving process and identified the stages he/she has experienced personally.

5. Assign Grief Books (5)

A. Several books on the grieving process were recommended to the patient.

B. The patient has read the material on the grieving process, and content from that material was processed.

C. The patient has not followed through on reading any of the grief material and was encouraged to do so.

D. The patient has shown an increased understanding of the steps of the grieving process as a result of reading the recommended grief material.

6. Assign *The Bereaved Parent* (6)

A. The parents were encouraged to read the book *The Bereaved Parent* (Schiff) to help them better understand grief related to a child's death.

B. The parents have followed through with reading the assigned book on parental grief, and themes from that reading were processed.

C. The parents have not followed through with reading the book on grieving parents and were encouraged to do so.

7. Assign Grief Journal (7)

A. It was recommended that the patient keep a daily grief journal to be shared in future sessions.

B. The patient has kept a grief journal on a daily basis and verbalized the feelings of grief that he/she has experienced.

C. Keeping a grief journal has helped the patient clarify and identify those feelings of grief and begin to resolve them.

8. Solicit Grief-Related Pictures/Mementos (8)

A. The patient was encouraged to bring to the session pictures or mementos connected with the loss.

B. The patient brought to the session pictures and mementos connected with his/her loss, and the feelings associated with these memories were processed.

C. The patient has failed to bring pictures and mementos associated with the loss to the session and was encouraged to do so.

9. Clarify Grief Feelings (9)

A. The patient was assisted in identifying, clarifying, and expressing those feelings associated with the loss.

B. The patient has become more open in expressing grieving feelings.

C. The patient minimizes and denies feelings of grief associated with the loss.

10. Assign Grief-Related Videos (10)

A. The patient was encouraged to watch videos dealing with themes of grief such as *Terms of Endearment, Dad,* or *Ordinary People.*

B. The patient has watched a grief-related video drama and discussed the feelings that were precipitated by watching these videos.

C. As a result of watching the videos on grief-related themes, the patient has identified his/her own patterns of avoidance of grief.

11. Grief Support Group Referral (11)

A. The patient was encouraged to attend a grief/loss support group.

B. The patient has followed through on attending a grief/loss support group and reported that it was a positive experience.

C. The patient has followed through on attending the grief/loss support group, but thought that it was a negative experience.

D. The patient has not followed through on attending the recommended grief/loss support group and was encouraged to do so.

12. List Grief Avoidance Consequences (12)

A. The patient identified ways that he/she has avoided the grief process and how this has had a negative impact on his/her life.

B. The patient has acknowledged that grief avoidance is not a productive way to cope with the loss.

13. Assess Substance Abuse (13)

A. The patient's use of mood-altering substances as an escape from the pain of grief was assessed.

B. The patient acknowledged that he/she has used substance abuse as an escape from the pain of grief.

C. The patient denied that his/her substance abuse is a problem and did not acknowledge that it plays a role in the escape from the pain of grief.

D. The patient did acknowledge that his/her substance abuse is a problem.

14. Chemical Dependence Referral (14)

A. The patient was referred for chemical dependence treatment since substance abuse has become a problem in and of itself.

B. The patient acknowledged a need for clean and sober living so that the grieving process can be faced directly, without escape into substance abuse.

C. The patient accepted the referral for chemical dependence treatment and has followed through on the referral.

D. The patient rejected the referral for chemical dependence treatment and would not acknowledge substance abuse as a problem.

15. Explore Anger Feelings (15)

A. The patient's feelings of anger or guilt that surround the loss were explored as to their depth and causes.

B. The patient verbalized feelings of anger and guilt focused on himself/herself that surround the grief experience of loss.

C. The patient has begun to resolve the feelings of anger and guilt that will allow the grieving process to continue.

16. Reinforce Forgiveness (16)

A. The patient was encouraged to forgive himself/herself and the deceased loved one rather than holding onto feelings of anger or guilt.

B. Books on forgiveness were recommended to the patient as a means of encouraging and understanding the forgiveness process.

C. The patient has followed through on reading books about forgiveness and has reported them to be beneficial.

D. The patient has not followed through on reading books about forgiveness and was encouraged to do so.

17. Assign Grief Letter (17)

A. The patient was assigned the task of writing a letter to the deceased person describing fond memories, painful and regretful memories, and how he/she currently feels.

B. The patient has followed through on writing a grief letter to the deceased loved one and this letter was processed within the session.

C. The patient has clarified and expressed his/her feelings to and about the lost loved one.

D. The patient has found some sense of relief at expressing thoughts and feelings that he/she had left unexpressed earlier.

18. Assign Last Contact Letter (18)

A. The patient was assigned to write a letter to the deceased loved one with a special focus on his/her feelings associated with their last meaningful contact.

B. The patient has followed through on writing a letter to the loved one regarding their contact and expressed strong feelings associated with that memory.

C. The patient has not followed through on writing a letter regarding the last contact with the loved one and was encouraged to do so.

19. Identify/Clarify Grief Feelings (19)

A. The patient was assisted in identifying and expressing the feelings of grief connected with the loss.

B. Writing letters to the lost loved one has helped the patient to identify and express his/her feelings of grief.

C. The patient has found it difficult to openly express his/her feelings regarding the loss and has continued the pattern of emotional avoidance.

20. Identify Dependency (20)

A. The patient was assisted in identifying his/her dependency on the significant other who has been lost.

B. The patient expressed his/her feelings of abandonment regarding the loss associated with the significant other.

C. The patient acknowledged dependency on the lost loved one and has begun to refocus his/her life on independent actions to meet emotional needs.

21. Assign List of Regrets (21)

A. The patient was assigned to make a list of all the regrets he/she has concerning the loss.

B. The patient identified the regrets that he/she has regarding the loss and also has clarified the causes for those feelings of regret.

22. Conduct Empty-Chair Exercise (22)

A. An empty-chair exercise was conducted with the patient in which he/she focused on expressing to the lost loved one what he/she never said while that loved one was present.

B. The patient expressed many thoughts and feelings that had been suppressed while the loved one was present.

23. Assign Grave Site Visit (23)

A. The patient was assigned to visit the grave of the lost loved one to express and ventilate feelings.

B. The patient reported that the visit to the grave site facilitated many thoughts and feelings that went unexpressed while the deceased was alive.

C. The patient has not followed through on the visit to the grave site and was encouraged to do so.

24. List Positive Memories (24)

A. The patient was asked to list the most positive aspects of and memories about the relationship with the lost loved one.

B. The patient identified the positive characteristics of the lost loved one and the positive aspects of the relationship.

25. Develop Memorial Rituals (25)

A. The patient was assisted in developing rituals that will allow the patient to celebrate the memorable aspects of the deceased loved one and his/her life.

B. The patient has followed through on developing rituals and implementing them to commemorate the memory of the lost loved one.

26. Use Rational Emotive Approach (26)

A. A rational emotive approach was used to confront the patient's statements of responsibility for the loss.

B. The patient was encouraged to consider the reality-based facts surrounding the loss and his/her distortion of those facts in accepting responsibility for the loss irrationally.

C. The patient has decreased his/her statements and feelings of being responsible for the loss.

27. Develop Grieving Ritual (27)

A. The patient was encouraged to develop a grieving ritual to be used while focusing on the feelings of sadness surrounding the anniversary of the loss.

B. The patient has followed through on implementing the grieving ritual surrounding the anniversary of the loss, and his/her experience with that ritual was processed.

C. The patient has not followed through on development of the grieving ritual and was encouraged to do so.

28. Suggest Time-Limited Mourning (28)

A. The patient was encouraged to set aside a specific time-limited period each day to focus on mourning the loss.

B. The patient has followed through on establishing a specific time each day to focus on the feelings of grief surrounding the loss and has been successful at compartmentalizing the grieving experience.

C. The patient has not followed through on grieving at a set time of day and instead is preoccupied with the feelings of grief throughout the day.

29. Develop Penitence Activity (29)

A. The patient was assisted in developing an act of penitence for the patient's feelings of having failed the departed loved one in some way.

B. The patient has begun to implement an activity of penitence for feelings of responsibility.

C. The patient reported that he/she is feeling relieved after participating in the activities of penitence.

30. Conduct Family Grieving (30)

A. A family therapy session was conducted, with all members of the family expressing their experience related to the loss.

B. Each family member has expressed his/her feelings of grief and how he/she is coping with their loss.

31. Encourage Spiritual Activity (31)

A. The patient was encouraged to rely upon his/her spiritual faith in terms of its promises and activities as a source of support.

B. The patient has implemented acts of spiritual faith as a source of comfort and hope to help deal with the feelings of grief.

IMPULSE CONTROL DISORDER

PATIENT PRESENTATION

1. Aggressive Impulsivity (1)

A. The patient described several incidences of loss of control over aggressive impulses that have resulted in acts of assault on other individuals.

B. The patient described several episodes of loss of control over impulses that have resulted in destruction of property.

C. The patient reported getting more control over aggressive impulses, although verbal aggression is still present.

D. The patient reported successful control over aggressive impulses with no recent incidences noted.

2. General Impulsivity (2)

A. The patient has a consistent pattern of acting before thinking that has resulted in numerous negative consequences on his/her life.

B. The patient is beginning to exercise better control over impulsivity.

C. The patient described instances when he/she thought before acting and controlled his/her impulsivity.

D. The patient reported no recent instances of impulsive behavior that have resulted in negative consequences.

3. Overreactivity (3)

A. The patient has a pattern of overreaction to mildly aversive stimulation.

B. The patient has a pattern of overreactivity to pleasure-oriented stimulation.

C. The patient has shown a regulation of his/her reactivity to stimulation.

4. Excessive Activity Shifting (4)

A. The patient has a pattern of excessive shifting from one activity to another and rarely completing anything that is started.

B. The patient is easily distracted from staying focused on and completing a task.

C. The patient has shown evidence of remaining more focused and completing tasks.

5. Lack of Organization (5)

A. The patient demonstrates a lack of organization in his/her personal life and environment.

B. The patient has become more focused on living by a schedule and organizing his/her environment.

C. As the patient has become more organized, he/she has also become more productive.

---

* The numbers in parentheses correlate to the number of the Behavioral Definition statement in the companion chapter with the same title in *The Complete Adult Psychotherapy Treatment Planner,* second edition (Jongsma and Peterson) by John Wiley & Sons, 1999.

6. Difficulty Waiting (6)

A. The patient reported a high degree of frustration whenever he/she must wait for others, such as standing in line or waiting for others to finish their conversation.

B. The patient has reported becoming more aware of his/her impatience and intolerance for waiting for others.

C. The patient has developed a more relaxed and patient attitude regarding having to wait for things.

7. Harmful Impulses (7)

A. The patient has a pattern of failure to resist impulses to perform acts that may be harmful to himself/herself or others.

B. The patient is showing more control over harmful impulses.

C. The patient reported that there have been no recent incidences of impulsive actions that are harmful to himself/herself or others.

INTERVENTION IMPLEMENTATION

1. Explore Impulsive Behavior (1)

A. The patient identified the impulsive behaviors that have been engaged in over the last six months.

B. The patient demonstrated limited insight into and awareness of his/her impulsive behaviors.

C. The patient has a good level of awareness of his/her pattern of impulsivity.

2. Teach Self-Observation (2)

A. A review of the patient's impulsivity was engaged in to heighten the patient's awareness of his/her impulsivity.

B. The patient demonstrated increasing awareness of his/her pattern of impulsivity.

C. The patient still has limited awareness of and insight into his/her patterns of impulsivity.

3. List Positive Consequences (3)

A. The patient was asked to make a list of positive consequences that result from his/her impulsive actions.

B. The patient's limited list of positive consequences that result from impulsivity was processed.

C. The patient could identify no positive consequences that result from impulsivity.

4. List Negative Consequences (4)

A. The patient was assigned the task of listing negative consequences that occurred because of his/her impulsivity.

B. The patient demonstrated good awareness of the negative consequences that are brought upon himself/herself and others as a result of his/her impulsivity.

---

* The numbers in parentheses correlate to the number of the Behavioral Definition statement in the companion chapter with the same title in *The Complete Adult Psychotherapy Treatment Planner,* second edition (Jongsma and Peterson) by John Wiley & Sons, 1999.

C. The patient minimizes and uses denial to avoid awareness of the negative consequences of his/her impulsivity.

5. Teach Awareness of Negative Consequences (5)

A. The patient was taught the connection between his/her impulsivity and the negative consequences that result from this behavior pattern.

B. The patient has demonstrated increased awareness of the negative consequences of his/her impulsivity.

6. Confront Responsibility Denial (6)

A. The patient was confronted about his/her denial of responsibility for impulsive behavior or the negative consequences of that behavior.

B. The patient accepted the confrontation of his/her impulsive behavior and the negative consequences of it.

C. The patient became defensive in the face of confrontation and continues to deny responsibility for his/her impulsive behavior.

7. Assign Impulsivity Journal (7)

A. The patient was asked to keep a log of impulsive behavior and its antecedents, mediators, and consequences.

B. The patient presented a log of his/her impulsive actions, and this material was processed in order to increase the patient's awareness of his/her behavior and the consequences of it.

C. The patient failed to keep a log of his/her impulsive behavior and was redirected to do so.

8. Reinforce Responsibility Acceptance (8)

A. The patient verbalized a clear connection between his/her impulsive behavior and negative consequences to himself/herself and others.

B. The patient was reinforced for acceptance of responsibility for and the connection between impulsive behavior and negative consequences.

9. Develop Feedback Contract (9)

A. A conjoint session was held to assist the patient in developing a contract for receiving feedback from others prior to engaging in impulsive acts.

B. The patient reported that he/she has implemented a review process with a trusted friend or family member for feedback regarding possible consequences of his/her impulsive behavior.

C. Reviewing behavior with others prior to engagement in that behavior has successfully reduced the patient's impulsivity.

10. Explore Impulsivity Triggers (10)

A. Past experiences the patient has had were explored in order to uncover triggers for his/her impulsive episodes.

B. The patient has identified the thoughts that trigger impulsive behavior.

11. Teach Cognitive Coping Methods (11)

A. The patient was taught cognitive methods such as thought stoppage, thought substitution, reframing for gaining and improving control over impulsive actions.

B. The patient reported that utilization of cognitive methods to control trigger thoughts and reduce impulsive behavior has been successful.

C. The patient reported specific instances of successful utilization of cognitive methods to control impulsive behavior.

12. Explore Anxiety Relief (12)

A. The role of anxiety reduction as a reward for impulsivity was explored.

B. The patient confirmed that as he/she becomes more anxious, impulsive behavior is triggered.

C. The patient denied any role of anxiety relief in maintaining impulsive behavior.

D. The patient cited specific instances of engaging in impulsive behavior to reduce stress and tension.

13. Teach Relaxation Methods (13)

A. The patient was taught relaxation techniques such as progressive relaxation and self-hypnosis to reduce tension levels and stress.

B. The patient reported implementation of relaxation exercises to control anxiety and to reduce impulsive behavior.

C. The patient has failed to use the relaxation techniques in his/her daily life and was redirected to do so.

14. Teach Behavioral Strategies (14)

A. The patient was taught behavioral methods to cope with anxiety, such as talking to others about stress, taking time out to relax, calling a friend or family member, or engaging in physical exercise.

B. The patient reported successful implementation of behavioral strategies to reduce tension and the consequent impulsive behavior.

C. The patient has failed to implement behavioral strategies and was encouraged to do so.

15. Teach Social Assertiveness (15)

A. Using modeling, role playing, and behavioral rehearsal, the patient was taught assertive techniques to express himself/herself.

B. The patient was taught the use of "I" messages as a way to express his/her thoughts and feelings directly and assertively.

C. The patient expressed anxiety about implementing assertiveness.

16. Review Assertiveness Implementation (16)

A. The patient identified situations in which assertiveness has been implemented and described his/her feelings associated with that behavior and the consequences of that behavior.

B. The patient expressed anxiety over the implementation of assertiveness, but was pleased with the consequences of it.

C. The patient was reinforced for successfully implementing assertiveness techniques.

D. The patient has failed to implement assertiveness consistently and was directed to do so.

17. Teach "Stop, Think, Listen, and Plan" (17)

A. Modeling, role playing, and behavior rehearsal were used to teach the patient the use of "stop, think, listen, and plan" in several life scenarios.

B. The patient was supported as he/she enacted "stop, think, listen, and plan" as applied to different current situations.

C. The patient was encouraged to use the "stop, think, listen, and plan" technique to control acting impulsively in his/her daily life.

18. Review Daily Use of "Stop, Think, Listen, and Plan" (18)

A. The patient was taught the use of "stop, think, listen, and plan" in day-to-day living.

B. The patient reported on the implementation of "stop, think, listen, and plan," as well as the positive consequences of this implementation.

19. Medication Evaluation Referral (19)

A. The patient was referred to a physician for a medication evaluation to help control impulsivity.

B. The patient has followed through on meeting with a physician for a medication evaluation and has begun to take prescribed medications.

C. The patient has not followed through on seeing a physician for a medication evaluation and was redirected to do so.

20. Monitor Medication (20)

A. The patent's compliance with taking the prescribed medication as well as the effectiveness and side effects of that medication were reviewed.

B. The patient reported taking all medications as ordered and indicated that the medication has been effective at reducing impulsivity.

C. The patient reported taking all medication as ordered, but that no positive effects have been noted.

21. Develop Behavior Modification Program (21)

A. The patient was assisted in identifying rewards that would be effective in reinforcing his/her suppression of impulsive behavior.

B. The patient agreed to implement a reward system that is contingent on suppression of impulsive behavior.

22. Implement Reward System (22)

A. The patient was encouraged to implement a reward system for replacing impulsive actions with reflection on consequences and choosing patient alternatives.

B. The patient has implemented a reward program for deterring impulsive actions, and the frequency of impulsivity has been reduced.

C. The patient has failed to consistently utilize the reward program for deterring impulsive behavior and was directed to do so.

INTIMATE RELATIONSHIP CONFLICTS

PATIENT PRESENTATION

1. Arguing with Partner (1)

A. The patient reported frequent or continual arguing with his/her partner.

B. The frequency of conflict between the partners has diminished.

C. The patient reported implementation of conflict resolution skills.

D. The patient reported that his/her relationship with the partner has improved significantly and arguing has become very infrequent.

2. Lack of Communication (2)

A. The patient complained of a lack of communication with his/her partner.

B. Communication between the patient and his/her partner has improved.

C. The patient cited instances of improved communication with his/her partner.

D. The patient reported being pleased with the amount and quality of the communication with his/her partner.

3. Projection of Responsibility (3)

A. The patient has a pattern of projecting the responsibility for conflict onto his/her partner.

B. The patient showed considerable anger at the partner, as he/she placed virtually all the responsibility for the problems between them on the partner.

C. The patient is beginning to take some of the responsibility for the conflict between himself/herself and his/her partner.

4. Marital Separation (4)

A. The patient and his/her partner have agreed to a marital separation.

B. The partner has initiated a separation from the patient.

C. The patient has initiated a marital separation from his/her partner.

D. The patient expressed feelings of hurt, disappointment, anxiety, and depression related to the marital separation.

5. Pending Divorce (5)

A. A divorce petition has been filed by the patient.

B. The patient's partner has filed for a petition of divorce.

C. The legal proceeding of a divorce has been finalized.

D. The patient expressed feelings of sadness surrounding his/her divorce.

E. The patient expressed feelings of anger and resentment over the divorce.

F. The patient places responsibility for the divorce on the partner.

* The numbers in parentheses correlate to the number of the Behavioral Definition statement in the companion chapter with the same title in *The Complete Adult Psychotherapy Treatment Planner,* second edition (Jongsma and Peterson) by John Wiley & Sons, 1999.

6. Multiple Intimate Relationships (6)

A. The patient described involvement in multiple intimate relationships concurrently.

B. The patient experiences emotional conflict regarding his/her engagement in multiple intimate relationships.

C. The patient feels no conflict over his/her concurrent involvement in multiple relationships.

D. The patient has acknowledged the need to terminate the multiple intimate relationships.

7. Abusive Relationship (7)

A. The patient reported incidences of verbal abuse that occur within the relationship.

B. The patient described incidences of physical abuse that have occurred within the relationship.

C. The patient has taken steps to remove himself/herself from the abusive relationship.

8. Avoidance of Closeness (8)

A. The patient described a pattern of superficial communication, infrequent or nonsexual contact, and excessive involvement in independent activities that contribute to the avoidance of closeness to his/her partner.

B. The patient and his/her partner have taken steps to spend more quality time together to increase the degree of intimacy between them.

C. The patient and his/her partner continue a pattern of involvement in independent activities that contributes to their distance from one another.

9. Broken Relationships Pattern (9)

A. The patient described a pattern of repeated broken or conflicted relationships due to a lack of problem-solving skills, recurrent distrust in the relationship, or choosing dysfunctional partners who may be abusive.

B. The patient has developed increased insight into his/her pattern of choosing dysfunctional partners with whom to become intimate.

INTERVENTIONS IMPLEMENTED

1. Plan Conjoint Sessions (1)

A. Both partners were asked to commit themselves to a series of conjoint sessions to address issues of communication and problem solving.

B. Both partners agreed to attend and actively participate in conjoint sessions.

2. Identify Relationship-Building Behaviors (2)

A. The partners were assisted in identifying behaviors that enhanced their relationship rather than contributing distancing and conflict.

B. Both partners agreed to commit themselves to working toward strengthening the relationship.

---

* The numbers in parentheses correlate to the number of the Behavioral Definition statement in the companion chapter with the same title in *The Complete Adult Psychotherapy Treatment Planner,* second edition (Jongsma and Peterson) by John Wiley & Sons, 1999.

3. Assign Positive Relationship Aspects Lists (3)

A. The partners were assigned to list, from each of their perspectives, the positive things about the relationship and about each other.

B. The partners have listed positive things about each other and the relationship, and it has taken their focus off of the negative aspects.

C. The partners have failed to follow through on completing the assigned list of positive relationship aspects and were encouraged to do so.

4. Assign Relationship Journaling (4)

A. Each partner was assigned the task of journaling about positive experiences regarding the relationship that occur between sessions.

B. The partners brought back to the session journal material relating positive interactions that occurred between them between sessions.

C. Neither partner has followed through on keeping a journal of positive interactions and both were encouraged to do so.

5. Explore Relationship Conflicts (5)

A. Each partner has identified the nature of the conflicts between them.

B. Each partner has demonstrated a tendency to project blame onto the other for their conflicts.

6. Assign *The Intimate Enemy* (6)

A. Both partners were assigned to read the book *The Intimate Enemy* (Bach and Wyden) to broaden their perspective on relationship dynamics.

B. The partners have read the assigned book on relationship dynamics, and key ideas were processed.

C. The partners have not followed through with reading the assigned book on relationship dynamics and were encouraged to do so.

7. Confront Responsibility Avoidance (7)

A. Both partners were confronted about avoiding responsibility for their own roles in the conflicts within the relationship.

B. Both partners tend to become defensive when pressed to acknowledge their own roles in the conflicts between them.

C. Each partner has become more open to identifying his/her own role in the conflicts and the changes that he/she must make to improve the relationship.

8. List Own Changes Needed (8)

A. Each partner was asked to list the changes that he/she must make to improve the relationship.

B. Each partner has followed through on listing the changes that he/she needs make to improve the relationship, and this list was processed in the contract session.

C. The partners have not followed through on listing their own changes that would improve the relationship and were encouraged to do so.

9. List Others' Changes (9)

A. Each partner was asked to list the changes the other partner needs to make to improve the relationship.

B. Each partner has identified changes the other needs to make, and these changes were processed in a conjoint session.

C. Each partner has failed to identify a list of changes the other needs to make to improve the relationship and both were encouraged to do so.

10. Solicit Change Commitment (10)

A. Each partner made a commitment to attempt to change specific behaviors that have been identified by himself/herself or the other partner.

B. Both partners were reinforced for their willingness to implement changes in themselves to improve the relationship.

C. Each partner's progress in making changes in himself/herself to improve the relationship were reviewed and processed.

11. Process Change Lists (11)

A. Within a conjoint session, each partner clarified his/her perspective on the changes that needed to be made to improve the relationship.

B. Each partner has begun to become more focused on noticing changes that need to be made within himself/herself rather than projecting blame onto the other.

12. Assign Specific Communication Time (12)

A. The partners were assigned the task of setting aside 10 minutes, two to three times each week, in which they communicate directly about conflict issues.

B. Practice at communication regarding conflict issues was done within the session, and the partners were assisted in communicating clearly and listening sensitively.

C. As the partners have implemented specific communication times regarding conflict issues, this experience was processed and reinforced.

D. The partners have not followed through on consistently implementing communication time regarding conflict issues and were encouraged to do so.

13. Recommend Relationship Seminar (13)

A. The partners were referred to a relationship seminar where communication and conflict resolution skills would be taught.

B. The partners have followed through on attending a relationship seminar and have begun to implement the skills within the home setting.

C. The partners reported success at implementing the communication and problem-solving skills that were learned within the relationship seminar.

14. Clarify Communication (14)

A. Both partners were assisted in clarifying their communication and their expression of feelings within conjoint sessions.

B. Both partners reported that they have increased the quality and frequency of communication with each other.

15. Assign Nonconflict Communication (15)

D. The partners were assigned to talk daily for a specific time with each other about pre-chosen, nonemotional, nonconflictual topics.

E. The partners reported success at implementing communication about nonconflictual topics.

F. The partners have not followed through on consistently talking on a daily basis about nonconflictual topics and were encouraged to do so.

16. Reframe Complaints into Requests (16)

A. The partners were taught to reframe their complaints about each other into requests for each other.

B. The partners have begun to reduce critical complaining about each other by reframing their complaints into polite requests for change.

C. Each partner reported specific instances of reframing complaints into polite requests and reported that this change was successful at reducing conflict.

17. Train in Assertiveness (17)

A. Modeling and role playing were used to teach the principles of assertiveness in communication.

B. The partners were referred to a seminar on assertiveness training.

C. The partners have begun to express thoughts and feelings regarding their relationship in a direct, nonaggressive manner.

18. Explore Relationship Expectations (18)

A. Each partner's expectations for the relationship were explored, and irrational, unrealistic expectations were noted.

B. The couple was assisted in developing realistic beliefs and expectations regarding the relationship.

19. Teach Mutual Satisfaction (19)

A. The partners were taught the key concept that each partner must be willing at times to sacrifice his/her own needs and desires to meet the needs and desires of the other.

B. The partners have verbally recognized their responsibility to meet some of the needs of the significant other in the relationship.

20. Teach Conflict Resolution Techniques (20)

A. The partners were taught conflict resolution techniques and these techniques were role-played within the session.

B. The partners reported implementation of the conflict resolution techniques to resolve issues reasonably between them.

21. Probe Family-of-Origin History (21)

A. Each partner's family-of-origin history was explored to identify patterns of destructive intimate relationship interaction.

B. The partners were encouraged to note the repetition of a family pattern of destructive intimate relationship interactions.

22. Gather Relationship History (22)

A. Each partner's personal history of previous dysfunctional intimate relationships was explored.

B. Each partner has indicated insight into past relationships as to causes for their failure and his/her own contribution to that failure.

C. Each partner identified a pattern of repeatedly forming destructive intimate relationships.

23. List Aggression-Escalating Behaviors (23)

A. Each partner was assisted in making a list of behaviors that escalate conflict between them and trigger abusive behavior.

B. The partners were asked to make special note of any conflict between them and the behaviors that contribute to that conflict escalating.

24. Develop Conflict Termination Signal (24)

A. The partners were assisted in identifying a clear verbal or behavioral signal to be used by either partner to terminate interaction immediately if either of them fears impending abuse.

B. Role playing and modeling were used to teach how the conflict termination signal could be used in future disagreements between them.

25. Solicit Conflict Termination Agreement (25)

A. Both partners were solicited for a firm agreement that the conflict termination signal would be responded to favorably and without debate.

B. The partners reported successful implementation of a conflict termination signal that has reduced incidences of abuse.

26. Explore Substance Abuse (26)

A. The role of substance abuse was explored as to its contribution to conflict and abuse in the relationship.

B. Substance abuse by one of the partners was acknowledged as a strong contributing factor to escalating conflict between the partners.

C. Although substance abuse appears to be a critical component of relationship conflict, neither partner was willing to acknowledge the fact of substance abuse being a factor.

27. Substance Abuse Treatment Referral (27)

A. The chemically dependent partner was referred for substance abuse treatment.

B. The chemically dependent partner has accepted a referral and followed through with obtaining substance abuse treatment.

C. The chemically dependent partner has refused to follow through with a referral to obtain substance abuse treatment.

28. Identify Infidelity Message (28)

A. The partners were assisted in clarifying the message that lies behind the infidelity within the relationship.

B. The unfaithful partner was unwilling to acknowledge any message behind his/her infidelity.

29. Assign *After the Affair* (29)

A. The partners were encouraged to read the book *After the Affair* (Abrahms-Spring) in order to help them identify the message behind the unfaithful partner's infidelity.

B. The couple has read the assigned book on marital affairs, and key concepts were processed together.

C. The partners have not followed through with reading the assigned book on marital affairs and were encouraged to do so.

30. Explore Need for Multiple Intimate Relationships (30)

A. The unfaithful partner's need for multiple intimate relationships was explored.

B. The unfaithful partner has very little insight into the causes of his/her infidelity.

C. The unfaithful partner tends to blame the multiple affairs on his/her partner.

D. The unfaithful partner takes full responsibility for his/her multiple affairs but has little insight into the causes of this behavior or the consequences of it.

31. Discuss Affair Consequences (31)

A. The consequences to self and others that result from multiple intimate relationships were discussed.

B. The unfaithful partner has expressed regret and remorse about his/her behavior.

C. The faithful partner expressed the pain of hurt, disappointment, and anxiety that has resulted from the unfaithful partner's affairs.

32. Assign *Getting the Love You Want* (32)

A. The partners were encouraged to read the book *Getting the Love You Want* (Hendrix) in order to learn more about intimate relationships and intimacy fears.

B. The couple has followed through with reading the recommended book on relationship intimacy, and key concepts were discussed and processed.

C. The recommended book on relationship intimacy was not read and the couple was encouraged to do so.

33. Explore Grief Feelings (33)

A. The feelings associated with the loss of the relationship were explored and clarified.

B. Each partner's desire for a level of intimacy was explored.

C. The factors that have contributed to the breakdown of this intimate relationship were explored, including the fear of getting too close.

34. Explore Closeness Vulnerability (34)

A. Each partner's fears regarding getting too close and feeling vulnerable to hurt, rejection, and abandonment were explored.

B. The partners have clarified their own fears of getting too close to each other out of fear of being hurt.

C. The partners identified experiences in their past that have contributed to their fear of closeness.

35. Assign Imago Exercises (35)

A. The couple was assisted in participating in an Imago exercise whereby each partner shared with the other childhood wounds that were experienced.

B. The partners have increased their skills at demonstrating understanding and empathy.

C. The partners have increased their skills at sharing feelings with each other.

36. Assign Genogram (36)

A. Each partner was assigned to complete his/her own genogram to be shared in future conjoint sessions.

B. The partners shared their individual genograms with each other and described family members and their patterns of interaction.

C. Sharing of genogram material has helped the partners share experience with each other and demonstrate understanding.

D. The partners have not completed the genograms to be shared and were encouraged to do so.

37. Identify Enjoyable Activities (37)

A. The partners were assisted in identifying and planning rewarding recreational activities that they could do together.

B. The partners have increased the time spent together in enjoyable contact.

C. The partners reported specific instances of recreational activities that they have enjoyed together.

D. The partners have failed to follow through on increasing their enjoyable recreational time together and were encouraged to do so.

38. Assign *Passionate Marriage* (38)

A. The partners were encouraged to read the book *Passionate Marriage* (Schnarch) in order to increase their awareness of the need for each of them initiating verbally and physically affectionate behaviors toward each other.

B. The partners have not followed through on reading the recommended material to increase the degree of passionate behaviors within their relationship and were encouraged to do so.

C. The partners have read the book on passionate marriage and increased the frequency of their verbally and physically affectionate behaviors toward each other.

D. Each partner reported specific instances of attempts to trigger and reinforce passion within the other partner.

39. Diffuse Passion Resistance (39)

A. The partners were encouraged to initiate affectionate and sexual interactions with each other without inhibition and resistance.

B. The partners reported specific instances of successful implementation of affection and sexual behaviors toward each other.

C. The partners continue to maintain patterns of sexual distance and a lack of passion within the relationship.

40. Explore Sexual Relationship (40)

A. The nature of the couple's sexual relationship was assessed for the presence of any sexual dysfunction or irrational sexual beliefs and attitudes.

B. The partners acknowledged sexual problems between them and have agreed to focus efforts on trying to resolve these problems.

C. The partners denied any sexual conflict between them.

41. Physician Evaluation Referral (41)

A. The couple was referred to a physician who specializes in sexual dysfunction to obtain an evaluation of any organic causes for their problems.

B. The couple has followed through on obtaining a physician evaluation of their sexual dysfunction.

C. The couple has not followed through on the recommended physician evaluation referral and was encouraged to do so.

D. The physician evaluation did not identify any organic basis for the couple's sexual dysfunction.

E. The medical problems identified by the physician as causes for the sexual dysfunction are being treated.

42. Gather Sexual History (42)

A. The sexual history of each partner was explored to determine areas of strength and to identify areas of dysfunction.

B. The sexual history information indicated a pattern of sexual dysfunction that predates the present relationship.

C. The sexual dysfunction that was identified seems to be associated with serious conflict within the relationship.

43. Create Sexual Genogram (43)

A. A sexual genogram was created with the couple, which identified the sexual patterns of behavior, activities, and beliefs for the couple and their extended family.

B. The sexual genogram was helpful in assisting the couple to see how their present sexual problems are related to extended family issues.

44. Solicit Commitment to Healthy Sexual Attitude/Behavior (44)

A. Each partner was asked to commit himself/herself to attempting to develop healthy, mutually satisfying sexual beliefs, attitudes, and behavior that is independent of previous childhood, personal, or family training or experience.

B. Each partner has verbalized a commitment to change his/her sexual attitudes and behavior to something healthier and gave evidence of that commitment through reporting implementation of healthier behavior and attitudes.

C. Each partner identified the difficulties that he/she is having separating himself/herself from previous dysfunctional sexual beliefs and attitudes.

45. Divorce Support Group Referral (45)

A. The partners were referred to a support group for divorced or divorcing people to assist them in resolving the loss and adjusting to a new life.

B. The partners verbalized the feelings associated with grieving the loss of a relationship, and those feelings were processed.

C. As the partners have participated in a divorce group, they have clarified and expressed their feelings associated with the loss of the relationship.

D. The partners have not followed through on attending a support group for divorcing people and were encouraged to do so.

46. Assign *How to Survive the Loss of a Love* (46)

A. The patient was encouraged to read *How to Survive the Loss of a Love* (Colgrove, Bloomfield, and McWilliams) in order to learn concepts related to dealing with the grief associated with the loss of a relationship.

B. The patient has followed through on reading the assigned grief material associated with the breaking of a relationship.

C. The patient has not read the grief material regarding the loss of a relationship and was encouraged to do so.

D. As the patient has read material on grief over the loss of a relationship, he/she has been able to verbalize various feelings associated with grieving this loss.

47. Provide Adjustment Support (47)

A. The patient was given support and encouragement in his/her adjustment to living alone and being single again.

B. The patient is beginning to express plans for how to cope with loneliness and is making plans for the future.

48. Recommend Community Resources (48)

A. The patient was informed about community resources and social opportunities that are available as sources of support during the adjustment period to being single.

B. The patient has begun to implement community resources and social opportunities that have helped him/her solve some of the loneliness in his/her life.

C. The patient has not reached out to community resources nor taken advantage of social opportunities but remains lonely and isolated.

49. Develop Social Network Plan (49)

A. The patient was assisted in developing a specific plan regarding building new social relationships to overcome withdrawal and fear of rejection.

B. The patient has begun to implement a plan to build a social network to help overcome loneliness.

LEGAL CONFLICTS

PATIENT PRESENTATION

1. Pending Legal Charges (1)
A. The patient has been arrested and has legal charges pending.
B. The patient's legal charges have been processed, and a sentence has been handed down.

2. Parole/Probation (2)
A. The patient is on parole subsequent to serving a sentence for legal charges.
B. The patient is on probation subsequent to arrest and conviction on legal charges.
C. The patient reported meeting regularly with his/her parole/probation officer.
D. The patient's parole/probation has ended.

3. Legal Pressure for Treatment (3)
A. The patient reported that due to legal pressure, he/she has entered treatment.
B. Reports must be made to the patient's legal authorities regarding the patient's cooperation with progress and treatment.
C. The patient has shown increased motivation to participate in treatment over and above that which comes from legal pressure.
D. The patient has been resistive to cooperation with treatment since his/her only motivation comes from legal pressure.

4. Extensive Criminal Record (4)
A. The patient has a long history of criminal activity leading to numerous incarcerations.
B. The patient projects responsibility for his/her behavior onto others.
C. The patient shows little remorse for his/her illegal activities.
D. The patient has recently been released from incarceration.

5. Chemical Dependence (5)
A. The patient's chemical dependence problem has resulted in several arrests and current court involvement.
B. The patient acknowledged that his/her chemical dependence has produced numerous negative consequences in his/her life.
C. The patient is in denial regarding his/her chemical dependence in spite of numerous legal problems.

6. Pending Divorce (6)
A. The patient reported legal complications secondary to a pending divorce.
B. The patient expressed frustration, anger, and sadness regarding the legal wrangling surrounding his/her divorce.
C. The patient reported a contentious custody battle over the children secondary to a divorce.

---

* The numbers in parentheses correlate to the number of the Behavioral Definition statement in the companion chapter with the same title in *The Complete Adult Psychotherapy Treatment Planner*, second edition (Jongsma and Peterson) by John Wiley & Sons, 1999.

7. Fear of Freedom Loss (7)

A. The patient is preoccupied with fear regarding the possibility that he/she may lose his/her freedom because of current legal charges.

B. The patient's anxiety has been predominant since legal charges have been filed.

C. The patient is beginning to cope more effectively with his/her anxiety associated with the potential loss of his/her freedom.

INTERVENTIONS IMPLEMENTED

1. Explore Legal Conflicts (1)

A. A history of the patient's behavior that led to his/her legal conflicts was gathered.

B. The patient's behavior and attitude fit a pattern of antisocial personality disorder.

C. The patient's legal conflicts do not have a chronic history to them and do not seem to fit a pattern of antisocial behavior.

D. The patient described the behavior that has led to his/her current involvement with the court system.

2. Encourage Attorney Representation (2)

A. The patient was encouraged to meet with an attorney to discuss plans for resolving his/her legal issues.

B. The patient has obtained counsel and has met with the attorney to make plans for resolving his/her legal conflicts.

C. The patient does not have financial resources to hire an attorney; therefore, a public defender has been appointed by the court.

3. Monitor Court Contact (3)

A. The patient was encouraged to keep his/her appointments with court officers as a fulfillment of sentencing requirements.

B. The patient reported consistent contact with his/her court officers as part of meeting the requirements of sentencing.

C. The patient has not been consistent in keeping contact with court officers as stipulated with sentencing requirements.

4. Explore Chemical Dependence (4)

A. The patient's pattern of using mood-altering drugs was explored as to how it has contributed to his/her legal conflicts.

B. The patient acknowledged that chemical dependence has played an important part in his/her legal problems.

C. The patient denied any chemical dependence problems.

5. Confront Chemical Dependence Denial (5)

A. The various negative consequences of chemical dependence were reviewed in an attempt to break down the patient's denial.

---

* The numbers in parentheses correlate to the number of the Behavioral Definition statement in the companion chapter with the same title in *The Complete Adult Psychotherapy Treatment Planner,* second edition (Jongsma and Peterson) by John Wiley & Sons, 1999.

B. The patient has acknowledged that drug and/or alcohol abuse have played a role in his/her legal problems.

C. The patient continues to deny any chemical dependence problems.

6. Reinforce the Need for Recovery (6)

A. A plan for substance abuse recovery was developed, and the patient was strongly encouraged to obtain substance abuse treatment.

B. The patient has stated a desire to remain abstinent and is seeking substance abuse treatment.

C. The patient continues to deny the need for substance abuse treatment and has not followed through on a referral for treatment.

7. Monitor Sobriety (7)

A. The patient's sobriety is being monitored through the use of verbal reports and periodic random urinalysis.

B. Monitoring of the patient's sobriety has indicated that he/she has been abstinent from mood-altering substances.

C. The patient has not been consistently abstinent from mood-altering substances.

D. The patient's consistent sobriety has been reinforced.

E. The patient's sobriety status has been reported to court officials.

8. Clarify Values (8)

A. The patient was assisted in clarifying values that allowed him/her to engage in an illegal activity.

B. The patient was encouraged to accept responsibility for the series of decisions and actions that eventually led to the illegal activity.

C. The patient was taught the value of mutual respect for the life and property of himself/herself and others.

9. Confront Responsibility Denial (9)

A. The patient was confronted on his/her denial of responsibility for his/her actions and projecting responsibility onto others for his/her own illegal actions.

B. The patient was encouraged to accept responsibility for the series of decisions and actions that eventually led to the illegal activity.

C. The patient has accepted responsibility for his/her behavior that led to illegal actions and legal conflicts.

D. The patient continues to deny responsibility for his/her behavior and project that responsibility onto others for decisions that led to illegal actions.

10. Teach Legal Boundary Values (10)

A. The patient was taught the values of legal boundaries and the rights of others, as well as the negative consequences of crossing these boundaries.

B. The patient has learned the values that affirm behavior that stays within the boundaries of the law.

11. Probe Emotional Triggers (11)

A. The patient's negative emotional states that have contributed to his/her illegal behavior were explored.

B. The patient verbalized how his/her emotional states of anger, frustration, helplessness, or depression have contributed to his/her illegal behavior.

C. The patient denied any role of negative emotional states acting as a trigger for the illegal activity.

12. Explore the Causes for Negative Emotions (12)

A. The patient was assisted in exploring the causes for his/her negative emotions that consciously or unconsciously foster criminal behavior.

B. The patient identified issues of neglect and abuse in his/her background that contribute to anger and illegal actions.

C. The patient identified role models within his/her extended family that influenced his/her decision to engage in an illegal activity.

13. Ongoing Counseling Referral (13)

A. The patient was referred for more in-depth counseling to deal with his/her emotional conflicts and antisocial impulses.

B. The patient has accepted a referral for counseling that will focus on the negative emotional states that have been associated with his/her illegal activities.

C. The patient has rejected the referral for ongoing counseling.

14. Interpret Antisocial Behavior (14)

A. The patient's antisocial behavior pattern was interpreted as being linked to past emotional conflicts and use of experiences.

B. The patient has accepted the interpretation of his/her antisocial behavior and is beginning to disclose feelings related to past abuse.

C. The patient has rejected any interpretation of his/her antisocial behavior.

15. Identify Cognitive Distortions (15)

A. The patient was assisted in identifying and clarifying cognitive belief structures that foster illegal behavior.

B. The patient has identified cognitive distortions that foster antisocial behavior and has indicated a willingness to revise these distortions.

C. The patient has been very resistive to identifying any cognitive belief structures that foster illegal behavior.

16. Restructure Cognitions (16)

A. The patient was assisted in restructuring his/her cognitions to those that foster the keeping of legal boundaries and respecting the rights of others.

B. The patient reported success at implementing positive self-talk that fosters positive behavior.

C. The patient has not implemented attempts at using restructured cognitions to foster positive behavior within legal boundaries.

17. Anger Management Group Referral (17)

A. It was recommended to the patient that he/she attend an anger management group.

B. The patient was referred to an impulse control group.

C. The patient has accepted the referral to an anger management group and has attended meetings consistently.

D. The patient has accepted the referral to a group to learn control over impulsivity and has attended meetings consistently.

18. Explore Prosocial Need Fulfillment (18)

A. The patient was assisted in identifying ways to meet social, emotional, spiritual, and financial needs without illegal activity.

B. The patient has begun to explore prosocial activities to meet his/her needs.

C. The patient has consistently rejected the idea of using prosocial means to meet his/her needs.

19. Teach Prosocial Behaviors (19)

A. The patient was taught the difference between prosocial and antisocial behaviors.

B. The patient was helped to make concrete plans on how to demonstrate respect for the law, being helpful toward others, and attending employment on a regular basis.

C. The patient has followed through on utilizing prosocial means to meet his/her life needs.

D. The patient consistently rejects prosocial behavior and attitudes for antisocial behavior and attitudes.

20. Ex-Offender Center Referral (20)

A. The patient was referred to an ex-offender center for assistance in obtaining employment and making an adjustment to society.

B. The patient has attended classes on how to successfully seek and maintain employment.

C. The patient has begun to seek employment on an active basis.

D. The patient has found gainful employment and has attended his/her job regularly.

21. Teach Honesty Value (21)

A. The patient was helped to understand the importance of honesty in building trust in others and self-esteem.

B. The patient has verbalized an understanding of the importance of honesty and building trustful relationships with others and self-respect.

C. The patient has rejected the importance of honesty and claims to have no interest in the trust of others.

22. Develop a Restitution Plan (22)

A. The patient was assisted in understanding the importance of restitution, and a plan for providing restitution was developed.

B. The patient has begun to implement and plan for restitution for his/her illegal activity and reported that he/she feels an increased sense of self-worth as a consequence of this.

C. The patient has not followed through on making restitution for his/her illegal activity and was encouraged to do so.

LOW SELF-ESTEEM

PATIENT PRESENTATION

1. Lack of Compliment Acceptance (1)

A. The patient described a pattern of discounting others when they give him/her a compliment.

B. The patient demonstrated within the session a pattern of rejecting compliments given.

C. The patient has begun to develop a more positive self-image and, therefore, does not reject compliments given to him/her.

D. The patient described situations in which he/she was given a compliment and it was accepted.

2. Self-Disparaging Remarks (2)

A. The patient displayed a pattern of being critical of himself/herself.

B. The patient described a pattern of making self-disparaging remarks on a frequent basis.

C. The patient has terminated the pattern of making self-disparaging remarks.

D. The patient has begun to make positive and realistic comments about himself/herself.

3. Poor Self-Image (2)

A. The patient verbalized seeing himself/herself as being unattractive, unimportant, and the feeling that he/she is worthless and a loser.

B. The patient has begun to develop a more positive self-image and has terminated verbalizing negative comments about himself/herself.

C. The patient has begun to make positive comments about himself/herself.

4. Self-Blame (2)

A. The patient displayed a pattern of blaming himself/herself for events that were out of his/her control.

B. The patient has a pattern of taking responsibility for other people's mistakes.

C. The patient described situations in which he/she would have previously taken blame for a situation but did not do so now.

D. The patient has begun to put boundaries on responsibility for behavior and not take blame for other people's actions.

5. Poor Grooming (3)

A. The patient came to the session poorly groomed.

B. The patient stated that others have complained about him/her not taking pride in his/her appearance.

---

* The numbers in parentheses correlate to the number of the Behavioral Definition statement in the companion chapter with the same title in *The Complete Adult Psychotherapy Treatment Planner,* second edition (Jongsma and Peterson) by John Wiley & Sons, 1999.

C. The patient has begun to show increased pride in his/her appearance as evidenced by proper grooming and hygiene.

6. Cannot Refuse Requests (4)

A. The patient described a pattern of difficulties in saying no to other people when he/she is presented with a request for a favor.

B. The patient has tried to ingratiate himself/herself to others by being eager to please them by meeting their needs.

C. The patient has been taken advantage of by others because he/she fears rejection if he/she refuses to comply with others' requests.

D. The patient has begun to set limits on doing things for others and complying with their requests.

7. Assumes Being Disliked (4)

A. The patient verbalized the assumption that others do not like him/her, even though there is little or no evidence to support this conclusion.

B. The patient's dislike for himself/herself is revealed in the fact that he/she believes that others do not like him/her.

C. As the patient's self-esteem has increased, he/she has begun to believe that others have a positive regard for him/her.

D. The patient described situations in which others' affection and caring has been accepted and noted.

8. Fear of Peer Rejection (5)

A. The patient verbalized a fear that others will reject him/her, and, therefore, he/she does virtually anything to please others.

B. The patient has been fearful of rejection of his/her peers for as long as he/she can remember.

C. The patient has begun to believe that others can and do accept him/her.

9. No/Low Goals (6)

A. The patient verbalized no or very low goals for himself/herself in terms of what he/she seeks from life.

B. The patient's lack of confidence in himself/herself is reflected in the fact that he/she has not set reasonable goals for his/her life.

C. As the patient's confidence has grown in himself/herself, he/she has begun to set reasonably high goals for future accomplishment.

10. No Positive Self-Statements (7)

A. The patient was unable to identify positive things about himself/herself.

B. The patient fails to make positive statements about himself/herself within the session.

C. The patient was able to identify some positive traits and accomplishments about himself/herself.

11. **Social Anxiety (8)**

A. The patient described a pattern of feeling uncomfortable in social gatherings because he/she believes others do not like him/her.

B. The patient's lack of confidence in himself/herself is reflected in anxiety and fear of rejection during social contact.

C. The patient has begun to feel more comfortable in social situations as he/she develops a more positive self-image.

D. The patient described incidents in which he/she was involved in social gatherings with little or no anxiety or assumptions that others do not like him/her.

INTERVENTIONS IMPLEMENTED

1. **Build Trust (1)**

A. Consistent eye contact, active listening, unconditional positive regard, and warm acceptance were used to help build trust with the patient.

B. The patient began to express feelings more freely as rapport and trust level increased.

C. The patient has continued to experience difficulty being open and direct in his/her expression of painful feelings.

2. **Explore Patient Self-Assessment (2)**

A. The patient was asked to describe his/her feelings about himself/herself and how he/she sees himself/herself as compared with others.

B. The patient acknowledged feeling less competent than most others and made many self-disparaging remarks.

3. **Confront/Reframe Self-Disparaging Remarks (3)**

A. The patient's self-disparaging remarks were confronted in order to increase his/her awareness of them.

B. The patient's self-disparaging remarks were reframed into more realistic self-assessment statements.

4. **Build an Awareness of Negative Self-Image (4)**

A. The patient was assisted in becoming aware of how he/she expresses or acts out negative feelings about himself/herself.

B. The patient was asked to journal all instances of making negative self-descriptive statements to others.

C. The patient's self-defeating behavior was interpreted as a reflection of his/her acting out feelings of low self-esteem.

D. The patient indicated that he/she has become increasingly aware of how he/she communicates his/her negative self-image.

---

* The numbers in parentheses correlate to the number of the Therapeutic Intervention statement in the companion chapter with the same title in *The Complete Adult Psychotherapy Treatment Planner,* second edition (Jongsma and Peterson) by John Wiley & Sons, 1999.

5. Build Rejection Fear Awareness (5)

A. The patient was assisted in becoming more aware of his/her fear of rejection and how that fear is connected with past experiences of rejection or abandonment.

B. The patient expressed insight into the historical and current sources of his/her low self-esteem.

6. Explore Abuse Experiences (6)

A. The patient's experiences of emotional, physical, and sexual abuse were explored.

B. The patient described his/her experiences of abuse and related how these experiences had a negative impact on his/her feelings of self-esteem.

C. The patient expressed increased insight into how his/her experiences of abuse and abandonment have resulted in low self-esteem.

D. The patient began to assert a positive feeling about himself/herself after understanding that he/she was unfairly victimized as a child.

7. Analyze Goals (7)

A. The patient was assisted in developing realistic goals for himself/herself instead of continuing a pattern of discounting his/her abilities and setting low goals.

B. The patient's goals for himself/herself were analyzed, and realistic, attainable goals were set.

C. The patient verbalized a plan of action that would result in the achievement of realistic goals.

D. The patient has begun to accomplish goals, and self-esteem has increased accordingly.

8. Assign Self-Esteem Exercises (8)

A. The patient was assigned cognitive and behavioral exercises designed to increase his/her self-esteem.

B. The patient was assigned self-esteem-building exercises from the book *The Building Blocks of Self-Esteem* (Shapiro).

C. The patient has followed through on implementing the self-esteem-building exercises and has reported positive results.

D. The patient has not followed through on implementing the self-esteem-building exercises and was encouraged to do so.

9. Assign *Ten Days to Self-Esteem!* (9)

A. The patient was assigned self-esteem-building exercises from the book *Ten Days to Self-Esteem!* (Burns).

B. The patient reported that he/she has begun to feel an increase in self-esteem since implementing the assigned exercises.

C. The patient has not followed through on completing the assigned self-esteem-building exercises and was encouraged to do so.

10. Identify Unmet Needs (10)

A. The patient was assisted in identifying his/her unmet emotional needs.

B. The patient was assisted in developing a plan for meeting his/her needs for self-fulfillment that would result in increased self-esteem.

C. The patient has begun to take actions that helped him/her meet his/her own unmet emotional needs.

11. Conduct a Conjoint Session (11)

A. A conjoint and/or family session was held to support the patient in expressing his/her unmet needs for self-fulfillment.

B. The patient has made reasonable requests of others to assist him/her in having his/her emotional needs met.

12. Plan Need Fulfillment (12)

A. The patient was assisted in developing a specific action plan to have his/her needs met that would result in increased feelings of self-esteem.

B. The patient articulated a plan to be proactive in having his/her identified needs met.

C. The patient has begun to implement a plan of action and has begun to realize fulfillment of unmet emotional needs.

D. The patient reported feelings of increased self-esteem as his/her needs were met through his/her proactive actions.

13. Assign Positive Self-Statements (13)

A. The patient was asked to make one positive statement about himself/herself on a daily basis and to record it on a chart or in a journal.

B. The patient has followed through on making positive self-statements on a daily basis and recording them.

C. The patient has developed a pattern of describing himself/herself more positively and is feeling an increased self-esteem from it.

D. The patient has not followed through on making one positive statement about himself/herself daily and was encouraged to do so.

14. Reinforce Positive Self-Statements (14)

A. The patient was reinforced for any and all statements that reflected confidence in himself/herself and/or a positive self-assessment.

B. The patient related incidents of accomplishment, and he/she was reinforced for these accomplishments.

C. The patient's frequency of making positive self-statements has increased as these statements have been reinforced.

15. Teach Positive Self-Talk (15)

A. The patient was taught how to positively and realistically assess his/her accomplishments and traits.

B. The patient was encouraged to note his/her accomplishments and traits in positive self-statements made on a regular basis.

C. The patient's fear of rejection has decreased, and his/her sense of confidence in himself/herself has increased as he/she has made a habit of complimenting himself/herself.

16. Assign Mirror Exercise (16)

A. The patient was assigned the task of looking at himself/herself in the mirror and talking positively about himself/herself.

B. The patient has increased his/her ability to identify positive traits and talents about himself/herself as a result of the implementation of the mirror exercise.

C. The patient has not followed through on implementation of the mirror exercise and was encouraged to do so.

17. Reinforce Positive Traits and Talents (17)

A. The patient's positive self-descriptive statements about his/her traits and talents were reinforced.

B. The patient's frequency of making positive self-descriptive statements has increased as a result of being reinforced for this behavior.

18. Confront Lack of Eye Contact (18)

A. The patient was confronted when he/she was observed avoiding eye contact with others.

B. The patient was confronted with any description of himself/herself that included a lack of eye contact within a social situation.

C. The patient's lack of eye contact within the session was confronted.

D. The patient was reinforced for maintaining reasonable eye contact during the session.

19. Assign Increased Eye Contact (19)

A. The patient was assigned to make eye contact with whomever he/she is speaking to.

B. The patient reported feeling very anxious while increasing his/her eye contact with others.

C. The patient has begun to feel more comfortable with reasonable eye contact with others during social interaction.

20. Assign a Feelings Journal (20)

A. The patient was asked to keep a daily journal of his/her emotions.

B. The patient has increased his/her ability to identify feelings as he/she has kept a daily journal of feelings.

C. The patient has not followed through on journaling his/her feelings and was encouraged to do so.

21. Identify Emotions (21)

A. The patient was assisted in clarifying, identifying, and labeling his/her feelings.

B. The patient demonstrated an increased ability to identify and express his/her personal feelings.

C. The patient continues to have difficulty in identifying and expressing his/her feelings.

22. Teach Secondary Gain (22)

A. The patient was taught the meaning and power of secondary gain in maintaining negative behavior patterns, especially as applied to his/her speaking negatively about himself/herself and refusing to take any risks.

B. The patient expressed an understanding of the power of secondary gain.

23. Apply Secondary Gain to Self-Disparagement (23)

A. The patient was assisted in identifying how self-disparagement and avoidance of risk taking have brought secondary gain.

B. The patient acknowledged that secondary gain has helped maintain his/her pattern of self-disparagement and refusal to take risks.

C. The patient identified the specific secondary gain that he/she has experienced as a result of his/her self-disparagement and refusal to take risks.

24. Monitor Grooming and Hygiene (24)

A. The patient's grooming and hygiene were monitored, and feedback was given to him/her as to when he/she was negligent and when he/she was acting responsibly in these areas.

B. The patient has pledged to take more responsibility for daily grooming and personal hygiene.

C. The patient has accepted the feedback about his/her hygiene and personal grooming and has shown improvement in these areas.

25. Assign Praise Acceptance (25)

A. The patient was assigned to be aware of and graciously acknowledge the praise and compliments of others.

B. The patient recalled incidences when he/she was complimented by others and was able to accept these compliments graciously.

C. The patient continues to discount the compliments of others and was confronted for doing so.

26. Teach Assertiveness (26)

A. The patient was referred to an assertiveness training group that will educate and facilitate assertiveness skills.

B. Role playing, modeling, and behavioral rehearsal were used to train the patient in assertiveness skills.

C. The patient has demonstrated a clearer understanding of the difference between assertiveness, passivity, and aggressiveness.

27. Assign Life Goals (27)

A. The patient was assigned to make a list of goals for various areas of his/her life and a plan for steps toward goal attainment.

B. The patient has followed through on making a list of goals for various areas of his/her life and has developed a plan for goal attainment.

C. The patient has formed appropriate, realistic, and attainable goals for himself/herself in many areas of his/her life and has begun to take steps to accomplish these goals.

D. The patient reported increased feelings of self-esteem as he/she has begun to accomplish goals set for life.

28. List Accomplishments (28)

A. The patient was asked to list his/her accomplishments, and these accomplishments were integrated into his/her self-concept.

B. The patient found it very difficult to identify accomplishments and, instead, discounted these.

C. The patient has become more adept at tuning into his/her accomplishments, and his/her self-esteem has increased.

29. Identify Negative Self-Talk (29)

A. The patient was assisted in identifying distorted negative beliefs about himself/herself and the world, which foster his/her low self-esteem.

B. The patient recalled instances of negative self-talk and thinking distorted thoughts about life, which have reinforced his/her feelings of low self-esteem.

30. Assign *What to Say When You Talk to Yourself* (30)

A. The patient was assigned to read the book *What to Say When You Talk to Yourself* (Helmstetter) in order to encourage him/her to use positive self-talk to build self-esteem.

B. The patient has followed through on reading the assigned book, and key ideas were processed.

C. The patient has not followed through on reading the assigned book on positive self-talk and was encouraged to do so.

D. As a result of reading the assigned book on positive self-talk, the patient has increased the frequency of positive self-descriptive statements given to himself/herself.

31. Reinforce Realistic Self-Talk (31)

A. The patient was reinforced for the use of realistic positive messages given to himself/herself in interpreting life events.

B. The patient is beginning to use positive self-talk messages to build his/her self-esteem on a consistent basis.

32. Role-Play Social Skills (32)

A. Role playing and behavioral rehearsal were used to teach the patient social skills in greeting people and carrying conversation.

B. The patient has increased the frequency of speaking up with confidence in social situations since using role playing to improve his/her social skills.

C. The patient finds it difficult to implement new social skills because of his/her fear of rejection and lack of confidence.

33. Assign *Shyness* (33)

A. The patient was assigned to read the book *Shyness* (Zimbardo) in order to help him/her learn social skills and increase his/her confidence in social interaction.

B. The patient has followed through on reading the assigned book, and key concepts were processed.

C. The patient has not followed through on reading the assigned book on social skills and was encouraged to do so.

MALE SEXUAL DYSFUNCTION

PATIENT PRESENTATION

1. Lack of Sexual Desire (1)

A. Patient describes a consistently very low desire for or pleasurable anticipation of sexual activity.

B. The patient's interest in sexual contact is gradually increasing.

C. The patient verbalized an increased desire for sexual contact, which is a return to previously established levels.

2. Avoidance of Sexual Contact (2)

A. The patient reported a strong avoidance of and repulsion for any and all sexual contact with his respectful partner.

B. The patient's repulsion for sexual contact has begun to diminish.

C. The patient no longer has a strong avoidance of sexual contact and, in fact, has expressed pleasure with such contact.

3. Lack of Physiological Sex Response (3)

A. The patient has experienced a recurrent lack of the usual physiological response of sexual excitement and arousal.

B. Instead of indicating an interest in sexual contact, the patient's physiological response to excitement is not present.

C. The patient is gradually regaining the usual physiological response of sexual excitement and arousal.

D. The patient reported that sexual contact resulted in a satisfactory level of physiological response of sexual excitement.

4. Lack of Subjective Enjoyment (4)

A. The patient reported a consistent lack of a subjective sense of enjoyment and pleasure during sexual activity.

B. The patient reported an increased sense of pleasure and enjoyment during recent sexual contact.

C. The patient reported a satisfactory level of enjoyment and pleasure during recent sexual activity.

5. Delay in/Absence of Reaching Ejaculation (5)

A. The patient reported a persistent delay in or absence of reaching ejaculation after achieving arousal and in spite of sensitive sexual pleasuring by a caring partner.

B. The patient reported an improvement in time to reach ejaculation during sexual contact.

* The numbers in parentheses correlate to the number of the Behavioral Definition statement in the companion chapter with the same title in *The Complete Adult Psychotherapy Treatment Planner,* second edition (Jongsma and Peterson) by John Wiley & Sons, 1999.

C. The patient reported a satisfactory response time to reaching ejaculation during sexual contact.

6. Genital Pain (6)

A. The patient reported persistent genital pain before, during, or after sexual intercourse.

B. The patient's genital pain associated with sexual intercourse has diminished.

C. The patient reported no experience of genital pain before, during, or after sexual intercourse.

INTERVENTIONS IMPLEMENTED

1. Assess Relationship (1)

A. The patient was asked to share his thoughts and feelings regarding his relationship with his sexual partner.

B. The patient described a lack of harmony and fulfillment within the relationship with his partner.

C. The patient outlined several areas of significant conflict that exist in the relationship with his partner.

2. Conjoint Sessions (2)

A. Conjoint sessions were held between the patient and his partner that focused on conflict resolution, expression of feelings, and sex education.

B. Both partners shared their thoughts and feelings regarding their perception of the relationship.

C. Both partners identified what each perceived as significant problems within their relationship that influenced their sexual activity.

3. Explore Family-of-Origin Sexual Attitudes (3)

A. The patient was asked to describe his perception of sexual attitudes that he learned from his family of origin.

B. The patient outlined what he saw as causes for his sexual inhibition and feelings of guilt, fear, and repulsion associated with sexual activity.

4. Gather Sexual History (4)

A. A detailed sexual history was gathered that examined current sexual functioning as well as childhood and adolescent experiences, level and sources of sexual knowledge, typical sexual practices, medical history, and use of mood-altering substances.

B. The patient provided detailed sexual history material regarding those things that he perceives had influence over his sexual attitudes, feelings, and behavior.

5. Explore Origin of Negative Sexual Attitudes (5)

A. The patient described his history of experiences within his family of origin that caused him to develop a negative attitude regarding sexuality.

* The numbers in parentheses correlate to the number of the Therapeutic Intervention statement in the companion chapter with the same title in *The Complete Adult Psychotherapy Treatment Planner,* second edition (Jongsma and Peterson) by John Wiley & Sons, 1999.

B. The patient outlined the family-of-origin experiences in which the subject of sexuality was taboo.

C. The patient described learning negative sexual attitudes from his mother, who shared his distaste for sexual interaction.

6. Explore Religious Training/Sexual Attitudes (6)

A. The roles of religious training and reinforcing feelings of guilt and shame surrounding sexual behavior and thoughts were explored with the patient.

B. The patient verbalized an understanding of how his religious training negatively influenced his sexual thoughts, feelings, and behavior.

7. Explore Sexual Abuse (7)

A. The patient's history was explored for sexual traumas or abuse.

B. The patient identified a history of sexual abuse as a child and acknowledged how this abuse has had a negative impact on sexual feelings and thoughts.

8. Process Sexual Trauma (8)

A. The patient's feelings surrounding an emotional trauma in the sexual arena were processed.

B. The patient verbalized a resolution of feelings regarding his sexual trauma.

C. The patient's childhood sexual abuse experiences have been resolved to the point that they no longer exercise a strong negative impact over current sexual attitudes, behavior, and feelings.

9. Teach Insight into the Past (9)

A. The patient was helped to develop insight into the role of past negative sexual experiences in creating current adult dysfunction.

B. The patient verbalized an understanding of the role of past negative sexual experiences and the development of dysfunctional sexual attitudes and responses in the present.

C. The patient made a commitment to put the negative attitudes and experiences in the past and to make a behavioral effort to become free from those influences.

10. Explore Sex Role Models (10)

A. The patient's sex role models who influenced him during his childhood or adolescence were explored.

B. The patient verbalized an understanding of the connection between the lack of positive sexual role models in childhood and his current adult sexual dysfunction.

11. Explore Automatic Thoughts (11)

A. The patient's automatic thoughts that trigger negative emotions before, during, and after sexual activity were explored.

B. The patient identified several negative cognitive messages that trigger feelings of fear, shame, anger, and grief during sexual activity.

12. Teach Healthy Self-Talk (12)

A. The patient was taught healthy alternative thoughts that will mediate pleasure, relaxation, and disinhibition during sexual activity.

B. The patient has begun to implement positive and healthy self-talk and reported that he is experiencing more relaxed feelings of pleasure during sexual activity.

13. Model Open Sexual Communication (13)

A. The patient was taught, through modeling, to talk freely and respectfully regarding sexual body parts, feelings, and behavior.

B. The patient is beginning to speak more freely and openly regarding his sexual feelings and behavior, as well as using anatomically correct labels for sexual body parts.

C. The patient has continued to show strong inhibition regarding talking openly and freely regarding sexual material.

14. Assign Sexuality Books (14)

A. The patient was assigned books on human sexuality that provide accurate sexual information and outline sexual exercises that disinhibit and reinforce sexual sensate focus.

B. The patient has followed through on reading the assigned books on human sexuality and has found them informative and healthy in reducing his inhibition in the sexual arena.

C. The patient has not followed through on reading the books on human sexuality and was encouraged to do so.

D. As a result of reading books on human sexuality, the patient has verbalized more positive and healthy attitudes regarding his sexual feelings and behavior.

15. Reinforce Open/Positive Sexual Communication (15)

A. The patient was reinforced for talking freely, knowledgeably, and positively regarding sexual thoughts, feelings, and behavior.

B. The patient has demonstrated healthy and accurate knowledge of sexuality by freely verbalizing adequate information of sexual functioning using appropriate terms for sexually related body parts.

C. The patient continues to experience strong inhibition regarding talking openly and knowledgeably regarding his experience of human sexuality.

16. Assess Biochemical Causes for Dysfunction (16)

A. The role that substance abuse, diabetes, hypertension, or thyroid disease may have on the patient's sexual functioning was identified and assessed.

B. The patient identified a pattern of substance abuse that could have a very negative effect on sexual functioning.

C. The patient identified a medical condition that may have an impact on sexual functioning, and he was referred to a physician for further evaluation.

17. Review Medications (17)

A. The patient's use of medication was reviewed as to the possible negative side effects on sexual functioning.

B. The patient was referred to his physician for a more comprehensive review of the impact on sexual functioning that the medication he is taking may have.

C. The patient acknowledged that medication side effects may be a powerful contributing factor to his sexual problems.

18. Physician Evaluation Referral (18)

A. The patient was referred to a physician for a complete physical to rule out any organic basis for his sexual dysfunction.

B. The patient has cooperated with a referral to a physician and has submitted to an examination to rule out any organic basis for his sexual dysfunction.

C. The patient's physical did identify medical conditions and or medications that may have a harmful effect on his sexual functioning.

D. An evaluation by a physician found no organic basis for the patient's sexual dysfunction.

19. Medication Referral (19)

A. The patient was referred to a physician to evaluate whether a prescription of medication may help him overcome his sexual arousal disorder.

B. The physician has prescribed medication in an attempt to increase the patient's sexual arousal response.

C. The patient reported that the medication prescribed by the physician to enhance his sexual arousal response has had a positive impact.

D. The patient reported that the medication prescribed by the physician to increase his sexual arousal response has not had any noticeable impact.

20. Assess Depression (20)

A. The patient's symptoms of depression were assessed for their frequency and severity.

B. The patient reported experiencing several key symptoms of depression and that depression of sexual desire coincided with the onset of the depression.

C. The patient reported that his feelings of depression began long after the depression of sexual desire and performance.

D. As the patient's depression has lifted, his sexual desire and performance have improved significantly.

21. Antidepressant Medication Referral (21)

A. The patient was referred for an evaluation for an antidepressant medication.

B. As the patient has consistently taken his antidepressant medication, he reported an improvement in mood and an increase in sexual desire.

C. Consistently taking antidepressant medication has not improved the patient's sexual dysfunction.

22. Explore Failed Relationships (22)

A. The patient's fears surrounding intimate relationships were explored along with his history of previously failed relationships.

B. The patient acknowledged that fear of intimacy was related to a history of painful, previously failed relationships.

C. As the patient has resolved some of his fears regarding intimate relationships, sexual dysfunction problems have dissipated.

23. Explore a Secret, Sexual Affair (23)

A. The patient identified a secret, sexual affair that has contributed to his sexual dysfunction with his partner.

B. The patient acknowledged his need to terminate one of his intimate relationships in order to focus emotional investment into the other intimate relationship.

C. The patient acknowledged that keeping a secret affair from his current partner has interfered with his ability to be sexually intimate.

24. Explore a Gay Interest (24)

A. The patient identified gay sexual urges that have predominated any heterosexual interests.

B. The patient acknowledged that his gay attraction is a major factor in his sexual dysfunction with his partner.

C. The patient has agreed to share his gay interest with his female partner and to discuss termination of their relationship.

25. Assign Sexual Awareness Exercises (25)

A. The patient was assigned body exploration and sexual awareness exercises to reduce his inhibition and to desensitize his sexual aversion.

B. The patient has followed through on body exploration and sexual awareness exercises and reports a reduction in sexual inhibitions.

C. The patient has not followed through on implementing the body exploration and sexual awareness exercises and was encouraged to do so.

26. Assign Sexual-Pleasuring Exercises (26)

A. The patient was assigned graduated steps of sexual-pleasuring exercises with his partner to reduce performance anxiety and focus on experiencing bodily arousal sensations.

B. The patient has followed through on practicing sensate focus exercises both alone and with his partner.

C. The patient shared his feelings associated with his sexual-pleasuring exercises and reports an increased satisfaction with the sexual activity.

D. The patient has not followed through on performing the graduated steps of sexual-pleasuring exercises and was encouraged to do so.

27. Reinforce Disinhibition (27)

A. The patient was given encouragement for less inhibited, less constricted sexual behavior with his partner.

B. The patient was assigned body-pleasuring exercises that would focus on decreasing inhibition and increasing the freedom of sexual behavior with his partner.

C. The patient has followed through on completing the body-pleasuring exercises and has reported an increased feeling of freedom to express himself sexually.

E. The patient has not followed through on the body-pleasuring exercises with his partner and was encouraged to do so.

28. Assign a Sexuality Journal (28)

A. The patient was encouraged to keep a journal of sexual thoughts and feelings to increase his awareness and acceptance of them as a normal occurrence.

B. The patient has followed through on keeping a journal of sexual thoughts and feelings, and the material was processed as the patient was reinforced for this normal experience.

C. The patient has failed to follow through on journaling his sexual thoughts and feelings, and his resistance to doing so was processed to resolution.

29. Encourage Sexual Fantasies (29)

A. The patient was encouraged to indulge himself in normal sexual fantasies that could mediate and enhance sexual desire.

B. The patient reported success at becoming aware of and indulging in sexual fantasies that have increased sexual desire.

C. The patient reported resistance to indulging sexual fantasies because feelings of guilt, embarrassment, and shame predominated.

30. Encourage Sexual Experimentation (30)

A. The patient was encouraged to experiment with coital positions and environmental settings for sexual play that could increase his feeling of security, arousal, and satisfaction.

B. The patient has implemented changes in coital positions and environmental settings for sexual play and reported increased feelings of security, arousal, and satisfaction.

C. The patient has been resistant to making changes in the pattern of sexual activity with his partner and was encouraged to do so.

31. Encourage Sexual Assertiveness (31)

A. The patient was encouraged to be more assertive in expressing his feelings of sexuality and sexual play with his partner.

B. The patient reported that he has engaged in more assertive behaviors that have allowed him to share his sexual needs, feelings, and desires with his partner.

C. The patient reported behaving in a more sensuous way and expressing pleasure more freely in sexual contact.

32. Explore Extrarelational Stressors (32)

A. Stressors that may interfere with the strength of sexual desire or performance were explored.

B. The patient identified stressors in the areas of work, social relationships, family responsibilities, and other areas that drain energy away from sexual desire.

C. The patient was assisted in developing coping strategies to reduce the degree of stress that interferes with sexual interest or performance.

D. The patient reported that sexual arousal and performance have increased as the degree of stress with other areas of life has been reduced.

33. Explore Fears of Sexual Inadequacy (33)

A. The patient's fear of inadequacy as a sexual partner was explored.

B. As the patient acknowledged his fears of inadequacy regarding sexual performance and body image, a connection to avoiding sexual activity with his partner was made.

C. An attempt was made to reduce the patient's fears of sexual inadequacy and to have his feelings of positive self-image associated with sexuality.

D. As the patient has developed a more positive self-image and increased his feelings of self-esteem, his interest in sexual activity has increased.

34. Explore Feelings of Threat (34)

A. The patient's feelings of threat, brought on by the perception of his partner as being sexually aggressive, were explored.

B. The patient has communicated his feelings of threat to his partner, which were based on a perception of his partner being too sexually aggressive or too critical of him.

C. As the patient has been freer to communicate his feelings of threat to his partner, sexual satisfaction has increased.

35. Teach the Squeeze Technique (35)

A. The patient was taught the penis squeeze technique to retard premature ejaculation.

B. The squeeze technique has been implemented by the patient during sexual intercourse, and premature ejaculation has been delayed.

C. The patient reported feelings of satisfaction with the delay in ejaculation produced by the squeeze technique and is now more desirous of sexual contact.

D. Implementation of the squeeze technique has not been successful at reducing the speed of ejaculation.

36. Reinforce Sexual Desire (36)

A. The patient's expressions of desire for, and pleasure with, sexual activity were strongly reinforced.

B. As the patient has made progress in resolving sexual dysfunction issues, he has reported an increased desire for, and pleasure with, sexual activity.

C. The patient was encouraged to express his renewed desire for, and pleasure with, sexual activity to his partner.

MANIA OR HYPOMANIA

PATIENT PRESENTATION

1. Pressured Speech (1)

A. The patient gave evidence of pressured speech within the session.

B. The patient reported that his/her speech rate increases as he/she feels stressed.

C. The patient's pressured speech has shown evidence of a decrease in intensity.

D. The patient showed no evidence of pressured speech in today's session.

2. Flight of Ideas/Racing Thoughts (2)

A. The patient demonstrated an inability to stay focused on one subject, but moved quickly from one topic to another.

B. The patient reported that he/she has difficulty concentrating on one thought, as other thoughts interfere.

C. The patient reported that at times of quiet reflection, he/she is disturbed by thoughts racing through his/her mind.

D. The patient's thoughts are not racing as they had been and he/she is able to stay focused on one topic in a conversation.

3. Grandiosity (3)

A. The patient gave evidence of grandiose ideas regarding his/her abilities, plans, and accomplishments.

B. In spite of attempts to try to get the patient to be more realistic, his/her grandiosity continued.

C. The patient's grandiosity has diminished and he/she has become more reality-based.

D. There has been no recent evidence of grandiosity in the patient's description of himself/herself or plans for the future.

4. Persecutory Beliefs (3)

A. The patient described feeling misunderstood and persecuted by others who do not acknowledge his/her grandiose ideas.

B. The patient described feelings of anger and persecution directed at those who discount his/her grandiosity.

C. As the patient's grandiosity has diminished, his/her feelings of persecution and low frustration threshold with others have also diminished.

5. Lack of Sleep/Appetite (4)

A. The patient described a pattern of attaining far less sleep than would normally be needed and also not eating on a regular basis.

* The numbers in parentheses correlate to the number of the Behavioral Definition statement in the companion chapter with the same title in *The Complete Adult Psychotherapy Treatment Planner,* second edition (Jongsma and Peterson) by John Wiley & Sons, 1999.

B. The patient has gone through periods of time when he/she did not sleep for 24 consecutive hours because his/her energy level was so high.

C. As the patient's mania has begun to diminish, he/she has begun to return to a more normal sleeping and eating pattern.

D. The patient is getting six to eight hours of sleep per night and is eating at least two meals per day.

6. Motor Agitation (5)

A. The patient was restless and agitated within the session and reports an inability to sit quietly and relax.

B. The patient's high energy level is reflected in increased motor activity, restlessness, and agitation.

C. The patient's motor activity has decreased and the level of agitation has diminished.

D. The patient demonstrated normal motor activity and reports being able to stay calm and relaxed.

7. Easily Distracted (6)

A. The patient gave evidence of a short attention span and a high level of distractibility.

B. The patient reported that he/she is unable to focus his/her thoughts on one topic.

C. The patient's attention shifted quickly from one stimulus to the next.

D. The patient has shown increased ability to focus attention and has reduced distractibility.

8. Disinhibition/Impulsivity (7)

A. The patient reported a behavior pattern that reflected a lack of normal inhibition and an increase in impulsivity without regard to potentially painful consequences.

B. The patient's impulsivity has been reflected in sexual acting out, poor financial decisions, and committing of social offenses.

C. The patient has gained more control over his/her impulses and has returned to a normal level of inhibition and social propriety.

9. Bizarre Dress/Grooming (8)

A. The patient's grooming and style of dress were outlandish.

B. The patient showed little comprehension of the impact of his/her outlandish and bizarre dress and grooming practices.

C. The patient has shown better judgment in dress and has become more conventional in grooming habits.

10. Expansive Moods/Irritability (9)

A. The patient gave evidence of a very expansive mood that can easily turn to impatience and irritability if his/her behavior is blocked or confronted.

B. The patient related instances of feeling angry when others tried to control his/her expansive, grandiose ideas and mood.

C. As the patient's expansive mood has been controlled, his/her impatience and irritable anger has diminished.

11. Lack of Follow-Through (10)

A. The patient described a behavior pattern that reflected a lack of follow-through on many projects, even though his/her energy level is high, since he/she lacks discipline and goal-directedness.

B. The patient's lack of follow-through on projects has resulted in frustration on the part of others.

C. The patient has begun to exercise more discipline and goal-directedness in his/her behavior, resulting in the completion of projects.

INTERVENTIONS IMPLEMENTED

1. Explore for Manic Signs (1)

A. The patient's thoughts, feelings, and behavior were explored for classic signs of mania such as pressured speech, impulsive behavior, euphoric mood, flight of ideas, high energy level, reduced need for sleep, and inflated self-esteem.

B. The patient described his/her feelings, thoughts, and behaviors, which confirm the presence of the classic signs of mania.

2. Assess Mania Intensity (2)

A. The patient was assessed for whether he/she was hypomanic, manic, or manic with psychotic features.

B. The patient was assessed to be hypomanic.

C. The patient was assessed to be manic.

D. The patient's mania was so severe as to evolve into periods of psychosis.

3. Arrange Hospitalization (3)

A. Arrangements were made for the patient to be hospitalized in a psychiatric setting based on the fact that his/her mania is so intense that he/she could be harmful to himself/herself or others or unable to care for his/her own basic needs.

B. The patient was not willing to voluntarily submit to hospitalization; therefore, commitment procedures were initiated.

C. The patient acknowledged the need for hospitalization and voluntarily admitted himself/herself to the psychiatric facility.

4. Psychiatric Evaluation (4)

A. The patient was referred for a psychiatric evaluation to consider psychotropic medication to control the manic state.

B. The patient has followed through with the psychiatric evaluation and pharmacotherapy has begun.

C. The patient has been resistive to cooperating with a psychiatric evaluation and was encouraged to follow through on this recommendation.

---

* The numbers in parentheses correlate to the number of the Therapeutic Intervention statement in the companion chapter with the same title in *The Complete Adult Psychotherapy Treatment Planner,* second edition (Jongsma and Peterson) by John Wiley & Sons, 1999.

5. Monitor Medication Reaction (5)

A. The patient's reaction to the medication in terms of side effects and effectiveness were monitored.

B. The patient reported that the medication has been effective at reducing energy levels, flight of ideas, and the decreased need for sleep.

C. The patient has been reluctant to take the prescribed medication for his/her manic state, but was urged to follow through on the prescription.

D. As the patient has taken his/her medication that has been successful in reducing the intensity of the mania, he/she has begun to feel that it is no longer necessary and has indicated a desire to stop taking it.

6. Pledge Support (6)

A. The patient was reassured on a regular basis that the therapist would be available to consistently listen to and support him/her.

B. The patient reacted favorably to the therapist's pledge of support and has begun to show trust in the relationship by sharing thoughts and feelings.

7. Explore Abandonment Fears (7)

A. The patient's fear of abandonment by sources of love and nurturance were explored.

B. The patient confirmed that he/she struggles with the fear that those who have provided love and nurturance to him/her will eventually abandon him/her.

C. The patient denied any fear of abandonment by sources of love and nurturance.

8. Probe Losses (8)

A. Real or perceived losses in the patient's life were explored.

B. The patient confirmed that he/she has unresolved feelings regarding losses that have been experienced.

C. The patient denied any significant losses in his/her life.

D. The patient's experience of loss has precipitated fears of abandonment in other relationships.

9. Explore Family-of-Origin History (9)

A. The patient shared experiences from his/her family-of-origin history that have caused feelings of low self-esteem and fear of abandonment.

B. The patient revealed experiences with critical and rejecting parents that led to feelings of low self-esteem.

C. The patient disclosed experiences of childhood abandonment by parent figures that have led to the fear of abandonment in current relationships.

10. Confront Grandiosity (10)

A. The patient's grandiosity and demandingness were gradually, but firmly, confronted.

B. The patient has become less expansive and more socially appropriate with the consistent confrontation of his/her grandiosity and demandingness.

C. The patient has reacted with anger and irritability when his/her grandiosity was confronted.

11. Process Losses (11)

A. The patient's experiences of loss were processed in an attempt to help him/her put them into proper perspective.

B. The patient was helped to identify adaptive ways to replace the losses that were experienced.

12. Differentiate Losses (12)

A. The patient was helped to differentiate between real and imagined, as well as actual and exaggerated, losses.

B. The patient verbalized grief, fear, and anger regarding real or imagined losses in life.

C. The patient was able to make a differentiation between his/her real and imagined losses, rejections, and abandonment.

13. Explore Stressors (13)

A. The patient was helped to identify current stressors that have precipitated an intensification of manic behavior.

B. The patient identified specific incidents that have increased his/her fear of rejection and abandonment.

C. The patient acknowledged that low self-esteem and fear of rejection do underlie the pattern of braggadocio.

D. As the patient was able to gain insight into the stressors that make him/her feel more fearful, he/she has reduced his/her level of braggadocio.

14. Focus on Impulsive Behavior Consequences (14)

A. The patient's impulsive behavior was repeatedly reviewed so as to help him/her identify the negative consequences that result from this pattern.

B. The patient's self-defeating and impulsive behavior was reviewed as to its negative consequences.

C. The patient has difficulty identifying negative consequences to his/her impulsive behavior as he/she is so focused on the here and now.

15. Facilitate Impulse Control (15)

A. Role playing, behavioral rehearsal, and role reversal were used to increase the patient's sensitivity to the consequences of his/her impulsive behavior.

B. The patient has significant difficulty identifying negative consequences for his/her impulsive behavior.

C. The patient is beginning to develop sensitivity to the negative consequences of his/her impulsivity.

16. Set Behavioral Limits (16)

A. The patient's expressions of hostility were listened to in a calm manner while limits were set on his/her aggressive or impulsive behavior on a consistent basis.

B. The patient's expressions of overt hostility or aggression have diminished in response to limit setting.

17. Set Limits on Manipulation (17)

A. The patient's attempts at manipulation or acting out of impulsive urges were directly confronted.

B. Clear rules have been established regarding manipulation and acting out such that consequences for breaking rules are clear.

18. Provide Structure and Focus (18)

A. Structure and focus were provided to the patient's thoughts and actions by regulating the direction of conversation and establishing plans for his/her behavior.

B. The patient's flight of ideas and pressured speech were countered by repeatedly bringing the patient back to the topic at hand and reminding him/her of the need for follow-through on his/her behavior.

19. Reinforce Slower Speech (19)

A. The patient was reinforced for reducing the rate of speech and becoming more deliberate in his/her thought process.

B. The patient responded favorably to reinforcement of slower speech and the introduction of more focus to his/her thought process.

C. The patient responded with anger and irritability when consistent focus was provided to slower speech.

20. Reinforce Appropriate Dress/Grooming (20)

A. The patient was encouraged in and reinforced for dressing appropriately and for responsible grooming.

B. The patient's dress and grooming have improved as encouragement and reinforcement were provided.

C. The patient has become less outlandish in his/her dress and neater in his/her grooming.

21. Assist in Self-Developed Limit Setting (21)

A. The patient was assisted in developing limits for himself/herself in regard to reasonable dress, grooming, and social behavior.

B. The patient has followed through on implementing his/her own limits for reasonable dress, grooming, and social behavior.

C. The patient has failed to follow through on implementing his/her own limits for dress, grooming, and social behavior, as his/her manic impulses predominate.

22. Interpret Dependency Fears (22)

A. The patient's braggadocio, hostility, and denial of dependency were interpreted as a fear of acknowledging dependency fears.

B. The patient has begun to verbalize acceptance of and peace with his/her dependency needs after he/she accepted the interpretation of his/her counterdependence behavior.

23. Identify Strengths (23)

A. The patient was assisted in identifying his/her strengths and assets that could build self-esteem and confidence.

B. The patient identified several strengths, assets, and accomplishments that could serve to build his/her self-esteem and self-confidence.

24. Encourage Realistic Sharing (24)

A. The patient was encouraged to share his/her feelings at a deep and realistic level to facilitate intimacy development in relationships.

B. The patient was encouraged to decrease grandiose statements and express himself/herself more realistically.

25. Reinforce Agitation Control (25)

A. The patient was reinforced for controlling his/her motor agitation and helped to set goals for and limits on this behavior.

B. The patient was taught relaxation techniques to help him/her reduce the level of agitation and restlessness.

26. Monitor Sleep (26)

A. The patient's sleep pattern was monitored and he/she was encouraged to return to a sleep pattern of five or more hours per night.

B. The patient has responded favorably to structure regarding sleep expectations and has increased his/her sleep to five or more hours per night.

C. The patient continues to function at a very high energy level and refuses to submit to sleep for five or more hours per night.

27. Monitor Energy Level (27)

A. The patient's energy level was monitored and he/she was reinforced for increased control over behavior, pressured speech, and expression of ideas.

B. The patient has responded favorably to placing more structure and control over his/her behavior and reported less agitation and flight of ideas.

28. Reinforce Focused Behavior (28)

A. The patient was reinforced for behavior that was more focused on goal attainment and is less distracted.

B. The patient reported staying more focused on a single activity to completion and was reinforced for this control.

29. Explore Illness Understanding (29)

A. The patient's understanding of his/her illness was explored and a realistic appraisal of his/her loss of judgment and increased impulsivity was given.

B. The patient verbalized a better understanding of his/her behavior, recognizing that poor judgment and control were a result of the manic illness.

30. Teach Need for Ongoing Care (30)

A. The patient was taught that his/her psychiatric condition calls for long-term, ongoing care and medication.

B. The patient was cautioned against believing that his/her condition is cured and therefore no further medication is necessary.

C. The patient was made aware of the high probability of relapse into a manic state if ongoing care and medication are not followed responsibly.

31. Explore Family's Feelings (31)

A. A family session was held to allow members to express their feelings of guilt, shame, fear, concern, confusion, or anger regarding the patient's manic behavior.

B. Family members have expressed their feelings openly regarding the patient's behavior and mental illness.

32. Educate Family Members (32)

A. The family members were taught the nature of the patient's serious mental illness, its behavioral manifestations, and the need for continuing treatment.

B. The family members expressed support for and commitment to the patient.

MEDICAL ISSUES

PATIENT PRESENTATION

1. Serious Medical Condition (1)

A. The patient presented with serious medical problems that are having a negative impact on his/her daily living.

B. The patient has pursued treatment for his/her medical condition.

C. The patient has refused treatment for his/her medical condition.

D. The patient has not sought treatment for his/her medical condition because of a lack of insurance and financial resources.

E. The patient's serious medical condition has been under treatment and is showing signs of improvement.

2. Chronic Pain (2)

A. The patient experiences chronic pain that is debilitating and results in depressed mood.

B. The patient has learned coping skills for adapting to his/her chronic pain.

C. The patient has learned to cope more effectively with the chronic pain and his/her mood has improved.

D. The patient's chronic pain continues and his/her mood has deteriorated, resulting in less adaptive behavior, more withdrawal, and significant depression.

3. Minor Medical Condition (3)

A. The patient has a medical condition that requires a physician's care.

B. The patient has obtained the necessary medical care and his/her condition is improving.

C. The patient's medical condition has worsened, since he/she has not cooperated with the physician's recommendations.

4. HIV Positive (4)

A. The patient reported that he/she has tested positive for the human immunodeficiency virus (HIV).

B. The patient has been HIV positive for many months but has had no serious deterioration in his/her condition.

C. The patient is obtaining consistent medical care for his/her HIV status.

D. The patient has refused medical care for his/her HIV-positive status and tends to be in denial about the seriousness of this situation.

5. AIDS (5)

A. The patient's HIV-positive status has resulted in the development of acquired immune deficiency syndrome (AIDS).

---

* The numbers in parentheses correlate to the number of the Behavioral Definition statement in the companion chapter with the same title in *The Complete Adult Psychotherapy Treatment Planner,* second edition (Jongsma and Peterson) by John Wiley & Sons, 1999.

B. The patient's medical condition resulting from AIDS has deteriorated and his/her anxiety and depression have increased.

C. Although the patient has serious AIDS complications, he/she remains at peace and is getting good medical care.

6. Chemical Dependence Complications (6)

A. Because of the patient's chronic chemical dependence history, he/she has developed medical complications.

B. The patient has accepted that he/she has deteriorated medically because of his/her chemical dependence pattern and has terminated substance abuse.

C. The patient is in denial about the effects of his/her substance abuse and continues this self-destructive pattern.

D. The patient's medical condition has improved subsequent to termination of substance abuse.

7. Psychological/Behavioral Complications (7)

A. The patient's current medical condition is complicated by psychological and behavioral factors that influence the course of the disease.

B. The patient is in denial about the psychological and behavioral factors that are having a negative impact on his/her medical condition.

C. The patient acknowledges that there are psychological and behavioral factors that are influencing his/her medical condition and is willing to seek treatment for these problems.

8. Health Neglect (8)

A. The patient described a history of neglecting his/her physical and medical problems.

B. The patient continues to refuse medical evaluation and treatment for physical problems.

C. The patient has agreed to seek medical treatment and has followed through on this recommendation.

D. After receiving medical treatment, the patient's physical and medical condition has improved significantly.

INTERVENTIONS IMPLEMENTED

1. Facilitate Medical Care (1)

A. The necessary arrangements were made for the patient to obtain needed medical services.

B. The patient has agreed to follow through with the recommendation for medical care.

C. The patient has continued to be resistive to obtaining medical care.

---

* The numbers in parentheses correlate to the number of the Therapeutic Intervention statement in the companion chapter with the same title in *The Complete Adult Psychotherapy Treatment Planner,* second edition (Jongsma and Peterson) by John Wiley & Sons, 1999.

2. Physician Referral (2)

A. The patient was referred to a physician for a complete physical to evaluate his/her medical condition.

B. The patient followed through with the referral to a physician for a medical evaluation.

C. The patient has failed to follow through on the recommendation to obtain a medical evaluation.

3. Encourage Medical Compliance (3)

A. The patient was given information about his/her medical condition and urged to cooperate with his/her doctor's recommendations.

B. The patient verbalized a more complete understanding of his/her medical problems and has stated a willingness to cooperate with medical care.

C. The patient does not demonstrate a good understanding of his/her medical condition and continues to refuse the necessary medical care.

4. Monitor Medical Treatment (4)

A. The patient was monitored for follow-through on physician's orders and on the effectiveness of the treatment.

B. The patient has failed to consistently follow through with the physician's orders regarding medical treatment and was encouraged to comply.

C. The patient has complied with the physician's recommendations for medical treatment and his/her condition has improved.

5. Physician Consultation (5)

A. The patient's physician has been contacted in order to review his/her orders for the patient.

B. The patient was encouraged to follow the physician's treatment orders as described by the patient's physician during a consultation contact.

C. The patient signed a release of information allowing the therapist to obtain medical information from his/her physician for the purposes of treatment coordination and follow-through monitoring.

6. Provide Medical Information (6)

A. The patient was provided appropriate literature and references to material that would increase his/her understanding of his/her medical condition.

B. The patient was encouraged to contact medical resources to obtain more information regarding his/her medical condition.

C. The patient has refused to seek further information regarding his/her medical condition, its treatment, and the prognosis.

7. Support Group Referral (7)

A. The patient was referred to a support group related to his/her physical condition.

B. The patient has attended a support group and reported it to be a positive experience.

C. The patient has learned more about his/her medical condition and has decreased his/her denial about the medical condition since attending a medical support group.

D. The patient has refused to attend a medical support group and was encouraged to do so.

8. Confront Denial (8)

A. The patient's denial of the seriousness of his/her medical condition was confronted and he/she was reinforced for showing any acceptance of the medical condition.

B. The patient accepted the confrontation regarding the seriousness of his/her medical condition and verbalized increased acceptance of the need for medical intervention.

C. The patient continues to be in denial regarding the seriousness of his/her medical condition in spite of confrontation and educational efforts.

9. Dietician Referral (9)

A. The patient was referred to a dietician who will explain proper nutrition that will enhance his/her medical recovery.

B. The patient accepted the dietician referral and attended an appointment.

C. The patient has verbalized an increased knowledge of how proper nutrition can have a positive impact on his/her medical condition.

D. The patient has refused to follow through on the referral to a dietician and was encouraged to do so.

10. Explore Chemical Abuse (10)

A. The role of chemical abuse in the patient's medical condition was explored.

B. The patient confirmed that he/she has a problem with chemical dependence and this has had a negative impact on his/her medical condition.

C. The patient denied any chemical dependence problems in spite of evidence that such a problem may exist.

11. Recommend Chemical Dependence Treatment (11)

A. A recommendation for chemical dependence treatment was given to the patient.

B. The patient has accepted the recommendation for chemical dependence treatment and has terminated his/her substance abuse.

C. The patient has refused chemical dependence treatment and continues to use substances that have a negative impact on his/her medical condition.

12. Assess STD Behaviors (12)

A. The patient's behavior was assessed for the presence of behaviors related to contracting sexually transmitted diseases and potentially contracting HIV.

B. The patient acknowledged that he/she does engage in high-risk behaviors that would increase the potential for contracting an STD and HIV.

C. The patient denied any high-risk behaviors associated with STDs.

D. The patient has agreed to terminate high-risk behaviors that increase the probability of contracting STDs.

13. Public Health/Physician Referral (13)

A. The patient was referred to the public health department or a private physician for testing, education, and treatment of an STD and/or HIV.

B. The patient accepted the referral to medical resources for STD and HIV testing, education, and treatment.

C. The patient refused to accept the referral to medical resources for STD and HIV testing, education, and treatment.

14. Monitor STD/HIV Follow-Through (14)

A. The patient has followed through with pursuing medical treatment for his/her STD.

B. The patient has followed through with obtaining medical treatment for his/her HIV condition.

C. The patient has not followed through with pursuing medical treatment and was strongly encouraged to do so.

15. HIV Treatment Referral (15)

A. The patient was referred to a program that specializes in treatment of patients with HIV/AIDS.

B. The patient has accepted the need for treatment for his/her HIV/AIDS and has followed through with medical treatment.

C. The patient continues to be in denial regarding his/her HIV status and refuses to accept the need for treatment.

16. Identify Emotional Reactions (16)

A. The patient was helped to identify, clarify, and express his/her feelings associated with the serious medical condition.

B. The patient denied any significant emotional reaction to his/her serious medical condition.

C. The patient openly expressed his/her feelings regarding the medical condition.

17. Identify Emotional Contribution (17)

A. The patient was taught how lifestyle and emotional distress can have a negative impact on his/her medical condition.

B. The patient's lifestyle and emotional state were reviewed in order to identify factors that may have a negative impact on his/her medical condition.

C. The patient acknowledged emotional stress and behavior patterns that probably had a negative impact on his/her medical condition.

D. The patient was in denial regarding the contribution of emotional status and behavior patterns to his/her medical condition.

18. List Supportive Health Behaviors (18)

A. The patient was assisted in making a list of things that he/she could do to help maintain his/her physical health.

B. The patient has listed changes in his/her behavior, nutrition, and emotional reactivity that could have a positive impact on his/her physical health.

C. The patient has implemented changes in his/her life that indicate an acceptance of holistic health principles.

19. Physical Therapist Referral (19)

A. The patient was referred to a physical therapist for an assessment and recommendations regarding an exercise plan that is appropriate for the patient's age and medical condition.

B. The patient has followed through with the recommendations to seek out a physical therapy evaluation regarding an exercise plan and has implemented this plan on a regular basis.

C. The patient has not followed through on a physical therapy evaluation for an exercise plan and was encouraged to do so.

D. Since the patient has begun a regular exercise program that is tailored to his/her medical condition, he/she has reported an increased feeling of well-being.

20. Explore Emotional Distress Sources (20)

A. The patient's sources of emotional distress were explored.

B. The patient acknowledged that the emotional distress that he/she is experiencing does increase his/her vulnerability to disease and reduces the efficacy of treatment.

C. The patient agreed to focus on the sources for emotional distress in his/her life so as to reduce this as a factor in trying to improve his/her medical status.

21. Develop Psychological Treatment Plan (21)

A. The patient was assisted in developing a treatment plan for his/her emotional problems that compromise medical treatment efforts.

B. The patient has accepted the need for treatment of concomitant emotional problems so as to increase the probability of successful medical treatment.

C. The patient has denied the need for treatment for emotional and/or behavioral problems that are related to his/her medical condition.

22. Identify Medical Treatment Fears (22)

A. The patient's fears regarding medical treatment and medical personnel were explored.

B. The patient was helped to process his/her fears regarding medical personnel and treatment so that he/she could obtain the necessary medical care.

C. The patient has successfully processed his/her fears and has implemented steps to obtain necessary medical treatment.

D. The patient continues to be so fearful as to refuse necessary medical care.

23. Plan Medical Attention (23)

A. As the patient's fears related to medical care were reduced, he/she was open to planning proper medical attention.

B. The patient has followed through with implementing a plan for obtaining proper medical attention.

C. The patient continues to resist following through with recommendations for proper medical treatment.

OBSESSIVE-COMPULSIVE DISORDER (OCD)

PATIENT PRESENTATION

1. Recurrent/Persistent Thoughts (1)

A. The patient described recurrent and persistent thoughts or impulses that are viewed as senseless, intrusive, and time-consuming and that interfere with his/her daily routine.

B. The intensity of the recurrent and persistent thoughts and impulses is so severe that the patient is unable to efficiently perform daily duties or interact in social relationships.

C. The strength of the patient's obsessive thoughts has diminished and he/she has become more efficient in his/her daily routine.

D. The patient reported that the obsessive thoughts are under significant control and he/she is able to focus attention and effort on the task at hand.

2. Failed Control Attempts (2)

A. The patient reported failure at attempts to control or ignore his/her obsessive thoughts or impulses.

B. The patient described many different failed attempts at learning to control or ignore his/her obsessions.

C. The patient is beginning to experience some success at controlling and ignoring his/her obsessive thoughts and impulses.

3. Recognize Internal Source of Obsessions (3)

A. The patient reported that he/she recognizes that the obsessive thoughts are a product of his/her own mind and are not coming from some outside source or power.

B. The patient acknowledged that the obsessive thoughts are related to anxiety and are not a sign of any psychotic process.

4. Compulsive Behaviors (4)

A. The patient described repetitive and intentional behaviors that are performed in a ritualistic fashion.

B. The patient's compulsive behavior pattern follows rigid rules and has many repetitions to it.

C. The repetitive and intentional behaviors of the patient are performed in response to obsessive thoughts.

D. The patient reported a significant decrease in the frequency of repetitive compulsive behaviors.

E. The patient reported very little interference in his/her daily routine from compulsive behavior rituals.

---

* The numbers in parentheses correlate to the number of the Behavioral Definition statement in the companion chapter with the same title in *The Complete Adult Psychotherapy Treatment Planner,* second edition (Jongsma and Peterson) by John Wiley & Sons, 1999.

5. Compulsive Prevention Behaviors (5)

A. The patient has engaged in repetitive compulsive behavior in an attempt to neutralize or prevent discomfort.

B. The patient's repetitive and compulsive behavior is engaged in to prevent some dreaded situation from occurring, which the patient is often not able to define clearly.

C. The patient's repetitive and compulsive behavior rituals are not connected in any realistic way with what the patient is trying to prevent or neutralize.

D. The patient's anxiety over some dreaded event has diminished significantly and his/her compulsive rituals have also decreased in frequency.

E. The patient has not engaged in any ritualistic behaviors designed to prevent some dreaded situation.

6. Sees Compulsions As Unreasonable (6)

A. The patient acknowledged that his/her repetitive and compulsive behaviors are excessive and unreasonable.

B. The patient's recognition of his/her compulsive behaviors as excessive and unreasonable has provided good motivation for cooperation with treatment and follow-through on attempt to change.

INTERVENTIONS IMPLEMENTED

1. Assess OCD History (1)

A. The patient described the nature, history, and severity of his/her obsessive thoughts and compulsive behaviors.

B. The patient described a severe degree of interference in his/her daily routine and ability to perform a task efficiently because of the significant problem with obsessive thoughts and compulsive behaviors.

C. The patient described many attempts to ignore or control the compulsive behaviors and obsessive thoughts, but without any consistent success.

D. The patient gave evidence of compulsive behaviors within the interview.

2. Conduct Psychological Testing (2)

A. Psychological testing was administered to evaluate the nature and severity of the patient's obsessive-compulsive problem.

B. The psychological testing results indicate that the patient experiences significant interference in his/her daily life from obsessive-compulsive rituals.

C. The psychological testing indicated a rather mild degree of Obsessive-Compulsive Disorder within the patient.

3. Medical Evaluation Referral (3)

A. The patient was referred to a physician for an evaluation for a medication prescription to aid in the control of his/her OCD.

---

* The numbers in parentheses correlate to the number of the Therapeutic Intervention statement in the companion chapter with the same title in *The Complete Adult Psychotherapy Treatment Planner*, second edition (Jongsma and Peterson) by John Wiley & Sons, 1999.

B. The patient has followed through with the referral for a medication evaluation and has been prescribed psychotropic medication to aid in the control of his/her OCD.

C. The patient has failed to comply with the referral to a physician for a medication evaluation and was encouraged to do so.

4. Monitor Medication Compliance (4)

A. The patient reported that he/she is taking the psychotropic medication as prescribed and that it is having a positive effect on controlling the OCD.

B. The patient reported complying with the psychotropic medication prescription, but that the effectiveness of the medication has been very limited or nonexistent.

C. The patient has not been consistent in taking the psychotropic medication as prescribed and was encouraged to do so.

5. Assign Thought Stopping (5)

A. The patient was taught the thought-stopping technique that will help him/her interfere with obsessive ruminations and replace them with thoughts of a pleasant scene.

B. The patient reported success at implementing the thought-stopping technique and stated that he/she spends less time ruminating over obsessive thoughts.

C. The patient has failed to consistently implement the thought-stopping technique and was encouraged to do so.

D. The patient reported that the thought-stopping technique was not effective at reducing his/her obsessive ruminations.

6. Train in Relaxation (6)

A. The patient was trained in deep muscle relaxation and positive imagery techniques as methods to use to counteract high anxiety.

B. The patient has implemented the relaxation methods within his/her daily routine and has reported a reduction in anxiety.

C. The patient has not implemented the relaxation methods within his/her daily life and was encouraged to do so.

D. As the patient has implemented relaxation methods to counteract high anxiety, his/her difficulties with OCD have diminished.

7. Administer Biofeedback (7)

A. The patient was administered biofeedback to help him/her learn to deepen the degree of relaxation that he/she is capable of.

B. The patient reported increased ability to develop deep relaxation and has implemented this skill within his/her daily life.

C. As the patient has utilized relaxation techniques successfully, the degree of obsessive-compulsive behavior has been reduced.

8. Explore Unresolved Conflicts (8)

A. As the patient's unresolved life conflicts were explored, he/she verbalized and clarified feelings connected to those conflicts.

B. The patient identified key life conflicts that raise his/her anxiety level and intensify the OCD symptoms.

C. As the patient clarified and shared his/her feelings regarding current unresolved life conflicts, his/her level of anxiety diminished and the OCD symptoms were reduced.

9. Read/Process Fables (9)

A. Fables from Friedman were read with the patient to help him/her gain perspective on unresolved life conflicts.

B. As the patient processed the content of the fables, he/she gained insight into the need to be less intense regarding life issues.

10. Assign *Stories for the Third Ear* (10)

A. Selections from the book *Stories for the Third Ear* (Wallas) were assigned to the patient to help him/her reduce the emotional intensity around life conflicts.

B. The patient followed through with reading the assigned stories by Wallas, and the material was processed to help increase insight into the need for less intensity to be attached to life conflicts.

C. The patient has not followed through with reading the selected and assigned readings and was encouraged to do so.

11. Encourage Feelings Sharing (11)

A. The patient was encouraged, supported, and assisted in identifying and expressing feelings related to key unresolved life issues.

B. As the patient shared his/her feelings regarding life issues, he/she reported a decreased level of emotional intensity around these issues.

C. It was difficult for the patient to get in touch with, clarify, and express emotions, as his/her pattern is to detach himself/herself from feelings.

12. Assign *Ten Days to Self-Esteem!* (12)

A. The patient was assigned to read "The Perfectionist's Script for Self-Defeat" in the book *Ten Days to Self-Esteem!* (Burns) to increase his/her awareness of how he/she believes and thinks in a self-defeating manner.

B. The patient has read the assigned material on perfectionism, and key concepts were discussed as they applied to his/her own experience.

C. The patient verbalized an increased awareness of his/her perfectionistic thought tendencies and how this is a self-defeating pattern.

13. Assign Perfectionism Exercises (13)

A. The patient was assigned to complete exercises from the book *Ten Days to Self-Esteem!* (Burns).

B. The patient has completed the perfectionism exercises, and the results of that exercise were processed.

C. The patient verbalized an increased awareness of his/her distorted thinking and belief errors, which have a negative effect on his/her daily functioning.

14. Identify Distorted Thoughts (14)

A. The patient was assisted in identifying his/her distorted automatic thoughts and beliefs that promote anxiety and OCD symptoms.

B. The patient verbalized specific distorted self-talk that he/she engaged in that supports and nurtures anxiety.

15. Develop Reality-Based Self-Talk (15)

A. The patient was assisted in developing reality-based self-talk as a strategy to help reduce his/her obsessive thoughts and compulsive behaviors.

B. The patient has begun to implement positive, reality-based self-talk that can reduce obsessive and perfectionist thoughts and compulsive behaviors.

C. As the patient is implementing cognitive techniques to reduce anxiety, his/her symptoms of OCD have been reduced.

16. Teach Rational Emotive Techniques (16)

A. The patient was taught the principles of a rational emotive therapy approach.

B. The patient was taught to analyze, attack, and destroy his/her self-defeating beliefs.

C. As the patient implemented rational emotive techniques, he/she has decreased ruminations about death and other perplexing life issues.

17. Develop Cognitive/Behavioral Intervention (17)

A. The patient was assigned the task of using a cognitive/behavioral intervention task that will help disrupt the obsessive-compulsive patterns.

B. As the patient has implemented the cognitive/behavioral intervention, he/she has decreased obsessive ruminations about unanswerable questions.

18. Assign Ericksonian Task (18)

A. The patient was assigned an Ericksonian task of performing a behavior that is centered around the obsession or compulsion instead of trying to avoid it.

B. As the patient has faced the issue directly and performed a task, bringing feelings to the surface, the results of this were processed.

C. As the patient has processed his/her feelings regarding the anxiety-provoking issue, the intensity of those feelings has diminished.

19. Create Strategic Ordeal (19)

A. A strategic ordeal (Haley) was created with the patient that offered a guarantee of cure for the obsession or compulsion.

B. The patient has engaged in the strategic ordeal to help him/her overcome the OCD impulses.

C. The strategic ordeal has been quite successful at helping the patient reduce OCD symptoms and feelings of anxiety.

D. The patient has not been successful at implementing the strategic ordeal consistently and was encouraged to do so.

20. Develop Ritual Interruption (20)

A. The patient was helped to develop a ritual of a very unpleasant task that he/she agrees to perform each time he/she experiences obsessive thoughts.

B. The patient has begun to implement the distasteful ritual at the times of experiencing obsessive thoughts.

C. The patient reports that engaging in the distasteful ritual has interrupted the obsessive thoughts and the current pattern of compulsion.

PARANOID IDEATION

PATIENT PRESENTATION

1. Extreme Distrust (1)

A. The patient described a pattern of consistent distrust of others generally.

B. The patient described an extreme distrust of a significant other in his/her life without sufficient basis.

C. The patient's level of distrust toward others has diminished.

D. The patient verbalized trust in the significant other that he/she had previously held in extreme distrust.

2. Expectation of Harm by Others (2)

A. The patient described an expectation of being exploited or harmed by others.

B. The patient's fear of being harmed by others has diminished.

C. The patient no longer holds to an irrational belief that he/she is being plotted against by others.

3. Misinterpretation of Benign Events (3)

A. The patient demonstrated a pattern of misinterpretation of benign events as having threatening personal significance.

B. The patient is beginning to accept a more reality-based interpretation of benign events as nonthreatening.

C. The patient no longer demonstrates a pattern of misinterpretation of benign events and has verbalized not feeling personally threatened.

4. Hypersensitivity to Criticism (4)

A. The patient described a pattern of hypersensitivity to any hint of personal criticism from others.

B. The patient showed defensive hypersensitivity to criticism within the session.

C. The patient has not reported any recent incidents of hypersensitivity to criticism from others.

D. The patient described incidents in which he/she was able to receive criticism without feeling personally threatened and defensive.

5. Keeps Distance from Others (5)

A. The patient acknowledged that he/she is inclined to keep emotional and social distance from others out of fear of being hurt or taken advantage of by them.

B. The patient is beginning to show some trust of others, as demonstrated by increased social interaction.

* The numbers in parentheses correlate to the number of the Behavioral Definition statement in the companion chapter with the same title in *The Complete Adult Psychotherapy Treatment Planner,* second edition (Jongsma and Peterson) by John Wiley & Sons, 1999.

C. The patient described a relationship with others that involves a degree of vulnerability and intimacy with which he/she has become comfortable.

6. Easily Offended/Quick to Anger (6)

A. The patient's history is replete with incidents in which the patient has become easily offended and was quick to anger.

B. The patient described a pattern of defensiveness in which he/she easily feels threatened by others and becomes angry with them.

C. The patient described a pattern of projection of threatening motivations onto others, to which the patient reacts with irritability, defensiveness, and anger.

D. The patient has become less defensive and has not shown any recent incidents of unreasonable anger.

7. Irrational Suspicion (7)

A. The patient described a pattern of being suspicious of the loyalty or fidelity of a significant other without reasonable cause.

B. The patient's unreasonable suspicion of his/her significant other has diminished.

C. The patient has verbalized trust in the loyalty and fidelity of his/her significant other.

8. Obsessional Mistrust (8)

A. The patient's level of distrust of others is so pervasive and obsessive that his/her daily functioning is disrupted.

B. The patient is unable to fulfill job and family responsibilities because of his/her preoccupation with issues of distrust.

C. The patient's level of trust has grown and he/she is more able to perform daily duties and responsibilities.

INTERVENTIONS IMPLEMENTED

1. Build Trust (1)

A. Consistent eye contact, active listening, unconditional positive regard, and warm acceptance were used to help build trust with the patient.

B. The patient began to express feelings more freely as rapport and trust level increased.

C. The patient has continued to experience difficulty being open and direct in his/her expression of painful feelings.

2. Demonstrate Calm Tolerance (2)

A. An effort was made to demonstrate calm tolerance toward the patient within the session in order to decrease his/her fear of others.

B. The patient has begun to demonstrate a level of trust within the session by disclosing some feelings and beliefs.

---

* The numbers in parentheses correlate to the number of the Therapeutic Intervention statement in the companion chapter with the same title in *The Complete Adult Psychotherapy Treatment Planner,* second edition (Jongsma and Peterson) by John Wiley & Sons, 1999.

3. Assess Paranoia (3)

A. The nature and extent of the patient's paranoia was assessed, with special attention to severely delusional components.

B. The patient identified those people and/or agencies that are distrusted and gave his/her irrational explanation for this distrust.

C. The patient demonstrated a pattern of severe delusional aspects to his/her paranoia.

D. The patient remained extremely guarded and defensive, refusing to openly describe the nature and severity of his/her distrust.

4. Explore Fear of Vulnerability (4)

A. The patient's fears of personal inadequacy and vulnerability were explored.

B. The patient described his/her feelings of vulnerability in cautious terms.

C. The patient refused to acknowledge any feelings of personal inadequacy or vulnerability.

5. Interpret Fear of Anger (5)

A. The patient's fear of his/her own anger was interpreted as a basis for the mistrust of others and the projection of anger coming from them.

B. The patient admitted feeling threatened by others and expressed some understanding of his/her own feelings of anger toward others as the basis for that feeling of threat.

6. Explore Family-of-Origin Experiences (6)

A. The patient's family-of-origin experiences were explored to uncover any historical sources of the feelings of vulnerability.

B. The patient identified a family pattern of distrust of others that has been reinforced within his/her own belief system.

C. The patient described experiences within his/her own childhood that have taught him/her to be mistrustful, as others have exploited or harmed him/her.

7. Explore Distorted Cognitions (7)

A. The patient's social interactions were reviewed, and his/her distorted cognitive beliefs that were operative during these interactions were explored.

B. The patient clearly holds to distorted cognitions that reinforce a fear of others.

C. The patient is beginning to express some openness toward other interpretations of people's motivations that are less threatening and more benign.

8. Assess Antipsychotic Medication Need (8)

A. The patient was assessed for the need for antipsychotic medication to counterattack significantly altered thought processes that are delusional and paranoid.

B. The patient's paranoid delusional system is so developed that antipsychotic medication appears to be necessary.

C. The patient's paranoid beliefs do not appear to be so severe as to need treatment with antipsychotic medication.

9. Medication Evaluation Referral (9)

A. Arrangements were made for the patient to have a medication evaluation by a physician to assess the need for an antipsychotic treatment regimen.

B. The patient has refused to follow a recommendation for psychiatric evaluation to assess the need for antipsychotic medication.

C. The patient has followed through on the recommendation for a psychiatric evaluation, and antipsychotic medication has been ordered.

D. The psychiatric evaluation results indicated that antipsychotic medication was not necessary.

10. Monitor Medication Compliance (10)

A. The patient described taking the prescribed medication on a consistent basis and reported that it has been helpful in reducing feelings of threat and delusional thinking.

B. The patient has not taken the antipsychotic medication consistently and was encouraged to do so.

C. The patient reported that side effects of the medication were such that he/she felt the need to terminate this medication, and he/she was referred to the psychiatrist for further evaluation.

D. The patient reported taking the medication as prescribed, but has not experienced any beneficial effects.

11. Psychological Evaluation (11)

A. Arrangements were made for a psychological evaluation to assess for a possible psychotic process underlying the paranoid thinking.

B. The patient completed the psychological evaluation to assess the depths of his/her paranoia, and a psychotic process was uncovered.

C. Psychological evaluation results indicated that the patient does not have a psychotic process present.

12. Neuropsychological Evaluation (12)

A. Arrangements were made for a neuropsychological evaluation to determine whether organic factors may be present and could account for the paranoid ideation.

B. The neuropsychological evaluation indicated a high probability of organic factors being present, and a neurological examination was recommended.

C. The neurological evaluation found no basis for organicity as an underlying factor in the paranoia.

D. The patient has refused to follow through on a neurological or neuropsychological evaluation and was encouraged to do so.

13. Relate Distrust to Inadequacy Feelings (13)

A. The patient was assisted in seeing the pattern of distrusting others as related to his/her own fears of inadequacy.

B. The patient is beginning to verbalize a connection between his/her fear of others and his/her own feelings of inadequacy.

C. The patient continues to refuse to acknowledge any feelings of inadequacy that could be the basis for a fear of others.

14. Provide Nonthreatening Interpretations of Others (14)

A. The patient was provided alternative explanations for the behavior and motivations of others that run counter to the patient's pattern of assumption that others have malicious intent.

B. The patient is beginning to accept alternative healthy explanations of others' benign behavior.

C. The patient continues to reject benign explanations for others' behavior and holds to a belief in their malicious intent.

D. The patient has acknowledged that his/her belief about others being threatening is based more on subjective interpretation than on objective data.

15. Develop Cost-Benefit Analysis (15)

A. The patient was asked to complete a cost-benefit analysis of his/her specific fears and to process the results of this in the session.

B. The patient has performed a cost-benefit analysis of his/her fears and has been able to identify the irrational basis for them and the high cost of continuing to hold them.

C. The patient has failed to follow through on the cost-benefit analysis assignment and was encouraged to do so.

16. Assess Trust of Significant Others (16)

A. A conjoint session was held to reinforce verbalizations of trust toward significant others.

B. The patient demonstrated within the conjoint session that he/she continues to hold irrational beliefs regarding the significant other's lack of loyalty and fidelity.

C. The patient verbalized trust toward the significant other within the conjoint session and this trust was reinforced.

17. Confirmed Irrational Distrust (17)

A. The patient's irrational distrust of others was confronted, and reality-based data was provided to support a belief of trust in others.

B. The patient has decreased the amount of accusations of others' plans of harm toward himself/herself, and he/she has begun to accept reality-based data that supports a feeling of trust.

C. The patient reacted with anger and irritability when his/her irrational feelings of distrust were challenged.

18. Assign "Porky, the Porcupine" (18)

A. The patient was asked to read the story "Porky, the Porcupine" from the book *Stories for the Third Ear* (Wallas).

B. The story "Porky, the Porcupine" was processed to help the patient understand the need for trust in others.

C. The patient verbalized an understanding that distrust of others leads to alienation and isolation.

19. Encourage Checking of Beliefs (19)

A. The patient was encouraged to check out his/her beliefs regarding others by assertively verifying his/her conclusions with others directly.

B. The patient is beginning to verbalize a sense of trust in significant others.

C. The patient has followed through on checking out his/her distrustful beliefs and has found that others do not share them, which has led to a reexamination by the patient of his/her unreasonable beliefs.

20. Utilize Role Playing to Increase Empathy (20)

A. Role playing, behavioral rehearsal, and role reversal were used to increase the patient's empathy for others and understanding of the impact of his/her behavior on others.

B. The patient has begun to increase his/her social interaction without fear or suspicion being reported.

C. The role-playing exercises have increased the patient's sense of understanding of the feelings of others.

D. The patient has begun to reduce his/her tendency to project malicious motivations onto others.

PHOBIA-PANIC/AGORAPHOBIA

PATIENT PRESENTATION

1. Unreasonable Fear of Object/Situation (1)

A. The patient described a pattern of persistent and unreasonable phobic fear that promotes avoidance behaviors because an encounter with the phobic stimulus provokes an immediate anxiety response.

B. The patient has shown a willingness to begin to encounter the phobic stimulus and endure some of the anxiety response that is precipitated.

C. The patient has been able to tolerate the previously phobic stimulus without debilitating anxiety.

D. The patient verbalized that he/she no longer holds fearful beliefs or experiences anxiety during an encounter with the phobic stimulus.

2. Severe Panic Symptoms (2)

A. The patient has experienced sudden and unexpected severe panic symptoms that have occurred repeatedly and have resulted in persistent concern about additional attacks.

B. The patient has significantly modified his/her normal behavior patterns in an effort to avoid panic attacks.

C. The frequency and severity of the panic attacks have diminished significantly.

D. The patient reported that he/she has not experienced any recent panic attack symptoms.

3. Fear of Environmental Situations Triggering Anxiety (3)

A. The patient described fear of environmental situations that he/she believes may trigger intense anxiety symptoms.

B. The patient's fear of environmental situations has resulted in his/her avoidance behavior directed toward those environmental situations.

C. The patient has a significant fear of leaving home and being in open or crowded public situations.

D. The patient's phobic fear has diminished and he/she has left the home environment without being crippled by anxiety.

E. The patient is able to leave home normally and function within public environments.

4. Interference with Normal Routines (4)

A. The patient's avoidance of phobic stimulus situations is so severe as to interfere with normal functioning.

B. The degree of the patient's distrust associated with avoidance behaviors related to phobic experiences is such that he/she is not able to function normally.

C. The patient is beginning to take on normal responsibilities and function with limited distress.

* The numbers in parentheses correlate to the number of the Behavioral Definition statement in the companion chapter with the same title in *The Complete Adult Psychotherapy Treatment Planner,* second edition (Jongsma and Peterson) by John Wiley & Sons, 1999.

D. The patient has returned to normal functioning and reported that he/she is no longer troubled by avoidance behaviors and phobic fears.

5. Recognition That Fear Is Unreasonable (5)

A. The patient's phobic fear has persisted in spite of the fact that he/she acknowledges that the fear is unreasonable.

B. The patient has made many attempts to ignore or overcome his/her unreasonable fear, but has been unsuccessful.

INTERVENTIONS IMPLEMENTED

1. Assess Phobic Fear (1)

A. The specifics regarding the patient's phobic fear were addressed.

B. The patient verbalized the specific stimuli for his/her phobic fear, the history of the fear, and the degree to which it interferes with his/her life.

2. Administer Fear Survey (2)

A. An objective fear survey was administered to the patient to assess the depth and breadth of his/her phobic fear.

B. The fear survey results indicated that the patient's phobic fear is extreme and severely interferes with his/her life.

C. The fear survey results indicate that the patient's phobic fear is moderate and occasionally interferes with his/her daily functioning.

D. The fear survey results indicate that the patient's phobic fear is mild and rarely interferes with his/her daily functioning.

3. Construct Anxiety Stimuli Hierarchy (3)

A. The patient was assisted in constructing a hierarchy of anxiety-producing situations associated with his/her phobic fear.

B. It was difficult for the patient to develop a hierarchy of stimulus situations, as the causes of his/her fear remain quite vague.

C. The patient was successful at creating a focused hierarchy of specific stimulus situations that provoke anxiety in a gradually increasing manner.

4. Train in Relaxation (4)

A. The patient was trained in progressive relaxation methods and deep breathing exercises.

B. The patient has become proficient in progressive deep muscle relaxation and the utilization of rhythmic deep breathing.

5. Utilize Biofeedback (5)

A. Biofeedback techniques were utilized to facilitate the patient's learning of deep muscle relaxation.

* The numbers in parentheses correlate to the number of the Therapeutic Intervention statement in the companion chapter with the same title in *The Complete Adult Psychotherapy Treatment Planner,* second edition (Jongsma and Peterson) by John Wiley & Sons, 1999.

B. The patient has developed a greater depth of relaxation as a result of the biofeedback techniques.

6. Train in Guided Imagery (6)

A. The patient was trained in the utilization of guided imagery to promote anxiety relief and deepen relaxation.

B. The patient was able to identify a nonthreatening, pleasant scene that was utilized to promote relaxation using guided imagery.

7. Direct Systematic Desensitization (7)

A. The patient was led in a systematic desensitization procedure in which imagery was used to prompt the anxiety response.

B. The patient cooperated with the systematic desensitization procedure and reported success at imagining anxiety-provoking scenes without feeling overwhelmed.

C. It was difficult for the patient to imagine phobic stimulus situations to a realistic enough degree to promote anxiety.

8. Assign In Vivo Desensitization (8)

A. The patient was assigned to complete in vivo desensitization contact with the phobic stimulus object or situation.

B. The patient was taught the principles of desensitization and encouraged to encounter the phobic stimulus in gradual steps, utilizing relaxation to counterattack any anxiety response.

9. Reinforce Progress (9)

A. The patient's encounters with the phobic stimulus object/situation were reviewed and successful experiences were reinforced.

B. The patient reported specific encounters with the phobic stimulus situation and reported feeling in control, calm, and comfortable.

10. Interpret Phobic Symbolism (10)

A. The patient was assisted in identifying the symbolic significance that the phobic stimulus may have as a basis for his/her fear.

B. The patient accepted the interpretation of the phobic stimulus situation as being representative of an unresolved conflict from the past.

C. The patient denied that the phobic stimulus situation had any symbolic significance.

11. Differentiate Current Fear from Past Pain (11)

A. The patient was taught to verbalize the separate realities of the current fear and the emotionally painful experience from the past that has been evoked by the phobic stimulus.

B. The patient was reinforced when he/she expressed insight into the unresolved fear from the past that is linked to his/her current phobic fear.

C. The irrational nature of the patient's current phobic fear was emphasized and clarified.

D. The patient's unresolved emotional issue from the past was clarified.

12. Encourage Sharing of Feelings (12)

A. The patient was encouraged to share the emotionally painful experience from the past that has been evoked by the phobic stimulus.

B. The patient was taught to separate the realities of the irrationally feared object or situation and the painful experience from his/her past.

13. Reinforce Insight (13)

A. The patient's insight into the link between his/her past emotional pain and present phobic anxiety was reinforced.

B. The patient has continued to deny any link between present phobic fear and his/her past painful experiences.

14. Identify Distorted Thoughts (14)

A. The patient was assisted in identifying the distorted schemas and related automatic thoughts that mediate anxiety responses.

B. The patient was taught the role of distorted thinking in precipitating emotional responses.

C. The patient verbalized an understanding of the cognitive beliefs and messages that mediate his/her anxiety responses.

15. Teach Cognitive Restructuring (15)

A. The patient was taught the need for revising core schemas using cognitive restructuring techniques.

B. The patient was assisted in identifying positive, healthy, and rational self-talk that reduces fear and allows behavioral encounters with the avoided stimuli.

C. The patient reported that the cognitive restructuring techniques have been successful at reducing the anxiety response to the phobic stimulus.

16. Medication Evaluation Referral (16)

A. Arrangements were made for the patient to have a physician evaluation for the purpose of considering psychotropic medication to alleviate phobic symptoms.

B. The patient has followed through with seeing a physician for an evaluation of any organic causes for the anxiety and the need for psychotropic medication to control the anxiety response.

C. The patient has not cooperated with the referral to a physician for a medication evaluation and was encouraged to do so.

17. Monitor Medication Compliance (17)

A. The patient reported that he/she has taken the prescribed medication consistently and that it has helped to control the phobic anxiety.

B. The patient reported that he/she has not taken the prescribed medication consistently and was encouraged to do so.

C. The patient reported taking the prescribed medication and stated that he/she has not noted any beneficial effect from it.

D. The patient was not prescribed any psychotropic medication by the physician after the evaluation.

18. Explore Panic Attacks (18)

A. The patient described the history and nature of his/her panic symptoms and the degree to which they interfere with his/her daily functioning.

B. The patient described frequent and severe panic symptoms and significant interference in his/her daily functioning.

C. The patient described moderate panic symptoms and a varying degree of interference in his/her daily functioning.

D. The patient described mild symptoms of panic and very little interference in his/her daily routine.

19. Explore Panic Stimulus Situations (19)

A. The patient described specific stimulus situations that precipitate panic symptoms.

B. The patient could not describe any specific stimulus situations that produce panic, but said that they occur unexpectedly and without any pattern to them.

C. The patient described that his/her panic symptoms occur when he/she leaves the confines of his/her home environment and enters public situations where there are many people.

20. Explore Secondary Gain (20)

A. Secondary gain was identified for the patient's panic symptoms because of his/her tendency to escape or avoid certain situations.

B. The patient denied any role for secondary gain that results from his/her modification of life to accommodate panic.

C. The patient was reinforced for accepting the role of secondary gain in promoting and maintaining the panic symptoms and encouraged to overcome this gain through living a more normal life.

21. Counteract Panic Myths (21)

A. The patient was consistently reassured of the fact that there is no connection between panic symptoms and heart attack, loss of control over behavior, or serious mental illness.

B. The patient verbalized an understanding that panic symptoms do not promote serious physical or mental illness.

22. Utilize Modeling/Behavioral Rehearsal (22)

A. Modeling and behavioral rehearsal were used to train the patient in positive self-talk that reassured him/her of the ability to work through and endure anxiety symptoms without serious consequences.

B. The patient has implemented positive self-talk to reassure himself/herself of the ability to endure anxiety without serious consequences.

23. Teach Coping Strategies (23)

A. The patient was taught behavioral and cognitive coping strategies such as diversion, deep breathing, positive self-talk, and muscle relaxation to alleviate panic symptoms.

B. The patient reported that implementation of the coping strategies has been successful in reducing the intensity of anxiety symptoms.

C. The patient has not implemented coping strategies consistently and was encouraged to do so.

24. Encourage Relaxation to Manage Panic (24)

A. The patient was encouraged to utilize deep muscle relaxation and deep breathing skills to manage panic symptoms.

B. The patient's use of relaxation skills has been successful at terminating panic symptoms and returning him/her to a feeling of peace.

25. Urge External Focus (25)

A. The patient was urged to keep his/her focus on external stimuli and behavioral responsibilities rather than being preoccupied with internal states and physiological changes.

B. The patient has made it a commitment to not allow panic symptoms to take control of his/her life and to not avoid and escape normal responsibilities and activities.

C. The patient has been successful at turning his/her focus away from internal anxiety states and toward behavioral responsibilities.

26. Reinforce Responsibility Acceptance (26)

A. The patient was supported and reinforced for following through with work, family, and social responsibilities rather than using escape and avoidance to focus on panic symptoms.

B. The patient reported performing responsibilities more consistently and being less preoccupied with panic symptoms or fear that panic symptoms might occur.

POSTTRAUMATIC STRESS DISORDER (PTSD)

PATIENT PRESENTATION

1. Exposure to Death/Injury to Others (1)

A. The patient has a history of having been exposed to the death or serious injury of others that resulted in feelings of intense fear, helplessness, or horror.

B. The patient's severe emotional response of fear has somewhat diminished.

C. The patient can now recall being a witness to the traumatic incident without experiencing the intense emotional response of fear, helplessness, or horror.

2. Exposure to Threatened Death/Injury to Self (1)

A. The patient has been a victim of a threat of death or serious injury to himself/herself that has resulted in an intense emotional response of fear, helplessness, or horror.

B. The patient's intense emotional response to the traumatic event has somewhat diminished.

C. The patient can now recall the traumatic event of being threatened with death or serious injury without an intense emotional response.

3. Intrusive Thoughts (2)

A. The patient described experiencing intrusive, distressing thoughts or images that recall the traumatic event and its associated intense emotional response.

B. The patient reported experiencing less difficulty with intrusive, distressing thoughts of the traumatic event.

C. The patient reported no longer experiencing intrusive, distressing thoughts of the traumatic event.

4. Disturbing Dreams (3)

A. The patient described disturbing dreams that he/she experiences and are associated with the traumatic event.

B. The frequency and intensity of the disturbing dreams associated with the traumatic event have decreased.

C. The patient reported no longer experiencing disturbing dreams associated with the traumatic event.

5. Flashbacks (4)

A. The patient reported experiencing illusions about or flashbacks to the traumatic event.

B. The frequency and intensity of the patient's flashback experiences have diminished.

C. The patient reported no longer experiencing flashbacks to the traumatic event.

---

* The numbers in parentheses correlate to the number of the Behavioral Definition statement in the companion chapter with the same title in *The Complete Adult Psychotherapy Treatment Planner,* second edition (Jongsma and Peterson) by John Wiley & Sons, 1999.

6. Distressful Reminders (5)

A. The patient experienced intense distress when exposed to reminders of the traumatic event.

B. The patient reported having been exposed to some reminders of the traumatic event without experiencing overwhelming distress.

7. Physiological Reactivity (6)

A. The patient experiences physiological reactivity associated with fear and anger when he/she is exposed to the internal or external cues that symbolize the traumatic event.

B. The patient's physiological reactivity has diminished when he/she is exposed to internal or external cues of the traumatic event.

C. The patient reported no longer experiencing physiological reactivity when exposed to internal or external cues of the traumatic event.

8. Thought/Feeling/Conversation Avoidance (7)

A. The patient described trying to avoid thinking, feeling, or talking about the traumatic event because of the associated negative emotional response.

B. The patient is making less effort to avoid thoughts, feelings, or conversations about the traumatic event.

C. The patient reported that he/she is now able to talk or think about the traumatic event without feeling overwhelmed with negative emotions.

9. Place/People Avoidance (8)

A. The patient reported a pattern of avoidance of activity, places, or people associated with the traumatic event because he/she is fearful of the negative emotions that may be triggered.

B. The patient is able to tolerate contact with people, places, or activities associated with the traumatic event without feeling overwhelmed.

10. Blocked Recall (9)

A. The patient stated that he/she has an inability to recall some important aspect of the traumatic event.

B. The patient's amnesia regarding some important aspects of the traumatic event has begun to lessen.

C. The patient can now recall almost all of the important aspects of the traumatic event, as his/her amnesia has terminated.

11. Lack of Interest (10)

A. The patient has developed a lack of interest and a pattern of lack of participation in activities that had previously been rewarding and pleasurable.

B. The patient has begun to show some interest in participation in previously rewarding activities.

C. The patient is now showing a normal interest in participation in rewarding activities.

12. Detachment (11)

A. The patient described feeling a sense of detachment from others.

B. The patient reported regaining a sense of attachment in participation with others.

C. The patient reported that he/she no longer feels alienated from others and is able to participate in social and intimate interactions.

13. Blunted Emotions (12)

A. The patient reported an inability to experience the full range of emotions, including love.

B. The patient reported beginning to be in touch with his/her feelings again.

C. The patient is able to experience the full range of emotions.

14. Pessimistic/Fatalistic (13)

A. Since the traumatic event occurred, the patient has had a pessimistic and fatalistic attitude regarding the future.

B. The patient is beginning to experience a somewhat hopeful attitude regarding the future.

C. The patient's pessimistic, fatalistic attitude regarding the future has terminated and he/she has begun to make plans and talk about the future with a more hopeful attitude.

15. Sleep Disturbance (14)

A. Since the traumatic event occurred, the patient has experienced a desire to sleep much more than normal.

B. Since the traumatic event occurred, the patient has found it very difficult to initiate and maintain sleep.

C. Since the traumatic event occurred, the patient has had a fear of sleeping.

D. The patient's sleep disturbance has terminated and he/she has returned to a normal sleep pattern.

16. Irritability (15)

A. The patient described a pattern of irritability that was not present before the traumatic event occurred.

B. The patient reported incidents of becoming angry and losing his/her temper easily, resulting in explosive outbursts.

C. The patient's irritability has diminished somewhat and the intensity of the explosive outbursts has lessened.

D. The patient reported no recent incidents of explosive, angry outbursts.

17. Lack of Concentration (16)

A. The patient described a pattern of lack of concentration that began with the exposure to the traumatic event.

B. The patient reported that he/she is now able to focus more clearly on cognitive processing.

C. The patient's ability to concentrate has returned to normal levels.

18. Hypervigilance (17)

A. The patient described a pattern of hypervigilance.

B. The patient's hypervigilant pattern has diminished.

C. The patient reported no longer experiencing hypervigilance.

19. Exaggerated Startle Response (18)

A. The patient described having experienced an exaggerated startle response.
B. The patient's exaggerated startle response has diminished.
C. The patient no longer experiences an exaggerated startle response.

20. Symptoms for One Month or More (19)

A. The patient stated that his/her symptoms of PTSD have been present for more than a month.
B. The patient's symptoms that have been present for more than a month have diminished.
C. The patient no longer experiences PTSD symptoms.

21. Depression (20)

A. The patient described experiencing sad affect, lack of energy, social withdrawal, and guilt feelings as part of a depressive reaction.
B. The patient's depression symptoms have diminished considerably.
C. The patient reported that he/she is no longer experiencing symptoms of depression.

22. Alcohol/Drug Abuse (21)

A. Since the traumatic experience, the patient has engaged in a pattern of alcohol and/or drug abuse as a maladaptive coping mechanism.
B. The patient's alcohol and/or drug abuse has diminished as he/she has worked through the traumatic event.
C. The patient reported no longer engaging in any alcohol or drug abuse.

23. Suicidal Thoughts (22)

A. The patient reported experiencing suicidal thoughts since the onset of PTSD.
B. The patient's suicidal thoughts have become less intense and less frequent.
C. The patient reported no longer experiencing any suicidal thoughts.

24. Interpersonal Conflict (23)

A. The patient described a pattern of interpersonal conflict, especially in regard to intimate relationships.
B. As the patient has worked through his/her reaction to the traumatic event, there has been less conflict within personal relationships.
C. The patient's partner reported that he/she is irritable, withdrawn, and preoccupied with the traumatic event.
D. The patient and his/her partner reported increased communication and satisfaction with the interpersonal relationship.

25. Violent Threat/Behavior (24)

A. The patient described having engaged in verbally violent threats since experiencing the traumatic event.
B. The patient's irritability has been magnified into physically violent behavior.

C. As the patient has worked through the emotions associated with the traumatic event, his/her verbal and physical violence has diminished.

D. The patient reported having no recent experiences with verbal or physical violence or threats of violence.

26. Employment Conflicts (25)

A. The patient has been unable to maintain employment due to authority/coworker conflict or anxiety symptoms.

B. As the patient has worked through the feelings associated with the traumatic event, he/she has been more reliable and responsible within the employment setting.

C. The patient has resumed his/her employment duties and attendance in a consistent and reliable manner.

INTERVENTIONS IMPLEMENTED

1. Psychological Testing (1)

A. Psychological testing was administered to assess for the presence and strength of the PTSD symptoms.

B. The psychological testing confirmed the presence of significant PTSD symptoms.

C. The psychological testing confirmed mild PTSD symptoms.

D. The psychological testing revealed that there are no significant PTSD symptoms present.

2. Identify Negative Impact (2)

A. The patient was asked to identify how the traumatic event has made a negative impact on his/her life.

B. The patient stated that he/she has been unable to function normally because of the PTSD symptoms interfering with his/her life.

C. The patient listed several PTSD symptoms that have caused significant interference in his/her life.

3. Administer CAPS-1 (3)

A. The Clinician Administered PTSD Scales (CAPS-1) were used to assess the patient's PTSD status.

B. The CAPS-1 results substantiated the patient's claim of significant PTSD and the impaired functioning that has resulted from it.

4. List/Rank PTSD Symptoms (4)

A. The patient was asked to list the specific PTSD symptoms that he/she experiences and to rank them according to the degree of distress they have caused.

---

* The numbers in parentheses correlate to the number of the Therapeutic Intervention statement in the companion chapter with the same title in *The Complete Adult Psychotherapy Treatment Planner,* second edition (Jongsma and Peterson) by John Wiley & Sons, 1999.

B. The patient has followed through with listing his/her PTSD symptoms and has ranked them according to their intensity and frequency of occurrence.

C. The patient had difficulty being specific regarding his/her PTSD symptoms in terms of listing them in rank order.

5. Explore Facts of Traumatic Event (5)

A. The patient was gently encouraged to tell the entire story of the traumatic event.

B. The patient was given the opportunity to share what he/she recalls about the traumatic event.

C. Today's therapy session explored the sequence of events before, during, and after the traumatic event.

6. Emotional Reaction during Trauma (6)

A. Today's therapy session explored the patient's emotional reaction at the time of the trauma.

B. The patient was able to recall the fear that he/she experienced at the time of the traumatic incident.

C. The patient was able to recall the feelings of hurt, anger, and sadness that he/she experienced during the traumatic incident.

D. The patient was unable to recall the emotions that he/she experienced during the traumatic incident.

E. A patient-centered therapy approach was used to explore the patient's emotional reaction at the time of the traumatic incident.

7. Explore Effects of PTSD Symptoms (7)

A. Today's therapy session explored the effects that the PTSD symptoms have had on the patient's personal relationships, functioning at home and work, and social/recreational life.

B. The patient acknowledged that his/her erratic and unpredictable shifts in mood have placed a significant strain on his/her personal relationships.

C. The patient identified how the traumatic event has had a negative impact on his/her functioning at work.

D. The patient verbally recognized how he/she has become more detached and engaged in significantly fewer social/recreational activities since the traumatic event.

8. Assess Chemical Dependence (8)

A. The patient was asked to described his/her use of alcohol and/or drugs as a means of escape from negative emotions.

B. The patient acknowledged that he/she has abused alcohol and/or drugs as a means of coping with the negative consequences associated with the traumatic event.

C. The patient was quite defensive about giving information regarding his/her substance abuse history and minimized any such behavior.

9. Gather Family/Personal Substance Abuse History (9)

A. The patient was asked to provide information regarding substance abuse patterns within his/her immediate and extended family of origin.

B. The patient confirmed that one or more members of his/her extended family have had difficulties with substance abuse and chemical dependence.

C. The patient stated that there have been no chemical dependence problems throughout his/her extended family.

D. The patient acknowledged that he/she has developed a pattern of substance abuse in re-action to the symptoms stemming from the traumatic event.

10. Probe Substance Abuse Negative Consequences (10)

A. The patient was asked to identify any feelings of shame, guilt, or low self-esteem that have resulted from his/her substance abuse and its consequences.

B. The patient verbalized a recognition that mood-altering chemicals were used as a pri-mary coping mechanism to escape from stress or pain and that their use has resulted in negative consequences.

C. The patient denied any negative consequences resulting from his/her substance abuse associated with the PTSD symptoms.

D. The patient's denial was such that he/she was not able to acknowledge a pattern of sub-stance abuse or the negative consequences of that substance abuse.

11. Teach Contributing Factors to Substance Abuse (11)

A. The patient was taught the familial, emotional, and social factors that have contributed to the development of his/her chemical dependence.

B. The patient verbalized an understanding of the factors contributing to his/her chemical dependence and acknowledged it as a problem.

C. The patient's denial led to a refusal to acknowledge his/her chemical dependence and any factors that have contributed to it.

12. Chemical Dependence Treatment Referral (12)

A. The patient was referred for chemical dependence treatment.

B. The patient consented to chemical dependence treatment, as he/she has acknowledged it as a significant problem.

C. The patient refused to accept a referral for chemical dependence treatment and contin-ued to deny that substance abuse is a problem.

D. The patient has followed through on obtaining chemical dependence treatment.

13. Assess Anger Control (13)

A. A history of the patient's anger control problems was taken in today's therapy session.

B. The patient shared instances in which poor control of his/her anger resulted in verbal threats of violence, actual harm or injury to others, or destruction of property.

C. The patient identified events or situations that frequently trigger a loss of control of his/her anger.

D. The patient was asked to identify the common targets of his/her anger to help gain greater insight into the factors contributing to his/her lack of control.

E. Today's therapy session helped the patient realize how his/her anger control problems are often associated with underlying, painful emotions about the traumatic event.

14. Teach Anger Management Techniques (14)

A. The patient was taught mediational and self-control strategies to help improve his/her anger control.

B. The patient was taught guided imagery and relaxation techniques to help improve his/her anger control.

C. Role playing and modeling techniques were used to demonstrate effective ways to control anger.

D. The patient was strongly encouraged to express his/her anger through controlled, respectful verbalizations and healthy physical outlets.

E. A reward system was designed to reinforce the patient for demonstrating good anger control.

15. Provide Trauma Reaction Education (15)

A. The patient was referred for didactic sessions that would focus on teaching him/her the facts about the effects of traumatic events on survivors and the survivors' subsequent adjustment.

B. The patient was taught within the session about the effects that trauma has on individuals and how their subsequent adjustment is affected by the trauma.

C. The patient was referred to books on traumatic reactions to help him/her understand trauma effects.

D. The patient has verbalized an awareness of how PTSD develops and its impact on himself/herself and others.

16. Teach Deep Muscle Relaxation (16)

A. The patient was taught deep muscle relaxation methods, along with deep breathing and positive imagery, to induce relaxation and decrease his/her emotional distress.

B. The patient reported a positive response to the use of deep muscle relaxation methods and positive imagery techniques to help him/her feel more relaxed and less distressed.

C. The patient appeared uncomfortable and unable to relax when being instructed in the use of deep muscle relaxation and guided imagery techniques.

17. Utilize EMG Biofeedback (17)

A. EMG biofeedback was utilized to help increase the depth of the patient's relaxation.

B. The patient reported a positive response to the use of EMG biofeedback to increase the depth of his/her relaxation and reduce the intensity of his/her emotional distress.

C. The patient reported little to no improvement in his/her ability to relax through the use of EMG biofeedback.

18. Encourage Physical Exercise (18)

A. The patient was assisted in developing a physical exercise routine as a means of coping with stress and developing an improved sense of well-being.

B. The patient has followed through on implementing a regular exercise regimen as a stress release technique.

C. The patient has failed to consistently implement a physical exercise routine and was encouraged to do so.

19. Recommend *Exercising Your Way to Better Mental Health* (19)

A. The book *Exercising Your Way to Better Mental Health* (Leith) was recommended to the patient as a means of encouraging physical exercise.

B. The patient has followed through with reading the book on exercise and mental health and has implemented a consistent exercise regimen.

C. The patient has not followed through with reading the book on exercise nor has he/she implemented a regular physical exercise regimen.

20. Utilize Systematic Desensitization (20)

A. Imaginal systematic desensitization was used to help the patient overcome emotional reactivity to the traumatic event by means of gradual exposure to a hierarchy of stimulus situations.

B. The patient is reacting positively to the imaginal systematic desensitization procedure and reports a decrease in emotional reactivity to stimulus items.

C. The patient reports that he/she has successfully overcome any significant emotional reactivity to stimulus items associated with the traumatic event.

D. The systematic desensitization techniques have not been successful at helping the patient reduce emotional reactivity to stimulus situations associated with the traumatic event.

21. Explore Feelings Surrounding Traumatic Event (21)

A. Today's therapy session explored the patient's feelings before, during, and after the traumatic event.

B. The patient was given support and affirmation when retelling the story of the traumatic event.

C. The retelling of the traumatic incident helped to reduce the patient's emotional distress.

D. The patient has continued to exhibit a significant amount of emotional distress when telling the story of the traumatic event.

22. Explore Negative Self-Talk (22)

A. Today's therapy session identified how the patient's negative self-talk and pessimistic outlook are associated with the trauma.

B. Today's therapy session focused on how the patient's pessimistic outlook and strong self-doubts interfere with his/her willingness to take healthy risks.

C. A cognitive-behavioral therapy approach was utilized to identify the patient's self-defeating thoughts.

D. The patient was helped to identify more adaptive ways to cope with the trauma instead of continuing to rely on unsuccessful coping strategies.

23. Replace Distorted, Negative, Self-Defeating Thoughts (23)

A. The patient was helped to replace his/her distorted, negative, self-defeating thoughts with positive, reality-based self-talk.

B. The patient was encouraged to make positive self-statements to improve his/her self-esteem and decrease his/her emotional pain.

C. The patient was given the homework assignment to make at least one positive self-statement daily around others.

D. The patient's distorted, negative, self-defeating thoughts were challenged to help him/her overcome the pattern of catastrophizing events and/or expecting the worst to occur.

E. The patient reported experiencing increased calm by being able to replace his/her distorted, cognitive self-defeating thoughts with positive, reality-based self-talk.

24. Develop Stimulus Approach Plan (24)

A. The patient was assisted in developing a plan to decrease his/her emotional reactivity by gradually approaching previously avoided stimuli that trigger thoughts and feelings associated with the trauma.

B. The patient developed a hierarchy of steps that he/she can take to gradually approach the previously avoided stimuli that trigger thoughts and feelings associated with the trauma.

C. The patient was trained in the use of relaxation, deep breathing, and positive self-talk prior to attempting to gradually approach the previously avoided stimuli.

D. The patient reported that the use of relaxation, deep breathing, and positive self-talk has helped him/her gradually approach the previously avoided stimuli without experiencing a significant amount of distress.

E. The patient failed to practice using the relaxation techniques and positive self-talk because of his/her fear of being overwhelmed by painful emotions.

25. Monitor Sleep Patterns (25)

A. The patient was encouraged to keep a record of how much sleep he/she gets every night.

B. The patient was trained in the use of relaxation techniques to help induce sleep.

C. The patient was trained in the use of positive imagery to help induce sleep.

D. The patient was referred for a medication evaluation to determine whether medication is needed to help him/her sleep.

26. Employ EMDR Technique (26)

A. The patient was trained in the use of the eye movement desensitization and reprocessing (EMDR) technique to reduce his/her emotional reactivity to the traumatic event.

B. The patient reported that the EMDR technique has been helpful in reducing his/her emotional reactivity to the traumatic event.

C. The patient reported partial success with the use of the EMDR technique to reduce emotional distress.

D. The patient reported little to no improvement with the use of the EMDR technique to decrease his/her emotional reactivity to the traumatic event.

27. Referral for Group Therapy (27)

A. The patient was referred for group therapy to help him/her share and work through his/her feelings about the trauma with other individuals who have experienced traumatic incidents.

B. The patient was given the directive to self-disclose at least once during the group therapy session about his/her traumatic experience.

C. The patient's involvement in group therapy has helped him/her realize that he/she is not alone in experiencing painful emotions surrounding a traumatic event.

D. The patient's active participation in group therapy has helped him/her share and work through many of his/her emotions pertaining to the traumatic event.

E. The patient has not made productive use of the group therapy sessions and has been reluctant to share his/her feelings about the traumatic event.

28. Referral for Medication Evaluation (28)

A. The patient was referred for a medication evaluation to help stabilize his/her moods and decrease the intensity of his/her feelings.

B. The patient and his/her parent(s) agreed to follow through with the medication evaluation.

C. The patient was strongly opposed to being placed on medication to help stabilize his/her moods and reduce emotional distress.

29. Monitor Effects of Medication (29)

A. The patient's response to the medication was discussed in today's therapy session.

B. The patient reported that the medication has helped to stabilize his/her moods and decrease the intensity of his/her feelings.

C. The patient reports little to no improvement in his/her moods or anger control since being placed on the medication.

D. The patient reports that he/she has consistently taken the medication as prescribed.

E. The patient has failed to comply with taking the medication as prescribed.

30. Conduct Family/Conjoint Session (30)

A. A conjoint session was held to facilitate healing the hurt that the patient's PTSD symptoms have caused to others.

B. The patient apologized to significant others for the irritability, withdrawal, and angry outbursts that are part of his/her PTSD symptom pattern.

C. Significant others verbalized the negative impact that the patient's PTSD symptoms have had on their life.

D. Significant others indicated support for the patient and accepted apologies for previous hurts that his/her behavior caused.

31. Assess Dissociative Symptoms (31)

A. An assessment of the patient's dissociative symptoms was employed to check for flashbacks, memory loss, identity disorder, and so on.

B. The patient identified dissociative symptoms as a part of his/her fear response, and treatment for this symptom pattern was recommended.

C. The patient denied that any dissociative symptom pattern was present.

32. Explore Vocational History (32)

A. The patient's vocational history was explored and the impact of the PTSD symptoms on his/her employment adjustment were noted.

B. The patient acknowledged that his/her PTSD symptom pattern has led to unreliable attendance and a lack of cooperation with coworkers and supervisors.

C. The patient denied that the PTSD symptoms have had any impact on his/her employment situation.

D. The patient's irritability, explosive temper, social withdrawal, and other PTSD symptoms have led to poor work adjustment.

33. Assess Depression (33)

A. The depth of the patient's depression and his/her suicide potential were assessed.

B. Since the patient has significant depression and verbalizes suicidal urges, steps were taken to provide more intense treatment and constant supervision.

C. The patient's depression was not noted to be particularly serious and he/she has denied any current suicidal ideation.

34. Identify Distorted Cognitive Messages (34)

A. The patient was assisted in identifying cognitive messages that reinforce his/her feelings of hopelessness and helplessness.

B. The patient has verbalized an increased awareness of his/her distorted cognitive messages and has agreed to try to replace them with more positive, reality-based self-talk.

C. The patient verbalized an understanding of how distorted cognitive messages can result in negative emotional states.

35. Reinforce Reality-Based Cognitions (35)

A. The patient was taught positive, reality-based self-talk to replace his/her distorted cognitive messages.

B. The patient was reinforced for implementing positive, reality-based cognitive messages that enhance self-confidence and increase adaptive action.

C. The patient has begun to verbalize hopeful and positive statements regarding the future and was reinforced for doing so.

PSYCHOTICISM

PATIENT PRESENTATION

1. Bizarre Thought Content (1)

A. The patient demonstrated delusional thought content.

B. The patient has experienced persecutory delusions.

C. The patient's delusional thoughts have diminished in frequency and intensity.

D. The patient no longer experiences delusional thoughts.

2. Illogical Thought/Speech (2)

A. The patient's speech and thought patterns are incoherent and illogical.

B. The patient demonstrated loose association of ideas and vague speech.

C. The patient's illogical thought and speech have become less frequent.

D. The patient no longer gives evidence of illogical form of thought and speech.

3. Perception Disturbance (3)

A. The patient has experienced auditory hallucinations.

B. The patient has experienced visual hallucinations.

C. The patient's hallucinations have diminished in frequency.

D. The patient reported no longer experiencing hallucinations.

4. Disturbed Affect (4)

A. The patient presented with blunted affect.

B. The patient gave evidence of a lack of affect.

C. At times, the patient's affect was inappropriate for the context of the situation.

D. The patient's affect has become more appropriate and energized.

5. Lost Sense of Self (5)

A. The patient has experienced a loss of ego boundaries and has a lack of personal identity.

B. The patient demonstrated blatant confusion and a lack of orientation as to his/her own person.

6. Volition Diminished (6)

A. The patient gave evidence of inadequate interest, drive, or ability to follow a course of action to its logical conclusion.

B. The patient has demonstrated pronounced ambivalence or cessation of goal-directed activity.

C. The patient has shown improvement in volitional behavior and has become more goal-directed in his/her actions.

* The numbers in parentheses correlate to the number of the Behavioral Definition statement in the companion chapter with the same title in *The Complete Adult Psychotherapy Treatment Planner,* second edition (Jongsma and Peterson) by John Wiley & Sons, 1999.

7. Relationship Withdrawal (7)

A. The patient has been withdrawn from involvement with the external world and has been preoccupied with egocentric ideas and fantasies.

B. The patient has shown a slight improvement in his/her ability to demonstrate relationship skills.

C. The patient has shown an interest in relating to others in a more appropriate manner.

8. Psychomotor Abnormalities (8)

A. The patient demonstrated a marked decrease in reactivity to his/her environment.

B. The patient demonstrated various catatonic patterns such as stupor, rigidity, posturing, negativism, and excitement.

C. The patient gave evidence of unusual mannerisms or grimacing.

D. The patient's psychomotor abnormalities have diminished, and his/her pattern of relating has become more typical and less alienating.

INTERVENTIONS IMPLEMENTED

1. Demonstrate Acceptance (1)

A. The patient was shown acceptance through a calm, nurturing manner, good eye contact, and active listening.

B. The patient responded to calm acceptance by beginning to describe his/her psychotic symptoms.

C. The patient remained agitated, tense, and preoccupied with his/her own internal stimuli.

2. Assess Thought Disorder Severity (2)

A. The severity of the patient's thought disorder was assessed through clinical interview.

B. Psychological testing was used to assess the patient's psychotic process.

C. The patient gave evidence of significant and pervasive psychotic disorder.

D. The patient's psychotic disorder seemed mild, and he/she demonstrated some capability to remain reality based and to relate appropriately.

3. Assess Psychosis History (3)

A. The history of the patient's illness revealed that the patient's symptom pattern is chronic with prodromal elements.

B. The patient's psychosis appears to be reactive and acute.

4. Explore Family History (4)

A. The patient's family history was assessed for serious mental illness.

B. It has been confirmed that severe and persistent mental illness does exist within the patient's extended family of origin.

C. There is no evidence of severe and persistent mental illness in the patient's extended family of origin.

---

* The numbers in parentheses correlate to the number of the Therapeutic Intervention statement in the companion chapter with the same title in *The Complete Adult Psychotherapy Treatment Planner,* second edition (Jongsma and Peterson) by John Wiley & Sons, 1999.

D. The patient and significant others were unable to provide sufficient information to determine if severe and persistent mental illness exists within the extended family of origin.

5. Provide Supportive Therapy (5)

A. The patient was provided emotional and social support in an understanding and accepting atmosphere in order to reduce his/her fears and feelings of alienation.

B. The patient seemed to relax and feel less agitated within an environment of acceptance.

6. Explain Psychotic Process (6)

A. The nature of the psychotic process was explained to the patient, as well as the biochemical causes and the confusing effect on rational thought.

B. The patient seemed to accept and understand that his/her distressing symptoms are due to mental illness.

C. The patient remains confused as to the basis for his/her thought disturbance.

7. Arrange Medication Evaluation (7)

A. Arrangements were made for the administration of appropriate psychotropic medications through a physician.

B. The patient has attended an appointment with a physician and has accepted the need for psychotropic medication.

C. Although the patient seems confused as to the need for medication, he/she is cooperative with taking it as directed.

8. Monitor Medication Compliance (8)

A. The patient is taking his/her antipsychotic medication consistently, but only under supervision.

B. The patient has been taking his/her antipsychotic medication consistently without supervision.

C. The patient was reinforced for taking medication consistently, and the need to continue to do so was stressed.

D. The patient is not at all consistent about taking his/her psychotropic medications, and more supervision of this is necessary.

9. Arrange Supervised Living (9)

A. Arrangements have been made for a supervised living situation to monitor the patient's medication compliance and ability to care for his/her own basic needs.

B. The patient is strongly resistive to placement in a supervised living situation, and commitment procedures have been initiated.

C. The patient has voluntarily cooperated with being placed in a supervised living situation.

10. Arrange Involuntary Commitment (10)

A. Since the patient has demonstrated an inability to care for his/her basic needs, commitment procedures to an inpatient psychiatric facility were initiated.

B. Since the patient has demonstrated the potential to be harmful to himself/herself, admission to an inpatient psychiatric facility was facilitated.

11. Probe Reactive Psychosis Causes (11)

A. The causes for the patient's reactive psychotic episode were explored.

B. The patient described recent severe stressors that may have precipitated the acute psychotic break.

C. Clearly, steps will need to be taken to reduce environmental stressors in order to facilitate recovery from the acute psychotic episode.

12. Explore Feelings Regarding Stressors (12)

A. The patient was encouraged to share his/her feelings associated with stressors present in his/her environment.

B. The patient shared feelings of fear, helplessness, and confusion associated with external stressors.

C. The patient was unable to articulate his/her feelings associated with the stressful environment.

13. Reduce Environmental Threat (13)

A. A plan was developed with the patient that focused on reducing the level of stress that he/she perceives in his/her environment.

B. Steps have been taken to change the environment in such a way as to reduce the patient's feeling of threat associated with it.

C. Arrangements have been made for the patient to be visited, monitored, supervised, and encouraged more frequently by supportive people.

14. Restructure Irrational Beliefs (14)

A. As the patient verbalized irrational beliefs, illogical thoughts, and perceptual disturbances, reality-based evidence was reviewed in an attempt to get the patient to restructure his/her irrational thoughts.

B. The patient was able to comprehend the reality-based evidence and modify his/her irrational beliefs.

C. The patient's psychotic process prohibited him/her from accepting reality-based evidence that would modify his/her irrational beliefs.

15. Encourage Reality Focus (15)

A. As the patient discussed and described his/her hallucinatory and delusional experience, an attempt was made to encourage a focus on the reality of the external world rather than the distortions of internal stimuli.

B. The patient reported hallucinations occurring with slightly less frequency and intensity.

C. The patient's hallucinatory and delusional experiences continue in spite of attempts to get him/her to focus on the reality of the external world.

D. As the patient takes his/her prescribed antipsychotic medication, he/she is more open to a reality focus rather than responding to internal stimuli.

16. Differentiate between Internal and External Stimuli (16)

A. The patient was helped to differentiate between self-generated internal messages and the reality of the external world.

B. The patient is beginning to understand and differentiate between self-generated messages and the reality of the external world.

C. Although the patient continues to experience hallucinations and delusions, he/she is able to understand that they are a product of his/her mental illness rather than reality based.

17. Reinforce Appropriate Social/Emotional Responses (17)

A. The patient was encouraged and reinforced for social and emotional responses to others that are typical and appropriate.

B. The patient is beginning to show limited social functioning by responding appropriately to friendly encounters.

C. The patient's relationship withdrawal is diminishing, and his/her emotional and social responses are becoming more normal.

18. Confront Illogical Thoughts/Speech (18)

A. The patient's illogical thinking and speech were gently confronted, and attempts were made to refocus the thinking toward a stronger reality basis.

B. The patient responded positively to the gentle confrontation of his/her illogical thoughts and speech and is speaking more logically and coherently.

C. As the patient has taken his/her antipsychotic medication more consistently, he/she is demonstrating more logical, coherent speech.

19. Reinforce Clarity/Rationality of Thought (19)

A. The patient's clear expression of thoughts and the reality basis to his/her thoughts were reinforced.

B. The patient is beginning to show more logical, coherent speech, and this pattern is being reinforced consistently.

20. Explore Underlying Needs/Feelings (20)

A. An attempt was made to explore the patient's underlying feelings and needs that may trigger irrational thought.

B. The patient expressed feelings of inadequacy, anxiety, and guilt, as well as fear of rejection.

C. The patient expressed an understanding that as his/her stress level increases, the psychotic symptoms increase in intensity.

21. Educate Family Members (21)

A. A family session was held to educate the family and significant others regarding the patient's illness, treatment, and prognosis.

B. Family members expressed their positive support of the patient and a more accurate understanding of his/her severe and persistent mental illness.

C. Family members were not understanding or willing to provide support to the patient in spite of his/her persistent mental illness.

22. Teach Double-Bind Avoidance (22)

A. Family members were taught the meaning of giving double-binding messages to the patient and that avoidance of this type of communication is important to reduce the patient's feelings of stress and anxiety.

B. Family members denied engaging in any double-binding messages and seemed defensive regarding any acknowledgment of this type of communication.

C. Family members were open to understanding the role of double-binding messages and committed themselves to more direct and honest communication.

23. Explore Family Members' Feelings (23)

A. Family members were encouraged to share their feelings of frustration, guilt, fear, or depression surrounding the patient's mental illness and behavior problems.

B. Family members shared their feelings of helplessness, embarrassment, and frustration surrounding the patient's behavior.

C. Although family members had been feeling frustrated and helpless at times, they also expressed feelings of empathy and support for the patient.

24. Family Support Group Referral (24)

A. Family members were referred to a community-based support group designed for families of psychotic patients.

B. Family members have been attending a support group for family members of severely mentally ill patients and have found it helpful.

C. Family members have not followed through on the recommendation that they attend a support group for family members of severely mentally ill patients.

25. Monitor/Redirect Patient Functioning (25)

A. The patient's level of functioning has been monitored as to the patient's providing care for his/her own basic needs.

B. As the patient's behavior deteriorates and his/her thought process slips into psychosis, support, encouragement, and redirection toward more intense treatment has been provided.

C. As the patient consistently takes his/her medication and follows the structured program of treatment and support provided, he/she is reinforced for follow-through.

SEXUAL ABUSE

PATIENT PRESENTATION

1. Vague Sexual Abuse Memories (1)

A. The patient has vague memories of inappropriate childhood sexual contact, and these memories are corroborated by significant others.

B. The patient has begun to recall more details of the sexual abuse of his/her childhood as the issue is being discussed within sessions.

C. The patient is unable to recall any specific details of the vague memories of inappropriate sexual contact in his/her childhood.

2. Detailed Sexual Abuse Memories (2)

A. The patient recalled with clear, detailed memories experiences of sexual abuse in childhood.

B. The patient's sexual abuse experiences cannot be corroborated by outside sources.

C. The patient's sexual abuse in childhood has been corroborated by outside sources.

D. The patient has experienced feelings of low self-esteem and shame related to his/her childhood sexual experiences.

E. The patient's feelings of shame and low self-esteem have diminished as he/she places responsibility on the perpetrator.

3. Inability to Recall Childhood (3)

A. The patient stated that he/she is unable to recall years of his/her childhood.

B. As the patient has begun to work through his/her childhood sexual abuse, recall of earlier years of abuse has increased.

4. Difficulty with Intimacy (4)

A. The patient has a pattern of extreme difficulty in forming intimate relationships with others.

B. As the patient begins to form intimate relationships with others, he/she experiences feelings of anxiety and avoidance.

C. As the patient has begun to work through his/her experiences of childhood sexual abuse, he/she reported less anxiety associated with current intimate relationships.

D. The patient no longer experiences anxiety and avoidance in current intimate relationships.

5. Sexual Dysfunction (5)

A. The patient reported an inability to enjoy sexual contact with a desired partner.

B. The patient experiences feelings of anxiety and tension when sexual contact with a desired partner is initiated.

* The numbers in parentheses correlate to the number of the Behavioral Definition statement in the companion chapter with the same title in *The Complete Adult Psychotherapy Treatment Planner,* second edition (Jongsma and Peterson) by John Wiley & Sons, 1999.

C. The patient reported that he/she has had a successful and satisfying enjoyable contact with a desired partner.

D. The patient no longer experiences feelings of anxiety during sexual contact with a desired partner and reported satisfaction in this area.

6. Unexplained Anger/Fear (6)

A. The patient described unexplainable feelings of anger, rage, or fear when coming into contact with a close family relative.

B. The patient has begun to identify a close family relative as the perpetrator of sexual abuse to him/her in his/her childhood.

7. Seduction/Promiscuity (7)

A. The patient described a pervasive pattern of promiscuity in his/her adolescent and adult history.

B. The patient has a pattern of seduction and sexualization of relationships since being a sexual abuse victim.

C. The patient acknowledged that he/she has developed an unhealthy sexualization of relationships as a result of his/her sexual abuse experiences.

D. The patient has terminated his/her pattern of sexual promiscuity and seduction.

INTERVENTIONS IMPLEMENTED

1. Build Trust (1)

A. Consistent eye contact, active listening, unconditional positive regard, and warm acceptance were used to help build trust with the patient.

B. The patient began to express feelings more freely as rapport and trust level increased.

C. The patient has continued to experience difficulty being open and direct in his/her expression of painful feelings.

2. Explore Sexual Abuse History (2)

A. The patient was encouraged to tell the entire story of the sexual abuse, giving as many details as he/she felt comfortable with.

B. The patient was overwhelmed with feelings of sadness and shame as he/she talked of his/her childhood sexual experiences.

C. The patient is now able to speak of the childhood sexual abuse without being emotionally overwhelmed.

3. Draw a House Diagram (3)

A. The patient was asked to draw a diagram of the house in which he/she was raised and to indicate where everyone slept, as well as where the abuse occurred.

B. The patient talked about the nature, frequency, and duration of the abuse as he/she worked with the diagram of the house he/she had created.

C. The patient continues to have difficulty talking about the details of the sexual abuse.

---

* The numbers in parentheses correlate to the number of the Therapeutic Intervention statement in the companion chapter with the same title in *The Complete Adult Psychotherapy Treatment Planner,* second edition (Jongsma and Peterson) by John Wiley & Sons, 1999.

4. Explore Feelings (4)

A. The patient was encouraged and supported in verbally expressing and clarifying his/her feelings associated with his/her experiences of childhood sexual abuse.

B. The patient identified feelings of shame, sadness, and anger associated with his/her experiences of childhood sexual abuse.

C. The patient described feelings of guilt and responsibility for his/her childhood sexual abuse experiences.

D. As the patient shared more freely details of his/her childhood sexual abuse experiences, the intensity of the feelings associated with those experiences was diminished.

5. Identify Supportive Individuals (5)

A. The patient was assisted in identifying those individuals who would be supportive in the process of resolving the sexual abuse issue.

B. The patient was encouraged to speak to those individuals whom he/she believed might be supportive and to enlist their support.

C. The patient could not identify anyone that he/she believed would be supportive if he/she made public the childhood sexual abuse.

6. Support Group Referral (6)

A. The patient was encouraged to attend a support group for survivors of sexual abuse.

B. The patient has followed through with attending a support group for survivors of sexual abuse and reported that it has been a positive experience.

C. The patient has not followed through on consistently attending a support group for survivors of sexual abuse and was encouraged to do so.

D. The patient reported that attending the group for survivors of sexual abuse has been a supportive experience.

7. Assign a Book on Sexual Abuse (7)

A. It was recommended to the patient that he/she read *The Courage to Heal* (Bass and Davis), *Betrayal of Innocence* (Forward and Buck), or *Outgrowing the Pain* (Gil).

B. The patient has read some of the recommended sexual abuse survivor material, and the content of that reading was processed.

C. The patient has not read any of the recommended sexual abuse material and was encouraged to do so.

D. The patient verbalized an increased knowledge of sexual abuse and its effects after reading the recommended sexual abuse material.

8. Assign *The Courage to Heal Workbook* (8)

A. The patient was assigned a written exercise from *The Courage to Heal Workbook* (Davis).

B. The patient has completed the exercise from *The Courage to Heal Workbook* and verbalized an increased knowledge of sexual abuse and its effects.

C. The patient has not completed the assigned written exercise from *The Courage to Heal Workbook* and was encouraged to do so.

9. Encourage Openness (9)

A. The patient was encouraged to be open in talking of the sexual abuse without shame, embarrassment, or the belief that he/she was responsible for the abuse.

B. The patient is beginning to demonstrate an increased ability to talk openly about the sexual abuse, reflecting acceptance of the experience without guilt.

C. The patient finds it difficult to talk of the sexual abuse experience and continues to experience feelings of guilt and shame.

10. Utilize the Empty-Chair Disclosure Technique (10)

A. The patient was guided in using an empty-chair conversation exercise with the nonabusive parent, telling them of the sexual abuse and its effects.

B. The empty-chair technique was used to assist the patient in becoming comfortable in sharing his/her sexual abuse experience with siblings and other members of the family.

C. The patient has agreed to share the sexual abuse experiences with key members of the family before the next session.

D. The patient has followed through with sharing the childhood sexual abuse experiences with members of the family and reported that it was a positive experience.

E. The patient reported that sharing the sexual abuse experiences with members of the family was not a positive experience and that he/she found no support from them.

11. Facilitate Telling Spouse of the Abuse (11)

A. A conjoint session was held wherein the patient told his/her spouse of the sexual abuse experience of his/her childhood.

B. The patient received empathetic support from his/her spouse after sharing the sexual abuse experience of his/her childhood.

C. The patient's spouse was rather detached and cold in response to his/her sharing his/her childhood sexual abuse experiences.

12. Facilitate Family Revelation (12)

A. The patient was supported in revealing the childhood sexual abuse to his/her parents.

B. The patient found his/her parents to be supportive and understanding when they were told about his/her childhood sexual abuse.

C. The patient's parents were rather detached upon hearing of his/her childhood sexual abuse experiences.

D. The patient's parents expressed disbelief at his/her revelation of his/her childhood sexual abuse experiences.

13. Process Guilt Feelings (13)

A. The patient was encouraged, supported, and assisted in identifying, expressing, and processing any feelings of guilt related to feelings of physical pleasure, emotional fulfillment, or responsibility connected with the sexual abuse events.

B. The patient expressed decreased feelings of shame and verbally affirmed himself/herself as not responsible for the abuse.

C. The patient continues to struggle with feelings of guilt and shame related to the childhood sexual abuse experiences.

D. The patient reported no longer feeling shame or guilt related to his/her childhood sexual abuse experiences.

14. Confront Taking Responsibility (14)

A. At any time that the patient indicated feelings of responsibility for the abuse, he/she was confronted and these feelings were processed.

B. The patient was assisted in working through issues of responsibility and guilt and coming to terms with himself/herself as a survivor of sexual abuse.

C. The patient continues to make statements that reflect responsibility for the abuse.

D. The patient continues to see himself/herself as a victim rather than empowering himself/herself as a survivor.

15. Arrange for Hypnosis (15)

A. Arrangements were made for the patient to undergo hypnosis in order to further uncover or to further clarify the nature and extent of the sexual abuse experiences in his/her childhood.

B. The patient recalled more details of the childhood sexual abuse while under hypnotic trance.

C. The hypnotic trance was not effective at helping the patient recall more details of the childhood sexual abuse experiences.

16. Assign a Journal (16)

A. To help the patient clarify memories of his/her childhood sexual abuse experiences, he/she was assigned to keep a journal of details recalled and to talk and think about the abuse incidences.

B. The patient was cautioned against embellishing his/her memories because of what he/she has read or seen in movies or video.

C. Care was used not to lead the patient, but to only allow him/her to recall on his/her own initiative details of his/her childhood sexual abuse experiences.

D. The patient has begun to recall more of the details of the childhood sexual abuse experiences because of keeping a journal and talking more freely about the incidences.

17. Assign a Letter to the Perpetrator (17)

A. The patient was assigned to write an angry letter to the perpetrator that expresses his/her feelings about the sexual abuse experiences.

B. The patient has followed through with writing the letter to the perpetrator of the sexual abuse and processed the content of the letter within the session.

C. The patient has decided to send the confrontational letter to the perpetrator of the sexual abuse.

D. The patient has decided to confront the perpetrator in person with the content of the letter that he/she has written.

E. The patient does not feel capable of confronting the perpetrator with the content of the letter.

18. Hold a Confrontational Conjoint Session (18)

A. The conjoint session was held wherein the patient confronted the perpetrator of the sexual abuse.

B. The patient expressed his/her feelings to the perpetrator and explained the negative impact that the abuse has had on his/her life.

C. The patient was overwhelmed with emotion as he/she confronted the perpetrator of the sexual abuse, but continued to put responsibility for the behavior on the perpetrator.

19. Develop a Symptom Line (19)

A. The patient was assisted in creating a line of symptoms that have developed since the experience of childhood sexual abuse.

B. The patient has verbalized the ways that the sexual abuse has impacted his/her life.

20. List Sexual Abuse Impact (20)

A. The patient was asked to make a list of the ways that the childhood sexual abuse has impacted his/her life.

B. The patient verbalized the ways that sexual abuse has impacted his/her life.

C. The patient listed difficulties with intimacy and sexual dysfunction as primary results of his/her childhood sexual abuse experience.

21. Explore Broken Boundaries in Family Pattern (21)

A. A genogram was developed with the patient to assist him/her in illuminating key family patterns of broken boundaries related to sex and intimacy.

B. The patient described how the sexual abuse experience is a part of a family pattern of broken boundaries through physical contact or verbal suggestiveness.

22. Read Books on Shame (22)

A. It was recommended to the patient that he/she read *Healing the Shame That Binds You* (Bradshaw), *Shame* (Kaufman), and *Facing Shame* (Fossum and Mason) in order to help him/her overcome feelings of shame related to childhood sexual abuse.

B. The patient has read the assigned sections in books dealing with shame and reported a better understanding of his/her feelings.

C. The patient reported less feelings of shame as a result of reading the recommended material.

D. The patient reported no longer feeling and experiencing shame related to the childhood sexual abuse experiences.

23. Distinguish between Victim and Survivor (23)

A. The patient was asked to complete an exercise that identified the positives and negatives of being a victim versus being a survivor of sexual abuse.

B. The patient has verbalized an understanding that he/she must no longer perceive himself/herself as a victim, but as a survivor.

C. The patient has expressed feelings of empowerment as a result of perceiving himself/herself as a survivor versus a victim.

24. Assign a "Cost-Benefit Analysis" Exercise (24)

A. The patient was assigned to complete a "Cost-Benefit Analysis" exercise from *Ten Days to Self-Esteem!* (Burns) on being a victim versus a survivor, or on holding on to anger versus forgiving the perpetrator.

B. The patient has completed the "Cost-Benefit Analysis" exercise and verbalized that there are considerable advantages to being a survivor and to beginning the process of forgiveness for the perpetrator.

C. The patient finds it difficult to give up the perception that he/she is a victim and needs to continue to feel rage toward the perpetrator.

25. Read "The Seedling" (25)

A. The story entitled "The Seedling," from the book *Stories for the Third Ear* (Wallas), was read and processed within the session to help the patient overcome the negative aspects of childhood sexual abuse.

B. The patient verbalized an understanding of the benefit of beginning a process of forgiveness toward the perpetrator of his/her childhood sexual abuse.

26. Recommend *Forgive and Forget* (26)

A. It was recommended that the patient read the book *Forgive and Forget* (Smedes) in order to help him/her understand the process of forgiveness as applied to the perpetrator of his/her childhood sexual abuse.

B. The patient has followed through with reading the book on forgiveness and has indicated a greater understanding of the benefit of forgiveness.

C. The patient has committed himself/herself to beginning the process of forgiveness of the perpetrator of the childhood sexual abuse.

D. The patient rejected the concept of forgiveness and continues to hold onto feelings of anger toward the perpetrator.

27. Assign a Forgiveness Letter (27)

A. The patient was assigned to write a forgiveness letter to the perpetrator of the childhood sexual abuse.

B. The patient was assigned to complete a forgiveness exercise from the book *Forgiving* (Simon and Simon).

C. The patient has followed through on the forgiveness exercise and has committed himself/herself to beginning the process of forgiving himself/herself, the perpetrator, and others connected with the sexual abuse.

D. The patient presented the completed forgiveness exercise, and the contents of that exercise were processed within the session.

28. Teach the Share-Check Method (28)

A. The patient was taught the share-check method of building trust in relationships.

B. The patient indicated a desire to increase the level of trust in others and has implemented the share-check method to do so.

C. The patient continues to be distrustful of others and has not implemented the share-check method to increase trust levels.

29. Role-Play Boundary Establishment (29)

A. Role playing and modeling were used to teach the patient how to establish reasonable personal boundaries that are neither too porous nor too restrictive.

B. As the patient has begun to feel confident in establishing boundaries in relationships, he/she has begun to show more trust in others, increased socialization, and greater intimacy tolerance.

C. The patient continues to have difficulty establishing boundaries and chooses to avoid relationships because of fear of intimacy.

30. Define Appropriate Touching (30)

A. The patient was encouraged to give and receive appropriate touching, and definitions of that appropriateness were developed.

B. The patient has begun to feel more comfortable with appropriate human touching.

C. The patient reported increased ability to accept and initiate appropriate physical contact with others.

D. The patient continues to experience anxiety and tension in whatever physical contact is initiated by others.

31. Assign Touch Initiation (31)

A. The patient was assigned to practice initiating touching in an appropriate manner with a trustworthy partner one or two times per week.

B. The patient has followed through with the touching exercise and reported an increased ability to accept and initiate appropriate physical contact.

C. The patient reported that he/she is now able to hug friends and give appropriate intimate touching to a partner.

SLEEP DISTURBANCE

PATIENT PRESENTATION

1. Sleep Initiation/Maintenance Problems (1)

A. The patient reported that he/she finds it very difficult to fall asleep within a reasonable period of time.

B. The patient reported that he/she can fall asleep within a reasonable period of time, but often awakens and is unable to return to sleep easily.

C. The patient reported that he/she awakens at a very early hour and is unable to return to sleep.

D. The patient reported that his/her sleep disturbance has diminished and that he/she is beginning to return to a normal sleep cycle.

E. The patient reported longer experiences without sleep disturbance symptoms and is sleeping fairly consistently.

2. Not Feeling Rested (2)

A. Although the patient reports getting an average amount of sleep per night, he/she is not feeling refreshed or rested upon awakening.

B. Despite sleeping more than seven to eight hours per night, the patient feels a need to take a nap during the day as he/she does not feel rested with a normal amount of sleep.

C. The patient reported that he/she is feeling more rested and refreshed upon awakening.

3. Daytime Sleepiness (3)

A. The patient reported that he/she feels very sleepy during the day and easily falls asleep, even while sitting in a chair.

B. The patient reported that he/she has fallen asleep in a chair in the presence of others in a social situation on many occasions.

C. The patient reported that he/she is beginning to feel more rested and alert during the day as his/her sleep pattern is returning to normal.

D. The patient reported no recent incidents of falling asleep too easily during the day.

4. Sleep-Wake Schedule Reversal (4)

A. Due to a reversal in the patient's normal sleep-wake schedule, he/she has experienced difficulty in staying asleep.

B. Because of a change in the patient's work schedule, he/she has had to reverse his/her sleep-wake schedule, and this has resulted in significant sleep disturbance.

C. The patient is beginning to adapt to the reversed sleep-wake schedule and obtain the necessary sleep required.

---

* The numbers in parentheses correlate to the number of the Behavioral Definition statement in the companion chapter with the same title in *The Complete Adult Psychotherapy Treatment Planner,* second edition (Jongsma and Peterson) by John Wiley & Sons, 1999.

D. The patient has not adapted to the reversal in his/her sleep-wake schedule and has changed his/her employment to be able to return to a normal sleep schedule.

5. Frightening Dreams Recalled (5)

A. The patient reported significant distress resulting from repeated awakening at night with detailed recall of extremely frightening dreams involving threats to himself/herself.

B. As the patient's daily life external stressors have increased, he/she has experienced repeated awakening and detailed recall of extremely frightening dreams involving threats to himself/herself.

C. As the patient has resolved external stressors, his/her incidents of experiencing nightmares has diminished significantly.

D. The patient reported that he/she no longer experiences extremely frightening dreams that awaken him/her in the night.

6. Abrupt Awakening without Dream Recall (6)

A. The patient reported that he/she has experienced abrupt awakening with a panicky scream followed by intense anxiousness and confusion or disorientation and no dream recall.

B. As the level of stress within the patient's life has decreased, his/her incidents of panic awakening have decreased.

C. The patient reported no recent incidents of panic awakening with confusion or disorientation.

7. Sleepwalking (7)

A. The patient reported incidents of sleepwalking accompanied by amnesia for the episode.

B. The frequency of the patient's sleepwalking experience has increased as stress levels within his/her life intensify.

C. As the patient has become more relaxed and less preoccupied with stress, the incidents of sleepwalking have diminished.

D. The patient reported no recent incidents of sleepwalking.

INTERVENTIONS IMPLEMENTED

1. Assess Sleep Disturbance (1)

A. The exact nature of the patient's sleep disturbance was assessed, including his/her bedtime routine, activity level while awake, nutritional habits, napping practice, actual sleep time, rhythm of time for being awake versus sleeping, and so on.

B. The assessment of the patient's sleep disturbance found a chronic history of this problem, which becomes exacerbated at times of high stress.

C. The assessment of the patient's sleep disturbance found that the patient does not practice behavioral habits that are conducive to a good sleep-wake routine.

---

* The numbers in parentheses correlate to the number of the Therapeutic Intervention statement in the companion chapter with the same title in *The Complete Adult Psychotherapy Treatment Planner,* second edition (Jongsma and Peterson) by John Wiley & Sons, 1999.

2. Assign a Stress Journal (2)

A. The patient was asked to keep a journal of his/her daily stressors and nightly sleep pattern and routine.

B. The patient has followed through on keeping a sleep journal, which also notes daily stressors, and this information was processed within the session.

C. The patient acknowledged that his/her sleep disturbance seemed clearly to be related to unresolved stressors in his/her daily life.

3. Assess Medication/Substance Abuse (3)

A. The patient was assisted in identifying any medication intake that may be related to his/her sleep disorder.

B. The degree of the patient's substance abuse and its relationship to his/her sleep disorder was assessed.

C. The patient was reinforced for acknowledging a relationship between his/her substance abuse and his/her sleep disturbance.

D. The patient was referred to treatment that was focused on substance abuse, which would secondarily improve his/her sleep.

E. The patient acknowledged that his/her sleep disturbance seemed related to a medication change, and he/she was referred to his/her physician for an evaluation of this relationship.

4. Physician Evaluation Referral (4)

A. The patient was referred to his/her physician to rule out any physical and/or pharmacological causes for his/her sleep disturbance.

B. The patient was referred to his/her physician to evaluate whether psychotropic medications might be helpful to induce sleep.

C. The physician has indicated that physical organic causes for the patient's sleep disturbance have been found, and a regimen of treatment for these problems has been initiated.

D. The physician ruled out any physical/organic, as well as medication, side effect causes for the patient's sleep disturbance.

E. The physician has ordered psychotropic medications to help the patient return to a normal sleep pattern.

5. Assess Depression (5)

A. The patient verbalized feelings of depression, and the onset of this mood disorder was related to his/her sleep disturbance.

B. The patient denied any feelings of depression and saw no relationship between the sleep disturbance and a mood disorder.

C. The patient identified several factors that had been contributing to several symptoms of depression, which include sleep disturbance.

6. Explore Traumatic Events (6)

A. The patient described experiences of emotional trauma that have disturbed his/her sleep since the incident occurred.

B. Because the patient shared the traumatic event and the feelings associated with it, he/she has reduced the amount of emotional reactivity and has increased a normal sleep pattern.

C. The patient described, in considerable detail and with significant emotion, traumatic events that have been disturbing to him/her.

7. Assign a Dream Journal (7)

A. The patient was assigned to keep a journal of disturbing dreams and how they may be related to current life stressors.

B. The patient described the material kept within his/her journal of disturbing dreams and also described the ongoing stressors within his/her life.

C. The patient acknowledged a relationship between the occurrence of disturbing dreams and unresolved conflicts in his/her life.

8. Explore Control Release Fears (8)

A. The patient described that he/she has difficulties relinquishing control and that this may be related to letting himself/herself fall into sleep.

B. The patient denied any issues of a high need to be in control.

C. As the patient's fears about relinquishing control have diminished, his/her sleep disturbance has also diminished.

9. Explore Death Fears (9)

A. The patient acknowledged having a strong fear of death that contributes to his/her sleep disturbance as he/she fears dying within sleep.

B. The patient's fears about dying in his/her sleep were processed.

C. The causes for the patient's fear of death while sleeping were explored and processed.

10. Identify Life Stressors (10)

A. The patient was assisted in identifying current life circumstances that are causing anxiety and may be interfering with sleep.

B. The patient identified several unresolved issues in his/her life that are causing stress and interfering with sleep.

C. The patient denied any current life stressors that may be interfering with sleep.

11. Formulate Stress Reduction Plan (11)

A. A stress reduction plan was formulated with the patient in order to modify his/her life situation to reduce stress and anxiety and increase normal sleep.

B. The patient has implemented the stress reduction plan and reported a reduction in anxiety and an increase in sleep.

C. The patient has not followed through on implementing the stress reduction plan and was encouraged to do so.

12. Explore Childhood Sleep Traumas (12)

A. The patient identified traumatic events that he/she experienced while sleeping, during childhood, that continue to interfere with normal sleep currently.

B. The patient talked in detail of the traumatic events that occurred during childhood sleep that continue to interfere with sleep currently.

C. As the patient has processed the traumatic events of childhood, his/her sleep has returned to a more normal cycle.

13. Explore Sexual Abuse (13)

A. The possibility of the patient having experienced sexual abuse in his/her bedroom before, during, or after sleep was explored.

B. The patient acknowledged that he/she has experienced sexual abuse and that the memory associated with these traumatic experiences continues to disturb his/her sleep.

C. The patient denied any sexual abuse incidents that may be interfering with his/her sleep.

14. Assign Sleep Induction Routine (14)

A. The patient was assigned a daily routine of exercise, low stimulation prior to sleep, relaxation training, consumption of a bland diet, taking a warm bath before sleep, reading neutral material, and other events that could promote relaxation and peace of mind.

B. The patient has followed through with the implementation of the sleep induction routine that was developed and has reported some success at increasing the initiation and maintenance of sleep.

C. The patient has not followed through with the implementation of the sleep induction routine that was developed and was encouraged to do so on a consistent basis.

D. The patient has followed through with implementing the sleep induction routine, but reported continuing sleep disturbance.

15. Teach Relaxation Skills (15)

A. The patient was trained in deep muscle relaxation and deep breathing exercises with and without the use of audiotape instruction.

B. The patient has implemented the deep muscle relaxation skills that were taught and has reported successful initiation of sleep.

C. The patient has not implemented the relaxation training skill on a consistent basis and was encouraged to do so.

16. Administer EMG Biofeedback (16)

A. The patient was administered electromyographic (EMG) biofeedback to reinforce successful relaxation responses.

B. The patient's ability to relax has increased as a result of the biofeedback training.

C. As the patient has increased his/her relaxation skills, he/she has been able to sleep better.

17. Arrange for Antidepressant Medication (17)

A. Arrangements were made for the patient to obtain a prescription for antidepressant medication in order to enhance restful sleep.

B. The patient reported taking antidepressant medication on a daily basis for the past three weeks and has found that sleep disturbance has diminished significantly.

C. The patient has taken the antidepressant medication consistently for the past three weeks, but reported a continuation of his/her sleep problems.

18. Monitor Medication Compliance (18)

A. The patient reported consistently taking the antidepressant medication and stated that it was effective at increasing normal sleep routines.

B. The patient reported not consistently taking his/her antidepressant prescription and was encouraged to do so.

C. The patient reported taking the antidepressant medication on a consistent basis for the past three weeks, but has not noted any positive effect on his/her sleep.

19. Sleep Clinic Referral (19)

A. The patient was referred to a sleep clinic for assessment of sleep apnea or other physiological factors that could interfere with normal sleep patterns.

B. The patient has followed through on the referral to a sleep clinic and reported that factors were found that have interfered with his/her sleep pattern.

C. The patient has followed through with the referral to the sleep clinic, but no physiological factors were found that have interfered with his/her sleep pattern.

D. The patient has not followed through with the referral to the sleep clinic and was encouraged to do so.

SOCIAL DISCOMFORT

PATIENT PRESENTATION

1. Social Anxiety/Shyness (1)

A. The patient described a pattern of social anxiety and shyness that presents itself in almost any interpersonal situation.

B. The patient's social anxiety presents itself whenever he/she has to interact with people whom he/she does not know or must interact in a group situation.

C. The patient's social anxiety has diminished, and he/she is more confident in social situations.

D. The patient has begun to overcome his/her shyness and can initiate social contact with some degree of comfort and confidence.

E. The patient reported that he/she no longer experiences feelings of social anxiety or shyness when having to interact with new people or group situations.

2. Disapproval/Hypersensitivity (2)

A. The patient described a pattern of hypersensitivity to the criticism or disapproval of others.

B. The patient's insecurity and lack of confidence has resulted in an extreme sensitivity to any hint of disapproval from others.

C. The patient has acknowledged that his/her sensitivity to criticism or disapproval is extreme and has begun to take steps to overcome it.

D. The patient reported increased tolerance for incidents of criticism or disapproval.

3. Social Isolation (3)

A. The patient has no close friends or confidants outside of first-degree relatives.

B. The patient's social anxiety has prevented him/her from building and maintaining a social network of friends and acquaintances.

C. The patient has begun to reach out socially and to respond favorably to the overtures of others.

D. The patient reported enjoying contact with friends and sharing personal information with them.

4. Social Avoidance (4)

A. The patient reported a pattern of avoiding situations that require a degree of interpersonal contact.

B. The patient's social anxiety has caused him/her to avoid social situations within work, family, and neighborhood settings.

---

* The numbers in parentheses correlate to the number of the Behavioral Definition statement in the companion chapter with the same title in *The Complete Adult Psychotherapy Treatment Planner,* second edition (Jongsma and Peterson) by John Wiley & Sons, 1999.

C. The patient has shown some willingness to interact socially as he/she has overcome some of the social anxiety that was formerly present.

D. The patient indicated that he/she feels free now to interact socially and does not go out of his/her way to avoid such situations.

5. Fear of Social Mistakes (5)

A. The patient reported resisting involvement in social situations because of a fear of saying or doing something foolish or embarrassing in front of others.

B. The patient has been reluctant to involve himself/herself in social situations because he/she is fearful of his/her social anxiety becoming apparent to others.

C. The patient has become more confident of his/her social skills and has begun to interact with more comfort.

D. The patient reported being able to interact socially without showing signs of social anxiety that would embarrass him/her.

6. Substance Abuse (6)

A. The patient has used alcohol and/or other chemicals to help ease the anxiety of becoming involved in social situations.

B. The patient reported that only when he/she is under the influence of a mood-altering substance is he/she able to relate to others comfortably.

C. The patient has acknowledged that his/her use of alcohol and/or other mood-altering chemicals to cope with social anxiety is not adaptive.

D. The patient has terminated the use of alcohol and/or other mood-altering chemicals to cope with social anxiety.

E. The patient reported being able to interact socially with others without anxiety in spite of not using alcohol or other mood-altering chemicals.

7. Solitary Activities (7)

A. The patient practices almost complete isolation or involvement in solitary activities during most of his/her waking hours.

B. The patient's lack of confidence in his/her social skills has resulted in avoidance of social contact and a predominance of isolation.

C. The patient is beginning to engage in activities that involve interacting with others.

D. The patient reported enjoying activities that required social interaction.

8. Physiological Anxiety Symptoms (8)

A. The patient has an increased heart rate, experiences sweating, dry mouth, muscle tension, and shakiness in most social situations.

B. As the patient has learned new social skills and developed more confidence in himself/herself, the intensity and frequency of physiological anxiety symptoms has diminished.

C. The patient reported engaging in social activities without experiencing any physiological anxiety symptoms.

INTERVENTIONS IMPLEMENTED

1. Identify Social Fears (1)

A. The patient identified and clarified the nature of the fears connected to associating with others.

B. The patient was assisted in clarifying the fears that are associated with interacting with others.

2. Explore Childhood Traumatic Experiences (2)

A. The patient was probed for childhood experiences of criticism, abandonment, or abuse that would foster low self-esteem, shame, and social insecurity.

B. The patient described experiences of frequent and severe parental criticism and mockery that have led to chronic feelings of low self-esteem and lack of social confidence.

C. The patient described experiences of abandonment and abuse that occurred within his/her childhood that have contributed to feelings of low self-esteem, shame, and social anxiety.

3. Explore Rejection Experiences (3)

A. The patient identified childhood and adolescent experiences of social rejection and neglect that have contributed to his/her current feelings of social anxiety.

B. The patient described in detail many incidences of feeling rejected by peers, which has led to social anxiety and social withdrawal.

4. Assign Books on Shame (4)

A. It was recommended to the patient that he/she read *Healing the Shame That Binds You* (Bradshaw) and *Facing Shame* (Fossum and Mason).

B. The patient has read the assigned books on shame and can now better identify how shame has affected his/her relating to others.

C. The patient has failed to follow through on reading the recommended materials on shame and was urged to do so.

D. As the patient has overcome his/her feelings of shame, he/she was asked to initiate one social contact per day for increasing lengths of time.

E. The patient reported success at initiating social contact once per day without debilitating anxiety.

5. List Positive Social Experiences (5)

A. The patient was asked to focus his/her attention on listing positive experiences of being involved in social activities and/or relating one-on-one with others.

B. The patient recalled experiences that have been positive in social interactions and was reinforced for his/her role in those interactions.

6. Identify Distorted Thoughts (6)

A. The patient was assisted in identifying his/her distorted automatic thoughts that are associated with anxiety over social interaction.

* The numbers in parentheses correlate to the number of the Therapeutic Intervention statement in the companion chapter with the same title in *The Complete Adult Psychotherapy Treatment Planner,* second edition (Jongsma and Peterson) by John Wiley & Sons, 1999.

B. The patient identified several specific negative self-talk messages that he/she engages in that contribute to social anxiety and social withdrawal.

C. The patient identified instances of reading other people's minds, projecting thoughts into them, catastrophizing situations, and judging himself/herself critically.

7. Develop Positive Self-Talk (7)

A. The patient was assisted in developing positive self-talk that will aid in overcoming fear of relating with others or participating in social activities.

B. The patient has implemented positive self-talk dialog that has been successful in helping him/her overcome fear of interacting with others.

C. The patient has not been consistent in implementing positive self-talk, but reverts to distorted negative messages.

8. Assign Conversation Initiation (8)

A. The patient was assigned to initiate one conversation daily, while increasing the time from one to five minutes per interaction.

B. Although the patient reported a strong desire to avoid social interaction, he/she agreed to attempt to initiate one conversation per day.

9. Monitor Conversation Initiation (9)

A. The patient was asked to relate his/her experience in initiating conversation with others and was given positive feedback regarding successful experiences.

B. The patient was encouraged and redirected when he/she indicated a desire to avoid initiating social contact one time per day.

10. Plan Social/Recreational Activities (10)

A. The patient was assisted in developing a plan of participation in social and recreational activities available within the community.

B. The patient reported positive experiences with reaching out and participating in social and recreational activities within the community.

C. The patient has failed to follow through with implementing social and recreational activities within the community and was urged to do so.

D. The patient reported on his/her attempts to participate in social and recreational activities within the community, but also indicated a strong degree of social anxiety being present during these experiences.

E. The patient was strongly reinforced for efforts to reach out for social and recreational contact within the community and was urged to continue in spite of feelings of anxiety.

11. Self-Help Group Referral (11)

A. A recommendation was made to the patient to participate in a self-help group that is appropriate to his/her situation.

B. The patient reported following through on becoming involved with a self-help group and described the experience as positive.

C. The patient's participation in a self-help group has reduced his/her social anxiety and increased social skills and social confidence.

D. The patient has not followed through with the recommendation to participate in a self-help group and was encouraged to do so.

12. Support Social Initiation (12)

A. The patient was encouraged and supported in any and all efforts that he/she made to initiate and build social relationships.

B. As the patient reported positive outcomes of participation in social and support groups, he/she was strongly encouraged to continue and was reinforced for his/her efforts.

13. Assign Self-Disclosure (13)

A. The patient was assigned to disclose his/her thoughts or feelings at least twice in each group session in which he/she participates.

B. The patient reported success at sharing his/her thoughts and feelings on two occasions within each group meeting.

C. The patient has failed to follow through with disclosing his/her own thoughts or feelings within a group situation and was encouraged to do so.

14. Communication Improvement Seminar Referral (14)

A. The patient was urged to attend a communication improvement seminar or a Dale Carnegie course.

B. The patient has followed through with the recommendation to attend a communications seminar to increase his/her social skills.

C. The patient has failed to follow through on the recommendation to attend a social skills–building seminar and was encouraged to do so.

15. Role-Play Conversation Initiation (15)

A. To facilitate the patient's social skills, role playing was used with the patient initiating conversation with another person for the first time.

B. The patient expressed more confidence in his/her social initiation ability after the role-playing experience.

C. The patient has followed through with implementing the initiation of a social contact and reported a feeling of success with this experience.

16. Utilize a Solution-Focused Approach (16)

A. The patient was asked to identify a time when he/she socialized with enjoyment and little anxiety.

B. The patient was urged to use this same skill that was previously successful in a similar social situation currently.

C. The patient reported success at implementing the previously successful social skills in a current situation.

17. Read *Friedman's Fables* (17)

A. "Jean and Jane" and "The Wallflower," from the book *Friedman's Fables* (Friedman), were read to the patient in order to help him/her identify ways that he/she is like other people and, therefore, acceptable to others.

B. The patient's questions and thoughts and reactions to the fables exercise were processed.

C. The patient indicated a deeper understanding of how he/she is similar to others.

18. Assign "Social Anxiety" (18)

A. The patient was assigned the "Social Anxiety" section in *The Feeling Good Handbook* (Burns).

B. The patient has followed through with completing the "Social Anxiety" section, and this assignment was processed to help the patient identify sources of his/her social anxiety and negative messages associated with that anxiety.

C. The patient reported a decrease in his/her feelings of fear associated with social contact as he/she has processed the "Social Anxiety" exercise.

19. Assign *Ten Days to Self-Esteem!* (19)

A. The patient was urged to complete and process the exercises on social anxiety and thought distortion within the book *Ten Days to Self-Esteem!* (Burns).

B. The patient has followed through on completing the social anxiety exercises within the book *Ten Days to Self-Esteem!*, and the exercise results were processed.

C. The patient has reported an increase in feelings of self-acceptance and has utilized positive self-talk to reduce feelings of anxiety.

20. Teach Similarity between Self and Others (20)

A. The patient was assisted in recognizing how he/she is like or similar to others and, therefore, acceptable to them.

B. The patient has tended to see himself/herself as different than and inferior to others in an irrational, unrealistic belief.

C. The patient has become more realistic in viewing himself/herself as similar to others with their flaws and shortcomings.

21. Assign Self-Acceptance Books (21)

A. Books on self-acceptance were recommended to the patient such as *Born to Win* (James and Jongeward), *Pulling Your Own Strings* (Dyer), or *I'm OK, You're OK* (Harris and Harris).

B. The patient reported reading material on self-acceptance and has been assisted in growing more confident in who he/she is.

C. The patient has increased his/her statements that reflect self-acceptance after reading the assigned material.

22. Use a Transactional Analysis Approach (22)

A. A transactional analysis (TA) approach was used to uncover and identify the patient's beliefs and fears that contribute to social anxiety.

B. The TA approach was used to alter the patient's beliefs and actions in a more adaptive and positive mode.

C. The patient reported successful social interactions after utilization of the TA approach.

23. Train in Assertiveness Skills (23)

A. The patient was trained in assertiveness skills that could be applied to various social situations.

B. The patient was referred to an assertiveness training class to build his/her confidence in social situations.

C. The patient reported implementation of assertiveness skills within social situations and was reinforced for this improvement.

24. Identify Defense Mechanisms (24)

A. The patient was assisted in identifying the defense mechanisms that he/she uses to avoid close relationships.

B. The patient was assisted in reducing his/her defensiveness so as to be able to build social relationships and not alienate himself/herself from others.

25. Reinforce Trust in Others (25)

A. The patient was reinforced for any statements that indicated an increased degree of trust that others are accepting of himself/herself.

B. The patient has demonstrated a renewed sense of trust in others and reported specific social interaction incidences that reflect his/her belief in that trust.

C. The patient reported social interaction instances that have reinforced his/her sense of trust in others as they have been accepting and supportive.

26. Plan Social and Solitary Activities (26)

A. The patient was assisted in developing a daily plan for nonworking hours that contains both social and solitary activities.

B. The patient has implemented a balanced plan for social and solitary activities and was reinforced for this follow-through.

C. The patient continues to isolate himself/herself more than the written plan for social interaction called for.

SOMATIZATION

PATIENT PRESENTATION

1. Preoccupation with Imagined Physical Abnormality (1)

A. The patient presented with a severe preoccupation with an imagined defect in his/her appearance when his/her actual appearance is quite normal.

B. The patient has an excessive concern regarding a small physical abnormality, which is probably unnoticeable to most other people.

C. The patient's preoccupation and excessive concern with insignificant or imagined physical abnormality has diminished.

D. The patient reported that he/she no longer is concerned about, or preoccupied with, the imagined physical abnormality.

2. Stress-Related Physical Malady (2)

A. The patient has experienced a physical malady caused by a psychosocial stressor triggering an internal psychological conflict.

B. As the patient has begun to resolve the psychological conflict, the physical problem has also ameliorated.

C. The patient reported no longer being troubled by the physical problem as the internal conflict over the psychosocial stressor has been resolved.

3. Fear of Physical Illness (3)

A. The patient is preoccupied with a fear of having a serious physical disease without any medical basis for this concern.

B. The patient's physician has been unable to reduce the patient's fears regarding his/her health through reassurances.

C. The patient's preoccupation with having a serious physical disease increases as his/her stress level increases.

D. The patient has become less preoccupied with the fear of having a serious physical disease.

E. The patient reported that he/she no longer experiences the fear of serious physical disease.

4. Many Physical Complaints (4)

A. The patient presented with a multitude of physical complaints that have no apparent or organic foundation and have caused the patient to change his/her life to accommodate these complaints.

B. The frequency and intensity of the patient's physical complaints have been reduced.

C. The patient is no longer preoccupied with physical complaints and is not altering his/her behavior to accommodate his/her physical concerns.

---

* The numbers in parentheses correlate to the number of the Behavioral Definition statement in the companion chapter with the same title in *The Complete Adult Psychotherapy Treatment Planner,* second edition (Jongsma and Peterson) by John Wiley & Sons, 1999.

5. Chronic Pain Preoccupation (5)

A. The patient presented with a history of preoccupation with pain that is beyond what is expected for his/her physical malady.

B. The patient is so pain focused that he/she is unable to carry on the responsibilities of day-to-day living.

C. The patient has learned management techniques and has become less preoccupied with the chronic pain problem.

6. Vague Physical Complaint (6)

A. The patient presented with a vague physical complaint that has no organic basis, and this preoccupation has impaired his/her life functioning.

B. The patient's preoccupation with his/her physical problems has resulted in a curtailment of normal functioning and an inability to focus on normal responsibilities.

C. The patient has terminated complaining about the physical problem and has resumed more normal functioning and performance of responsibilities.

7. Pain Related to Psychological and Medical Conditions (7)

A. The patient is preoccupied with pain in one or more anatomical sites with both psychological factors and a medical condition as the basis for that pain.

B. Although a medical condition does contribute to the patient's pain, his/her fixation with the pain and exaggerated complaints are based in psychological causes.

C. As the patient has resolved his/her psychological problems, he/she has become less preoccupied with pain complaints.

D. The patient no longer is preoccupied with pain.

INTERVENTIONS IMPLEMENTED

1. Explore Complaints (1)

A. A nonjudgmental attitude and unconditional positive regard were used to explore the patient's physical complaints.

B. The patient verbalized negative feelings regarding his/her body and discussed his/her preoccupation with the catastrophized consequences of his/her perceived body abnormality.

2. Refocus Physical Complaints to Emotional Conflict (2)

A. An effort was made to refocus the patient's discussion from physical complaints to emotional conflicts and expression of feelings.

B. It has been difficult for the patient to stay focused on emotional issues and expression of feelings rather than becoming preoccupied with his/her physical complaints.

C. The patient was led to understand that his/her physical problems are related to unresolved emotional issues.

---

* The numbers in parentheses correlate to the number of the Therapeutic Intervention statement in the companion chapter with the same title in *The Complete Adult Psychotherapy Treatment Planner,* second edition (Jongsma and Peterson) by John Wiley & Sons, 1999.

3. Explore Emotional Conflicts (3)

A. The patient's sources of emotional conflict were explored, including feelings of fear, feelings of inadequacy, and experiences of rejection or abuse.

B. As the patient talked about his/her negative emotional experiences, he/she has become less preoccupied with physical complaints.

4. Teach Secondary Gain (4)

A. The patient was assisted in understanding the role of secondary gain in maintaining physical illness and somatic complaints.

B. The patient verbalized an understanding that he/she has been excused from responsibilities because of his/her excessive physical complaints.

5. Connect Somatic Focus to Emotional Conflicts (5)

A. The patient was assisted in understanding the connection between his/her physical problems and preoccupations and the avoidance of facing emotional conflicts that are unresolved.

B. The patient accepted that there is a relationship between his/her emotional conflicts and physical complaints.

C. The patient resisted and rejected the idea of a connection between his/her physical problems and emotional conflicts.

6. Explore Anger Causes (6)

A. Current and historical experiences that have triggered feelings of anger within the patient were explored.

B. The patient identified several issues that cause him/her to feel anger.

C. The patient was led to see a connection between his/her suppression of anger and physical preoccupation.

D. The patient expressed an understanding of the connection between unresolved feelings of anger and physical symptoms.

7. Teach Anger Expression (7)

A. Using role playing and behavioral rehearsal, the patient was taught assertive and respectful expression of angry feelings.

B. As the patient has begun to express his/her angry feelings respectfully, assertively, and directly, his/her preoccupation with physical complaints has diminished.

8. Train in Assertiveness (8)

A. The patient was trained in the concept of assertiveness behavior.

B. The patient was referred to an assertiveness training class to increase his/her expression of feelings in a respectful manner.

C. The patient has begun to assert himself/herself and to express feelings of anger as well as other emotions.

D. As the patient has become more assertive in expression of feelings, his/her physical complaints have diminished.

9. Reinforce Assertiveness (9)

A. The patient's practice of assertiveness was reinforced as a means of attaining healthy need satisfaction in contrast to his/her pattern of helplessness and complaining.

B. As the patient has become more appropriately assertive, his/her degree of whining, complaining, and helplessness has diminished.

10. Plan Pleasurable Activities (10)

A. In an attempt to get the patient to divert his/her attention away from bodily focus, a list of pleasurable and rewarding activities was developed.

B. The patient listed several pleasurable and constructive activities that could serve as a diversion from self-preoccupation.

11. Assign Diversion Activities (11)

A. The patient was assigned to engage in pleasurable and rewarding activities that will take the focus off himself/herself and redirect it toward such things as hobbies, social activities, assisting others, completing projects, or returning to work.

B. The patient has followed through with engaging in diversion activities and has found success in resuming these rewarding activities.

C. The patient has resisted becoming involved in pleasurable and constructive activities and remains preoccupied with his/her somatic complaints.

12. Explore Somatic Family History (12)

A. The patient's family history of modeling and reinforcement of physical complaints was explored.

B. The patient identified a family pattern that has existed around an exaggerated focus on physical maladies.

C. The patient verbalized an understanding of the fact that his/her family of origin has reinforced a preoccupation with physical complaints.

13. Probe Low-Self-Esteem Causes (13)

A. The patient identified experiences within his/her childhood that have contributed to feelings of low self-esteem and inadequacy.

B. The patient's negative childhood experiences were explored and the feelings about those experiences were processed.

14. Connect Low Self-Esteem to Negative Body Image (14)

A. The patient was taught the connection between his/her low self-esteem and his/her preoccupation with a negative body image.

B. The patient verbalized an understanding of the connection between his/her negative body image and general low self-esteem that emanates from early family experiences.

15. Reinforce Body Acceptance (15)

A. The patient was reinforced for verbalizing any and all acceptance of his/her body as normal in function and appearance.

B. The patient's frequency of verbalizing acceptance of his/her body is increasing and his/her frequency of physical complaints is decreasing.

16. Convert Illness Preoccupation to Health Interest (16)

A. The patient was helped to focus on his/her health rather than illness.

B. The patient was issued a prescription for increased pleasurable and healthy activities such as physical exercise, sexual interaction, or other enjoyable activities.

C. As the patient has learned to focus on health rather than illness, he/she has become less preoccupied with physical complaints.

17. Train in Relaxation (17)

A. The patient was trained in relaxation techniques using biofeedback, deep breathing, and positive imagery methods.

B. The patient was encouraged to implement the use of relaxation skills to reduce tension in response to stress in his/her daily life.

18. Assign Daily Exercise (18)

A. A daily exercise routine was developed, and the patient was assigned to implement it consistently.

B. The patient was encouraged to increase his/her daily exercise regimen to reduce tension and to increase a sense of self-confidence in his/her own body.

19. Reinforce Empowerment (19)

A. The patient was taught to empower himself/herself with a sense of control over environmental events rather than to continue his/her perspective of being a victim of events.

B. The patient was encouraged to develop an assertive internal focus of control over the environment rather than viewing himself/herself as controlled by events around himself/herself.

C. The patient was encouraged to develop a perspective of empowered control rather than continuing a perspective of helplessness, frustration, anger, and "poor me."

20. Limit Preoccupation Times (20)

A. The patient was encouraged to develop specific times each day to think about, talk about, and write down his/her physical problems, and not focus on his/her physical condition at any other time.

B. The patient has begun to set aside a specific, limited time each day to focus on, talk about, and journal the details of his/her physical complaints.

C. The patient reported on the success of limiting his/her preoccupation to specific times of the day, allowing energy to be more constructively utilized at other times.

21. Utilize Ordeal Technique (21)

A. The patient was assisted in creating an ordeal to be enacted each time the symptom of physical complaining occurs.

B. The patient was taught the effectiveness of following through on a prescription of enacting an ordeal as a punishment for the focus on physical symptoms.

C. Though it has been difficult for the patient, he/she has followed through with the ordeal technique and reported that the frequency of physical complaints has diminished.

D. The patient has not followed through with implementing the ordeal technique and was encouraged to do so.

22. Plan Coping Techniques (22)

A. The patient was asked to list coping behaviors that will be implemented when his/her physical symptoms reappear.

B. The patient was asked to predict when the next attack of pain or physical problems may occur and then to plan a specific coping behavior to respond with.

C. The patient reported that he/she has implemented the coping behavior that was planned and that this has reduced his/her preoccupation with the physical problem.

23. Assign a Survey of Others (23)

A. The patient was assigned to a ritual of surveying his/her partner, friends, neighbors, pastors, and so on about how concerned they feel he/she should be about his/her physical problem.

B. The patient was asked to poll others about how concerned they would be and what they would recommend he/she do each time a physical complaint occurs.

C. The patient has followed through with this surveying, and the results of this assignment were processed.

D. The patient has come to realize that others react much less seriously than he/she does to the relatively minor physical preoccupations.

24. Challenge Pain Endurance (24)

A. The patient was challenged to endure pain and carry on with responsibilities so as to build self-esteem and a sense of contribution to life.

B. The patient was encouraged to decrease physical complaints, doctor visits, and reliance on medication while increasing verbal assessment of himself/herself as able to function normally and productively.

C. The patient was confronted with avoiding responsibilities through physical complaint preoccupation and taught the value of resuming normal functioning.

25. Teach the Negative Impact of Complaining (25)

A. The patient was assisted in identifying the negative and destructive social impact on friends and family of consistent complaintive verbalizations or negative body focus.

B. The patient was encouraged to engage in normal responsibilities vocationally and socially without complaints or withdrawal into avoidance by using physical preoccupation as an excuse.

26. Pain Clinic Referral (26)

A. The patient was referred to a pain clinic for learning pain management techniques, as well as obtaining medical support for pain relief.

B. The patient has followed through with obtaining a pain clinic appointment.

C. The patient has not followed through on obtaining an appointment at a pain clinic and was encouraged to do so.

SPIRITUAL CONFUSION

PATIENT PRESENTATION

1. Desire for Higher Power Relationship (1)

A. The patient verbalized a desire for a closer relationship with God.

B. The patient stated that he/she has not felt a close relationship with a higher power and would like to develop this in his/her life.

C. The patient has begun to utilize spiritual practices that have increased a sense of relationship with God.

D. The patient reported feeling more in touch with, understood by, and supported by a higher power.

2. Negative Attitudes about a Higher Power (2)

A. The patient reported feelings and attitudes about God that are characterized by fear, anger, and distrust.

B. As the patient has processed his/her feelings of fear, anger, and distrust, a more positive attitude about God has developed.

C. The patient verbalized positive feelings toward God as being a part of his/her life.

3. Feelings of Emptiness (3)

A. The patient verbalized a feeling of emptiness and lack of direction to his/her life as if some important part were missing.

B. The patient verbalized the lack of meaning that life has, but recognized that he/she needs to discover the meaning of a spiritual journey.

C. The patient has begun to explore spiritual beliefs and to engage in faith practices that have reduced the feeling of emptiness and meaninglessness.

4. Bleak Outlook on Life (4)

A. The patient verbalized a bleak, negative outlook on life and other people.

B. The patient verbalized an understanding that he/she lacks a spiritual focus that allows for perceiving life in a positive, meaningful way.

C. As the patient has deepened his/her spiritual focus, he/she has found a positive perspective on life and other people.

5. Lack of Religious Training (5)

A. The patient complained about having no religious education or training during his/her childhood, and now he/she feels lost as to how to begin to understand the role of God in his/her life.

B. The patient has begun to explore religious belief systems and to engage in faith practices in order to deepen spiritual focus.

---

* The numbers in parentheses correlate to the number of the Behavioral Definition statement in the companion chapter with the same title in *The Complete Adult Psychotherapy Treatment Planner,* second edition (Jongsma and Peterson) by John Wiley & Sons, 1999.

C. The patient reported that a new sense of meaning has entered his/her life as he/she engages in spiritual growth.

6. Painful Religious Experiences (6)

A. The patient described painful religious experiences that resulted in feelings of hurt and anger.

B. The patient's painful religious experiences have resulted in the patient feeling distrustful of and alienated from God.

C. As the patient has processed his/her painful religious experiences, he/she has been freer to explore religious beliefs and practice his/her faith.

7. Resistance to AA Concepts (7)

A. The patient verbalized a struggle with understanding and accepting Steps 2 and 3 of the Alcoholics Anonymous program, which direct the patient to a belief in a higher power.

B. The patient has resolved many of his/her concerns regarding a higher power and has begun to understand the need for this power in his/her life.

C. The patient has found a meaningful relationship with God that brings comfort, support, encouragement, and direction.

INTERVENTIONS IMPLEMENTED

1. Assign a Written Spiritual Journey (1)

A. The patient was asked to write out a story of his/her spiritual quest and to bring the story to a later session for processing.

B. The patient was encouraged to summarize the highlights of his/her spiritual journey up to this date.

C. The patient has followed through on the assignment of writing about his/her spiritual journey and the content of this journaling was processed.

D. The patient listed several experiences within his/her life that have caused alienation from God.

2. Clarify Higher Power Beliefs (2)

A. The patient was assisted in processing and clarifying his/her own ideas and feelings regarding the existence of a higher power.

B. The patient was encouraged to describe his/her beliefs about the idea of a higher power.

3. List Higher Power Beliefs (3)

A. The patient was assigned to list all of his/her beliefs related to a higher power and to process these beliefs at a later session.

B. The patient processed his/her beliefs around the idea of a higher power and developed reasons to explore his/her spiritual journey.

* The numbers in parentheses correlate to the number of the Therapeutic Intervention statement in the companion chapter with the same title in *The Complete Adult Psychotherapy Treatment Planner,* second edition (Jongsma and Peterson) by John Wiley & Sons, 1999.

4. Review Early-Life Religious Experiences (4)

A. The patient's early-life experiences involving religion were reviewed.

B. The patient was encouraged to describe his/her early-life training and spiritual concepts and to identify the impact of this training on his/her current beliefs.

5. Assign a Talk with a Spiritual Leader (5)

A. The patient was encouraged to talk with a chaplain, pastor, rabbi, or priest regarding his/her spiritual struggles, issues, or questions.

B. Regarding his/her spiritual struggles, the patient processed the experience of talking to a religious leader.

C. The patient verbalized an increased understanding of the concept of a higher power as a result of talking with this spiritual leader.

6. Read Books about God (6)

A. The patient was encouraged to read books such as *God: A Biography* (Miles) or *The History of God* (Armstrong) to build his/her knowledge and understanding of a higher power.

B. The patient has followed through on reading the books about God, and concepts from those readings were processed.

C. The patient has not followed through on reading the books about God and was encouraged to do so.

7. Explore Emotional Components (7)

A. The patient was asked to identify and verbalize feelings related to his/her understanding of God.

B. The patient verbalized feelings of fear, rejection, and abandonment that are associated with his/her understanding of God.

C. The patient verbalized feelings of peace, acceptance, and love that are associated with his/her understanding of God.

8. Explore Religious Distortions (8)

A. The patient was asked to describe any religious distortions and judgmental attitudes that he/she was subjected to by others.

B. The patient described negative life experiences that are associated with religious faith within his/her family.

C. The patient described being subjected to rejection within the community because of religious belief practices.

9. Identify Spirituality Blocks (9)

A. The patient was assisted in identifying specific issues that block or prevent the development of his/her spirituality.

B. The patient discussed specific experiences that have worked against his/her deepening of faith in God.

10. Assign Books on Conversion (10)

A. The patient was encouraged to read books dealing with the conversion experiences of significant people, such as *Surprised by Joy* (Lewis), *Confessions of St. Augustine* (Augustine), *The Seven Storey Mountain* (Merton), or *Soul on Fire* (Cleaver).

B. The patient has read material on conversion experiences, and content from that reading was processed.

C. The patient has not followed through on reading the material on conversion experiences and was encouraged to do so.

D. The patient reported that reading the books that detail the experience of others who have had spiritual struggles was enlightening to his/her own spiritual journey.

11. Recommend Daily Meditation (11)

A. It was recommended to the patient that he/she implement daily prayer and meditation on God to increase his/her contact with a higher power.

B. The patient reported that he/she has found meaning and peace from implementing daily meditation and prayer.

C. The patient has failed to implement daily meditation and prayer and was encouraged to do so.

12. Assign a Letter to the Higher Power (12)

A. The patient was encouraged to write a note on a daily basis to his/her higher power as a means of increasing the sense of contact and meaningful communication.

B. The patient was encouraged to implement daily contact with his/her higher power as a means of building on his/her spiritual journey.

13. Develop Devotional Rituals (13)

A. The patient was assisted in developing and implementing a daily spiritual devotional time.

B. The patient was encouraged to implement faith practices common to his/her belief system that will foster spiritual growth.

C. The patient reported that implementation of faith practices has deepened his/her spirituality.

14. Differentiate between Religion and Spirituality (14)

A. The patient was taught the difference between formalized religion belief and practice and spiritual faith on a more personal, individualized level.

B. As the patient has grown to understand the difference between religion and spiritual faith, he/she has been freer to explore the latter.

15. Emphasize the Higher Power's Forgiveness (15)

A. An emphasis was placed on the higher power as being characterized by love and gracious forgiveness rather than harsh judgmentalism.

B. The patient was encouraged to accept the higher power's forgiveness as he/she has expressed remorse and seeking of forgiveness.

16. Differentiate between Earthly Father and Higher Power (16)

A. The patient was asked to compare his/her beliefs in a higher power with attitudes and feelings that he/she has regarding his/her earthly father.

B. The patient verbalized an insightful understanding of how he/she has converted feelings about his/her earthly father to feelings and attitudes regarding God.

17. Separate Beliefs (17)

A. The patient was urged to separate feelings and beliefs regarding his/her earthly father from those that he/she holds toward a higher power in order to allow for his/her own spiritual growth and maturity.

B. The patient was reinforced for verbalizing a separation between beliefs and feelings toward his/her earthly father from those toward a higher power.

18. Separate Painful Religious Experiences from Religious Tenets (18)

A. The patient was assisted in evaluating religious belief systems separate from the painful emotional experiences that he/she has had with "religious people" in the past.

B. The patient was reinforced when he/she separated the negative experiences with "religious people" from current spiritual issues and evaluations.

19. Read Books on Serenity (19)

A. The patient was encouraged to read such books as *Serenity* (Helmfelt and Fowler), *Alcoholics Anonymous (AA) Big Book Steps 2 and 3* (Alcoholics Anonymous), *The Road Less Traveled* (Peck), and *Search for Serenity* (Presnall).

B. The patient has followed through on reading material on serenity and has verbalized increased acceptance of forgiveness from a higher power.

C. The patient's reading of books on serenity was processed.

D. The patient has failed to follow through on reading the material on serenity and was encouraged to do so.

20. Explore Shame/Guilt Feelings (20)

A. The patient's feelings of shame and guilt were explored that have led to his/her feeling unworthy to a higher power and to other people.

B. The patient was encouraged to accept forgiveness from a higher power and himself/herself as a step toward overcoming shame and guilt.

21. Encourage Spiritual Mentoring (21)

A. The patient was encouraged to search for and find a spiritual mentor to guide his/her spiritual development.

B. The patient reported that he/she asked a respected person who has apparent spiritual depth to serve as his/her mentor.

C. The patient's experience with his/her spiritual mentor was processed.

22. Spiritual Group Referral (22)

A. The patient was made aware of opportunities to join groups of people who are dedicated to deepening their spiritual faith, and he/she was encouraged to pursue those that were appealing to him/her.

B. The patient reported that he/she has attended groups dedicated to enriching spirituality and has found those experiences to be rewarding.

23. Spiritual Retreat Referral (23)

A. The patient was made aware of opportunities for a spiritual retreat such as De Colores or the Course in Miracles and was encouraged to explore these if they appealed to him/her.

B. The patient has attended a spiritual retreat experience, and his/her feelings associated with that were processed.

24. Recommend Spiritual Communication Books (24)

A. The patient was recommended to read books on ways to expand his/her spirituality and depth of communicating with a higher power, such as *Cloistered Walk* (Norris), *Hymns to an Unknown God* (Keen), and *The Care of the Soul* (Moore).

B. The patient reported that he/she has begun to read books on spirituality and communication with God and has found them rewarding.

SUICIDAL IDEATION

PATIENT PRESENTATION

1. Death Preoccupation (1)

A. The patient reported recurrent thoughts of his/her own death.

B. The intensity and frequency of the recurrent thoughts of death have diminished.

C. The patient reported no longer having thoughts of his/her own death.

2. Suicidal Ideation without Plan (2)

A. The patient reported experiencing recurrent suicidal ideation, but denied having any specific plan to implement suicidal urges.

B. The frequency and intensity of the suicidal urges have diminished.

C. The patient stated that he/she has not experienced any recent suicidal ideation.

D. The patient stated that he/she has no interest in causing harm to himself/herself any longer.

3. Suicidal Ideation with Plan (3)

A. The patient reported experiencing ongoing suicidal ideation and has developed a specific plan for suicide.

B. Although the patient acknowledged that he/she has developed a suicide plan, he/she indicated that the suicidal urge is controllable and promised not to implement such a plan.

C. Because the patient had a specific suicide plan and strong suicidal urges, he/she willingly submitted to a supervised psychiatric facility and more intensive treatment.

D. The patient stated that his/her suicidal urges have diminished and he/she has no interest in implementing any specific suicide plan.

E. The patient reported no suicidal urges.

4. Recent Suicide Attempt (4)

A. The patient has made a suicide attempt within the last 24 hours.

B. The patient has made a suicide attempt within the last week.

C. The patient has made a suicide attempt within the last month.

D. The patient denied any interest in suicide currently and promised to engage in no self-harm behavior.

5. Suicide Attempt History (5)

A. The patient reported a history of suicide attempts that have not been recent, but did require professional and/or family/friend intervention to guarantee safety.

B. The patient minimized his/her history of suicide attempts and treated the experience lightly.

---

* The numbers in parentheses correlate to the number of the Behavioral Definition statement in the companion chapter with the same title in *The Complete Adult Psychotherapy Treatment Planner,* second edition (Jongsma and Peterson) by John Wiley & Sons, 1999.

C. The patient acknowledged the history of suicide attempts with appropriate affect and explained the depth of his/her depression at the time of the attempt.

D. The patient indicated no current interest in or thoughts about suicidal behavior.

6. Family History of Depression (6)

A. There is a positive family history of depression.

B. There is a positive family history of suicide.

C. The patient acknowledged the positive family history of depression/suicide and indicated concern about the impact of this tendency on himself/herself.

7. Hopeless Attitude and Life Stressors (7)

A. The patient displayed a bleak, hopeless attitude regarding life, linked to recent stressful experiences that are overwhelming him/her.

B. The patient described a hopeless attitude related to a recent divorce proceeding.

C. The patient displayed a hopeless attitude related to the death of a family member.

D. The patient displayed a hopeless attitude related to the recent loss of employment.

E. The patient's hopeless attitude about life has diminished and he/she has begun to make more hopeful statements about the future.

F. The patient no longer has a hopeless attitude about life and has demonstrated a normal attitude of hope and planning for the future.

8. Social Withdrawal (8)

A. The patient has withdrawn from his/her usual social network and become preoccupied with his/her depressive and suicidal thoughts.

B. The patient has not responded to overtures from others who have tried to be encouraging and supportive.

C. The patient has begun to respond favorably to others and to show an interest in social contact.

D. The patient has returned to normal levels of social interaction and is no longer preoccupied with depression and suicide.

9. Lethargy/Apathy (8)

A. The patient reported no longer having the energy for or the interest in activities that he/she formerly found challenging and rewarding.

B. The patient reported a pattern of engaging in little or no constructive activity and often just sitting or lying around the house.

C. The patient has begun to demonstrate increased energy and interest in activity.

D. The patient has returned to normal levels of energy and has also shown renewed interest in enjoyable and challenging activities.

10. Premature Demonstrations of Being at Peace (9)

A. The patient has made a sudden change from being depressed to being upbeat and at peace, but there has been no genuine resolution of conflict issues.

B. The patient has taken actions that seem to indicate that he/she is "putting his/her house in order."

C. The patient acknowledged that the core depression is still very much present and a death wish exists.

D. The patient has made genuine progress toward resolution of the conflict issues in his/her life and has a more genuine feeling of serenity.

INTERVENTIONS IMPLEMENTED

1. Assess Suicidal Ideation (1)

A. The patient was asked to describe the frequency and intensity of his/her suicidal ideation, the details of any existing suicide plan, the history of any previous suicide attempts, and any family history of depression or suicide.

B. The patient was encouraged to be forthright regarding the current strength of his/her suicidal feelings and the ability to control such suicidal urges.

2. Monitor Suicide Potential (2)

A. The patient was monitored on an ongoing basis for his/her suicide potential.

B. The patient was asked to describe his/her current suicidal urges and the degree to which he/she felt they could be controlled.

3. Notify Significant Others (3)

A. Significant others were notified of the patient's suicidal ideation and they were asked to form a 24-hour suicide watch until the patient's crisis subsides.

B. The follow-through of significant others in providing supervision of the patient during this suicide crisis was monitored.

C. Significant others were contacted to make sure that the patient was receiving adequate supervision.

4. Administer Psychological Testing (4)

A. Psychological testing was administered to the patient to evaluate the depth of his/her depression and the degree of suicide risk.

B. The psychological test results indicate that the patient's depression is severe and the suicide risk is high.

C. The psychological test results indicate that the patient's depression is moderate and the suicide risk is mild.

D. The psychological test results indicate that the patient's depression level has decreased significantly and the suicide risk is minimal.

5. Elicit Promise of No Self-Injurious Behavior (5)

A. The patient was asked to make a verbal commitment that he/she will initiate contact with the therapist or a helpline if the suicidal urge becomes strong and before any self-injurious behavior occurs.

---

* The numbers in parentheses correlate to the number of the Therapeutic Intervention statement in the companion chapter with the same title in *The Complete Adult Psychotherapy Treatment Planner,* second edition (Jongsma and Peterson) by John Wiley & Sons, 1999.

B. The patient was asked to sign a suicide prevention contract that stipulated that he/she would contact the therapist or some other emergency helpline if a serious urge toward self-harm arose.

C. The patient has made a commitment to not engage in any self-injurious behavior.

6. Provide Helpline Information (6)

A. The patient was provided with an emergency helpline telephone number that is available to him/her 24 hours per day.

B. The patient was asked to promise to use the emergency helpline before engaging in any self-injurious behavior, and he/she agreed to do so.

7. Develop Suicide Prevention Contract (7)

A. A suicide prevention contract was developed with the patient that stipulated what he/she will and will not do when experiencing suicidal thoughts or impulses.

B. The patient was asked to make a commitment to agree to the terms of the suicide prevention contract and did make such a commitment.

8. Offer Telephone Availability (8)

A. The patient was given the therapist's telephone number and the patient agreed to make contact at any time if a suicide urge becomes unmanageable.

B. The patient was asked to attempt to contact the therapist if suicide urges become strong and, if the therapist is not available, to contact an emergency helpline service with the telephone numbers provided.

9. Remove Lethal Weapons (9)

A. Significant others were encouraged to remove firearms and other potentially lethal means of suicide from the patient's easy access.

B. Contact was made with significant others within the patient's life to monitor the patient's behavior and to remove potential means of suicide.

10. Encourage Honesty (10)

A. The patient was encouraged to be open and honest regarding his/her suicidal urges.

B. The patient was reassured regularly of the caring concern of the therapist and significant others.

11. Arrange for Hospitalization (11)

A. Because the patient was judged to be uncontrollably harmful to himself/herself, arrangements were made for psychiatric hospitalization.

B. The patient cooperated voluntarily with admission to a psychiatric hospital.

C. The patient refused to cooperate voluntarily with admission to a psychiatric facility, and therefore commitment procedures were initiated.

12. Explore Emotional Pain Sources (12)

A. The patient was asked to explore and identify life factors that preceded the suicidal ideation.

B. The patient was supported as he/she identified the sources of emotional pain and hope-lessness that precipitated the suicidal crisis.

13. Encourage Feelings Expression (13)

A. The patient was encouraged to express rather than suppress the feelings that led to his/her suicide crisis in order to clarify those feelings and increase insight into the causes for them.

B. The patient was supported and reinforced as he/she began to open up about the feelings behind the suicidal ideation.

C. The patient was led to develop insight into his/her feelings of hopelessness and helpless-ness.

14. Explore Significant Others' Understanding (14)

A. The patient's significant others were interviewed about their understanding of the causes for the patient's deep distress.

B. Significant others were encouraged to communicate their understanding, support, and concern for the patient.

15. Probe Family Conflict (15)

A. The patient's feelings of despair related to his/her conflicted family relationships were explored.

B. The patient was supported as he/she identified feelings of sadness, anger, and hopeless-ness related to a conflicted relationship with significant others.

16. Promote Family Communication (16)

A. A family therapy session was held to promote communication of the patient's feelings of sadness, hurt, and anger.

B. The family members were encouraged to communicate their respect and understanding of the patient's feelings.

C. Family members were encouraged to process the conflicts and feelings between them so as to find a resolution and to express a commitment to an ongoing relationship.

17. Medication Evaluation Referral (17)

A. An assessment was made about the patient's need for antidepressant medication, and arrangements were made for a prescription.

B. The patient agreed to accept a prescription for antidepressant medication.

C. The patient refused to accept a prescription for antidepressant medication.

D. The patient cooperated with a referral to a physician who evaluated him/her for antide-pressant medication and provided a prescription for this medication.

18. Monitor Medication Compliance (18)

A. The patient has been monitored for compliance with the prescribed antidepressant med-ication, and the effects of that medication were assessed.

B. The patient has been taking the medication as prescribed and reported that it has pro-duced a reduction in the depth of depression and suicidal ideation.

C. The patient has not been taking the antidepressant medication consistently and was urged to do so.

D. The patient reported taking the antidepressant medication consistently, but said that no positive effects from this medication have been noted.

E. The patient's prescribing physician has been contacted regarding the patient's medication compliance and the effect of the medication on the depression and suicidal ideation.

19. Identify Suicidal Ideation Precursors (19)

A. The patient was assisted in becoming aware of life factors that were significant precursors to the beginning of his/her suicidal ideation.

B. The patient was supported as he/she identified unresolved issues in his/her life and shared the feelings that underlie the suicidal thoughts.

20. Explore Relationship Grief (20)

A. The patient was encouraged to share feelings of grief related to the breaking up of a close relationship.

B. The patient was supported as he/she disclosed the distress caused by a broken romantic relationship that has led to feelings of abject loneliness and rejection.

C. The patient was supported as he/she shared the feelings of hopelessness associated with an impending divorce.

D. The patient was encouraged to share feelings associated with the death of a loved one, which has left him/her feeling abandoned.

21. Review Problem-Solving Skills (21)

A. The patient's problem-solving attempts were reviewed and new skills were taught as they could be applied to the current interpersonal crisis.

B. The patient was reinforced as he/she identified how his/her previous attempts to solve interpersonal problems have failed, resulting in feelings of helplessness.

C. The patient was urged to implement new problem-solving skills to resolve the current interpersonal crisis.

22. Monitor Eating/Sleeping Patterns (22)

A. The patient was encouraged to resume normal eating and sleeping patterns.

B. The patient was given relaxation training to facilitate sleep.

C. The patient was encouraged to take medications consistently to get sleep and return to normal eating patterns.

23. Develop Coping Strategies (23)

A. The patient was assisted in developing coping strategies for suicidal ideation that include physical exercise, reduced internal focus, increased social involvement, and increased expression of feelings.

B. The patient was reinforced when he/she reported a decrease in the frequency and intensity of suicidal ideation as a result of implementing new coping strategies.

24. Promote Hopeful Attitude (24)

A. The patient was assisted in identifying positive and hopeful things in his/her life at the present time.

B. The patient identified positive aspects, relationships, and achievements in his/her life, and these positive things were supported and reinforced.

C. The patient was supported as he/she reported and demonstrated an increased sense of hope for himself/herself and the future.

25. Identify Sources of Support (25)

A. The patient was assisted in reviewing the successes that he/she has had and the sources of love, compassion, and concern that continue to exist in his/her life.

B. The patient was asked to compile a list of people who have been and will continue to be supportive of and encouraging to him/her.

C. The patient was strongly reinforced as he/she identified the positive relationships and achievements in his/her life.

26. Identify Distorted Cognitions (26)

A. The patient was assisted in developing an awareness of the negative and distorted cognitive messages that reinforce hopelessness and helplessness.

B. The patient has identified several distorted self-talk messages that he/she engaged in that are counterproductive and precipitate feelings of low self-esteem, hopelessness, and helplessness.

27. Confront Catastrophizing (27)

A. The patient's tendency to catastrophize in his/her cognitive processing was confronted.

B. The patient was taught a more realistic perspective of hope in the face of pain, rather than pessimism and catastrophizing.

28. Use Cognitive Restructuring Techniques (28)

A. The patient was taught cognitive restructuring techniques to revise distorted negative core schemas.

B. The patient was reinforced for modifying his/her negative automatic thoughts and replacing them with more realistic positive thoughts that produce feelings of hope and empowerment.

29. Assign Journaling (29)

A. The patient was asked to keep a daily record of his/her self-defeating thoughts and to bring them to sessions for review.

B. The patient's record of self-defeating thoughts was reviewed, and each thought was challenged for accuracy and identified as distorted and unrealistic.

C. The patient was taught to replace each dysfunctional thought with one that is positive and self-enhancing.

D. The patient was reinforced for implementing positive cognitive processing patterns that maintain a realistic and hopeful perspective.

30. Develop Penitence Ritual (30)

A. The patient was assisted in developing a penitence ritual in which he/she could express grief for others who have died and absolve himself/herself of guilt for continuing to live.

B. The patient was supported and encouraged to implement the penitence ritual connected with being a survivor.

C. The patient's feelings regarding implementation of the penitence ritual were processed.

31. Explore Spiritual Support System (31)

A. The patient's spiritual belief system was explored to discover whether it could be a source of reassurance, support, and peace.

B. The patient was encouraged to engage in the faith practices that nurture and strengthen his/her spiritual belief system.

C. The patient was reinforced for verbalizing the feeling of support that results from his/her spiritual faith.

32. Spiritual Leader Referral (32)

A. The patient was encouraged to meet with his/her identified spiritual leader to obtain support, encouragement, and strengthening of spiritual tenets.

B. The patient's meeting with his/her spiritual leader was processed and support for continued involvement in his/her faith network was encouraged.

TYPE A BEHAVIOR

PATIENT PRESENTATION

1. Time Pressure (1)

A. The patient described a pattern of pressuring himself/herself and others to accomplish more within a limited amount of time.

B. The patient frequently complains about not having enough time to accomplish what he/she wants to do.

C. The patient is beginning to place less of an emphasis on the limitations of time.

D. The patient has become more relaxed and less intense about accomplishing so much within a limited time frame.

2. Competitive Spirit (2)

A. The patient displayed an intense, competitive spirit in describing all of his/her activities.

B. The patient has alienated others from himself/herself because of his/her intense competitive spirit.

C. The patient has begun to realize that he/she must reduce the degree of competitiveness in all of his/her activities.

D. The patient has developed a much more cooperative and collegial attitude regarding working in and around others.

3. Compulsion to Win (3)

A. The patient demonstrated an intense compulsion to win at all costs, regardless of the type of activity or who else is competing.

B. The patient has alienated himself/herself from others because of his/her intense compulsion to win at all costs.

C. The patient has begun to realize the need to temper his/her competitive spirit and to consider the feelings of others and the nature of the situation.

D. The patient has become much more considerate of others' feelings and is less compelled to win at all costs.

4. Dominating/Controlling Behavior (4)

A. The patient described an inclination to dominate all social and business situations by being too direct and overbearing.

B. The patient has alienated himself/herself from others because of his/her dominating and controlling manner.

C. The patient has become more considerate of other people's opinions and feelings and has reduced his/her degree of control over situations.

D. The patient has yielded control to others and has solicited leadership from others.

---

* The numbers in parentheses correlate to the number of the Behavioral Definition statement in the companion chapter with the same title in *The Complete Adult Psychotherapy Treatment Planner,* second edition (Jongsma and Peterson) by John Wiley & Sons, 1999.

5. Easily Irritated with Others (5)

A. The patient has a propensity to become easily irritated by the actions of others who do not conform to his/her sense of propriety or correctness.

B. When others do not meet the patient's standards, he/she becomes critical, frustrated, and overly reactive.

C. The patient is becoming more tolerant of other people's standards and behavior.

6. Perpetual Impatience (6)

A. The patient described a pattern of perpetual impatience with any waiting, delay, or interruptions.

B. The patient becomes easily irritated with others who cause him/her to have to wait.

C. The patient is intolerant of any need to stand in line or wait his/her turn.

D. The patient is beginning to practice relaxation techniques to improve and increase his/her tolerance for waiting.

E. The patient reported a significant increase in his/her ability to tolerate waiting or interruptions.

7. Difficulty Relaxing (7)

A. The patient described having difficulty in quietly relaxing and reflecting.

B. The patient is restless and agitated.

C. The patient has to be on the move and doing something active.

D. The patient has improved his/her ability to sit quietly and relax.

E. The patient reported being comfortable sitting quietly and reflecting.

8. Facial Signs of Intensity (8)

A. The patient demonstrated facial signs of intensity and pressure such as muscle tension, scowling, glaring, or tics.

B. The patient expressed a lack of awareness of the facial signs of intensity and pressure that he/she projects to others.

C. The patient has become more aware of his/her facial signs of intensity and pressure and has begun to modify them.

D. The patient has developed the ability to relax and now projects an image of increased serenity rather than intensity.

9. Verbal Signs of Intensity (9)

A. The patient demonstrated verbal signs of intensity and pressure such as forceful speech or laughter and rapid and intense speech.

B. The patient displayed verbal signs of intensity such as the frequent use of obscenities to attempt to emphasize his/her points.

C. The patient has become more aware of his/her verbal signs of intensity and has begun to modify them.

D. The patient no longer demonstrates verbal signs of intensity, as his/her speech is slower and quieter.

INTERVENTIONS IMPLEMENTED

1. Explore Pressured Lifestyle (1)

A. The patient was asked to give examples of indications of pressure in his/her lifestyle.

B. The patient was supported in describing the pattern of pressure-driven living that he/she experiences.

C. The patient listed examples of pressured living such as impatience, domination, competitive spirit, inability to relax, and time frustration.

2. Promote Self-Awareness (2)

A. The patient was asked to list the traits and characteristics that he/she believes other people see in him/her.

B. Role playing and role reversal were used to assist the patient in becoming more aware of the impact of his/her behavior on others.

C. The patient was reinforced for demonstrating increased insight into the impact of his/her behavior on others.

3. Psychological Testing (3)

A. The patient was administered psychological testing to assess him/her for any psychopathology and to further delineate personality patterns.

B. The patient agreed to and cooperated with psychological testing to evaluate personality patterns.

C. The patient refused to cooperate with psychological testing, stating that it would be a waste of time.

4. Process Psychological Testing Results (4)

A. The results of the psychological testing were presented to the patient and processed.

B. The psychological testing results confirmed a lack of any serious psychopathology, but the presence of a high level of energy and a tendency to control others.

C. The psychological testing results showed the presence of a bipolar disease pattern and the need for psychological and psychopharmacological treatment.

5. Explore Family History (5)

A. The patient's family-of-origin history was explored for role models of or parental pressure for high achievement and compulsive drive.

B. The patient identified a family pattern that fostered a driven lifestyle.

6. Assign Books on Type A Attitudes (6)

A. It was recommended to the patient that he/she read books on Type A behavior and attitudes such as *Positive Addiction* (Glasser) and *Overdoing It* (Robinson).

B. The patient has read the assigned material on Type A behavior, and key ideas were processed within the session.

---

* The numbers in parentheses correlate to the number of the Therapeutic Intervention statement in the companion chapter with the same title in *The Complete Adult Psychotherapy Treatment Planner,* second edition (Jongsma and Peterson) by John Wiley & Sons, 1999.

C. The patient has failed to read the recommended material on Type A behavior and was encouraged to do so.

D. The patient was encouraged and supported for developing insight into the specific beliefs that support his/her driven, overachieving behavior.

7. Explore Beliefs about Worth (7)

A. The patient was asked to make a list of his/her beliefs about what contributes to his/her own worth and the worth of others.

B. The patient's list of beliefs regarding self-worth and the worth of others was processed.

8. Train in Relaxation (8)

A. The patient was trained in deep muscle relaxation and breathing techniques to help him/her slow the pace of his/her life.

B. The patient was encouraged to implement deep muscle relaxation on a daily basis to relieve tension and reduce the intensity of his/her life.

C. The patient was reinforced when he/she reported an increased use of relaxation techniques to reduce intensity and pressure.

9. Reduce Work Hours (9)

A. The patient's pattern of hours spent working was reviewed and recommendations were given regarding a significant reduction.

B. The patient was supported and reinforced for reporting a decrease in the number of hours worked on a daily basis.

10. Assign Recreational Activity (10)

A. The patient was assigned to do one noncompetitive recreational activity each day for a week and to process this experience within the next session.

B. The patient was encouraged to continue the time spent in relaxing activities.

11. Assign Hobby Activity (11)

A. Nonvocational interests of the patient were explored and listed.

B. The patient was assigned to spend time and energy involved in a nonvocational interest activity two times per week for one month.

C. The patient's response to involvement in nonvocational activities was processed and reinforced.

12. Clarify Value System (12)

A. An exploration of the patient's value system was performed and he/she was assisted in developing priorities based on the importance of relationships, recreation, spiritual growth, reflection time, giving to others, and so on.

B. The patient was helped to critically examine values that provide motivation for an overemphasis on accomplishment, achievement, and success.

C. The patient was supported in verbalizing a desire to reprioritize values to focus less on himself/herself and more on others.

13. Assign Biographies (13)

A. The patient was encouraged to read biographies or autobiographies of altruistic or spiritual individuals such as Thomas Merton, Albert Schweitzer, C.S. Lewis, or St. Augustine.

B. Key concepts from the books about altruistic or spiritual people were reviewed and processed.

C. The patient was reinforced for identifying and applying more humanitarian values to his/her life.

14. Enforce Single-Activity Focus (14)

A. The patient was encouraged and reinforced for focusing on one activity at a time without a sense of urgency.

B. The patient reported success at performing one task at a time with less emphasis on feeling pressured to complete it quickly, and this accomplishment was strongly reinforced.

15. Assign Comedy Movies (15)

A. The patient was assigned to watch comedy movies and identify the positive aspects of this activity.

B. The patient was reinforced for identifying the benefits of balancing time spent on daily activities of work and leisure.

C. The patient was reinforced for watching the assigned comedy movies and identifying the benefits of this activity.

16. Reinforce Life Balance (16)

A. The patient was reinforced for demonstrating and verbalizing changes in his/her life that reflect a greater sense of balance among work, recreation, spiritual growth, and giving to others.

B. The patient reported a sense of enjoyment and fulfillment in incorporating more balance into his/her life.

17. Explore Intolerance/Impatience (17)

A. The patient acknowledged a pattern of intolerance and impatience with other people, and the depth and causes for this lack of understanding were explored.

B. The patient was reinforced for acknowledging that he/she has been unreasonable in his/her intolerance and impatience with others.

C. The patient was supported as he/she set a goal of becoming more compassionate, understanding, and patient with others.

18. Identify Standards of Criticism (18)

A. The patient was assisted in identifying his/her critical beliefs about other people and connecting them to his/her behavior patterns in daily life.

B. The patient was supported in verbalizing a recognition that he/she is too critical of others and impatient with them.

C. The patient was reinforced for reporting a more tolerant, accepting attitude toward others instead of his/her previous approach to hostile criticism.

19. Reflect Hostility (19)

A. An effort was made to reflect the patient's hostility so as to assist him/her in becoming more aware of it.

B. The patient was assisted in identifying sources of hostility toward and impatience with others.

C. The patient was helped to process his/her hostile feelings toward others and to resolve them so as to develop a more accepting attitude.

20. Assign Ericksonian Task (20)

A. The patient was assigned an Ericksonian task of performing a neutral activity and then simply reflecting about a subject for a preestablished length of time.

B. The patient's performance of the Ericksonian task was processed with the goal of helping him/her recognize impatience and difficulty with quiet reflection.

21. Train in Assertiveness (21)

A. The patient was trained in the principles of assertive behavior as contrasted with aggressive behavior that tramples on the rights of others.

B. The patient was encouraged to implement assertiveness without becoming aggressive in his/her interaction with others.

C. The patient was reinforced for understanding and implementing the distinction between respectful assertiveness and insensitive directness or verbal aggression that is controlling of others.

22. Confront Self-Centeredness (22)

A. The patient's actions and/or verbalizations that indicate a self-centered, insensitive attitude toward others were confronted and reframed.

B. Role playing and role reversal exercises were used to attempt to increase the patient's empathy for others.

C. The patient was reinforced for any statements that indicated an increased sensitivity to others.

23. Explore Family Pressure to Achieve (23)

A. The patient's family-of-origin history was explored for the experience of being pressured to achieve but never succeeding at satisfying a parental figure.

B. The patient was encouraged to discuss his/her feelings regarding a parent figure pressuring him/her for success that never seemed to be attainable.

24. Assign Active Listening (24)

A. The patient was assigned to talk to an associate or a child, focusing on listening to the other person and learning several key things about that person.

B. The patient was taught the principals of active listening that included eye contact, quiet patience, and reflection of content.

C. The patient was reinforced for reporting success at the implementation of active listening skills in conversation with others.

25. Identify Distorted Thoughts (25)

A. The patient was assisted in identifying distorted automatic thoughts that lead to feeling pressured to achieve.

B. The patient was supported as he/she identified specific distorted automatic thoughts that are engaged in on a repeated basis and that motivate pressured living.

26. Teach Positive Self-Talk (26)

A. The patient was trained in replacing distorted automatic thoughts with more realistic, positive self-talk that will assist in promoting a slower pace, greater self-acceptance, and sensitivity to others.

B. The patient was reinforced for reporting implementation of positive self-talk that has altered beliefs that fostered compulsive achievement-oriented behaviors.

27. Assign Experiential Weekend (27)

A. The patient and significant others were assigned to attend an experiential weekend that promotes cooperation and self-awareness.

B. The patient was supported for verbalizing decreased impatience with others and increased appreciation and understanding of the good qualities of others.

28. Assign Camping/Volunteering Project (28)

A. The patient was assigned to select a weekend experience that reflects a total break from pressured living and vocational achievement such as a camping and canoeing trip or a work camp project or volunteering with the Red Cross.

B. The patient was reinforced for demonstrating and implementing a more humanitarian approach to life.

29. Encourage Nonprofit Volunteering (29)

A. The patient was encouraged to volunteer for a nonprofit social agency, school, or the like for one year, doing direct work with people.

B. The patient was supported and reinforced for his/her report on performing volunteer activities at a nonprofit social agency.

C. The patient was reinforced for reporting rewards that were inherent in serving others and demonstrating compassion, kindness, and forgiveness in dealing with others.

30. Encourage Spontaneous Kindness (30)

A. The patient was assisted in identifying a multitude of spontaneous acts of kindness that he/she could perform.

B. The patient was encouraged to enact one random, spontaneous act of kindness on a daily basis and to explore the positive feelings associated with this.

C. The patient's experience with performing a random act of kindness on a daily basis was processed and reinforced.

31. Assign *The Road Less Traveled* (31)

A. The patient was assigned to read the book *The Road Less Traveled* (Peck) and to process key ideas in subsequent therapy sessions.

B. The patient has read the book *The Road Less Traveled* and key ideas from that were processed.

C. The patient has failed to follow through with reading the recommended book *The Road Less Traveled* and was encouraged to do so.

D. The patient's reading of the book *The Road Less Traveled* has helped him/her develop a balance between the quest for achievement and the appreciation of aesthetic things.

32. Encourage Expression of Appreciation (32)

A. The patient was encouraged to express warmth, appreciation, affection, and gratitude toward others.

B. The patient was reinforced for reports of his/her success at expressing appreciation and gratitude to others.

33. Assign "List of Aphorisms" (33)

A. The patient was assigned to read "List of Aphorisms" in the book *Treating Type A Behaviors and Your Heart* (Friedman and Olmer) three times daily for at least one week.

B. The patient was encouraged to pick several aphorisms to incorporate into his/her daily life.

C. The patient was reinforced for the incorporation of aphorisms into his/her daily life that resulted in a reduction in the quest for achievement.

34. List Aesthetic Enjoyment Activities (34)

A. The patient was assisted in listing activities he/she could engage in for purely aesthetic enjoyment such as visiting an art museum, attending a symphony concert, taking a hike in the woods, or taking painting lessons.

B. The patient was reinforced for incorporating purely aesthetically enjoyable activities into his/her daily routine.

VOCATIONAL STRESS

PATIENT PRESENTATION

1. Coworker Conflict (1)

A. The patient reported feelings of anxiety and depression secondary to experiencing perceived harassment, shunning, and confrontation from coworkers.

B. The patient has become more withdrawn and isolated within the work environment due to coworker conflict.

C. The patient has begun to resolve conflicts with coworkers, and this has resulted in an improved emotional state.

D. The patient reported feeling comfortable with and enjoying interaction with his/her coworkers.

2. Severe Business Losses (2)

A. The patient described feelings of inadequacy, fear, and failure secondary to his/her severe business losses.

B. The financial and economic stress is resulting in feelings of failure and anxiety.

C. The patient has begun to develop a sense of empowerment and a plan to overcome recent financial setbacks.

3. Fear of Failure (3)

A. Since receiving a promotion with increased responsibility and expectations, the patient has experienced a fear of failure.

B. As the patient has become more successful, he/she has developed a sense that failure is right around the corner.

C. The patient has begun to accept his/her success as earned and warranted rather than fearing that he/she will not be able to live up to the expectations.

D. The patient is beginning to feel challenged and confident regarding future expectations.

4. Authority Conflict (4)

A. The patient described a pattern of rebellion against and conflict with authority figures within the employment situation.

B. The patient's rebellion against authority has resulted in being dismissed from employment on more than one occasion.

C. The patient's authority conflicts within the employment situation have resulted in failure to achieve promotions.

D. The patient has developed a more accepting attitude toward authority and is willing to take direction within the employment arena.

---

* The numbers in parentheses correlate to the number of the Behavioral Definition statement in the companion chapter with the same title in *The Complete Adult Psychotherapy Treatment Planner,* second edition (Jongsma and Peterson) by John Wiley & Sons, 1999.

5. Loss of Employment (5)

A. The patient reported feelings of anxiety and depression secondary to losing his/her employment.

B. The patient has been fired due to poor work performance and a negative attitude.

C. The patient has been laid off from his/her employment due to a downsizing within the company.

D. The patient's feelings of anxiety and depression related to loss of employment have diminished as he/she has developed a plan of seeking new employment.

6. Job Jeopardy (6)

A. The patient reported severe feelings of anxiety related to perceived job jeopardy.

B. The patient's perception of his/her job jeopardy has been reversed as he/she has consulted with a supervisor and has been reassured of job security.

C. The patient has begun to develop an alternate plan of reaction if the job jeopardy results in a loss of employment.

7. Job Dissatisfaction (7)

A. The patient described feelings of depression and anxiety related to being dissatisfied with his/her job responsibilities.

B. The patient feels depressed and anxious due to the stress of his/her employment responsibilities.

C. The patient's feelings of depression and anxiety have diminished as he/she has developed new coping skills to apply to the employment situation.

D. The patient has been assigned to different work responsibilities, and this has resulted in a resolution of the feelings of depression and anxiety.

INTERVENTIONS IMPLEMENTED

1. Clarify Work Conflicts (1)

A. The patient was asked to describe the nature of his/her conflicts with coworkers and/or supervisor.

B. The patient was supported as he/she described the history and nature of the conflicts with his/her coworkers.

2. Identify Patient Role in Conflict (2)

A. The patient was helped to identify his/her own role in the coworker conflict.

B. Role playing and role reversal were used to help the patient understand the coworker's point of view within the employment conflict situation.

C. The patient was reinforced for identifying and accepting his/her own role within the conflict with coworkers rather than projecting all of the blame and responsibility onto others.

---

* The numbers in parentheses correlate to the number of the Therapeutic Intervention statement in the companion chapter with the same title in *The Complete Adult Psychotherapy Treatment Planner,* second edition (Jongsma and Peterson) by John Wiley & Sons, 1999.

3. Explore Substance Abuse (3)

A. The possible role of substance abuse as a contributing factor to the employment problems was explored.

B. The patient acknowledged that his/her substance abuse is a problem and that it does contribute to vocational conflicts.

C. The patient denied any substance abuse problems as having a role in his/her employment problems.

4. Explore Personal Problems (4)

A. The patient was assisted in identifying personal problems that may be contributing to conflicts within the employment situation.

B. The patient was supported for acknowledging problems in his/her personal life that are having a negative influence on his/her work performance and coworker relationships.

C. Attention was given to the personal problems that the patient has identified, and suggestions were made toward resolution of those problems in order to improve employment performance and coworker relationships.

D. The referral was given to the patient to seek treatment for his/her personal problems in order to improve his/her employment situation.

5. Confront Projection of Responsibility (5)

A. The patient was confronted for projecting responsibility for his/her behavior and feelings onto others.

B. The patient was supported and reinforced for replacing projection of responsibility for conflict feelings or behavior with acceptance of responsibility for his/her own behavior feelings and role in the conflict.

6. Reinforce Responsibility Acceptance (6)

A. The patient was reinforced for accepting responsibility for his/her feelings and behavior without projecting responsibility for them onto others.

B. As the patient accepted responsibility for his/her own behavior and feelings, he/she was reinforced for identifying behavioral changes that he/she could make to improve his/her employment situation.

7. Assign a Written Action Plan (7)

A. The patient was assigned to write a plan for constructive action that contains various alternatives to resolve the coworker or supervisor conflict.

B. The patient's action plan was reviewed and processed.

C. The patient's action plan for resolving conflict within the employment situation included complying with authority, initiating pleasant greetings, complimenting others' work, and avoiding critical judgments of others.

8. Role-Play Social Skills (8)

A. Role playing, behavioral rehearsal, and role reversal were used to teach the patient social skills that would increase the probability of positive encounters within the employment situation.

B. The patient was reinforced for reporting interpersonal encounters that promoted harmony with coworkers and supervisors.

9. Train in Assertiveness Skills (9)

A. The patient was trained in assertiveness skills as they could be applied to the employment situation.

B. The patient was referred to an assertiveness training class to learn skills that could be applied to the employment situation.

C. The patient was reinforced for implementing assertiveness that increased effective communication of needs and feelings without aggression or defensiveness.

10. Process Corrective Action Plan (10)

A. The patient's plan for correcting problems that exist within the employment situation was reviewed and processed.

B. The patient was supported and encouraged in taking responsibility for proactive action to resolve employment conflicts.

C. The patient's implementation of a proactive plan to resolve employment conflicts was reinforced.

11. Explore Interpersonal Conflict Patterns (11)

A. The patient's pattern of interpersonal conflict beyond the workplace was explored.

B. The patient was supported and reinforced for accepting the fact that he/she has similar patterns of conflict with people outside of the work environment.

C. The patient acknowledged responsibility for the need to change his/her style of interacting with others to reduce interpersonal conflict generally.

12. Explore Family Patterns of Conflict (12)

A. The patient's family-of-origin history was reviewed to determine roots for interpersonal conflict that are being reenacted within the work setting.

B. The patient was encouraged and supported for his/her insight into a reenactment of family-of-origin conflicts within the work setting.

C. The patient's work adjustment has improved and was reinforced, and he/she has addressed family-of-origin conflicts.

13. Probe Childhood History (13)

A. The patient's childhood history was reviewed for the origin of feelings of inadequacy, fear of failure, or fear of success.

B. The patient was supported for identifying childhood experiences that have contributed to his/her fear of failure.

C. The patient was assisted in working through childhood experiences that have contributed to his/her feelings of inadequacy.

14. Clarify Emotional Reactions (14)

A. The patient's feelings associated with the vocational stress were explored and clarified.

B. The patient was supported and reinforced for openly sharing feelings of fear, anger, and helplessness associated with the vocational stress.

15. Identify Distorted Cognitions (15)

A. The patient was helped to identify the distorted cognitive messages and schema that are connected with his/her feelings of vocational stress.

B. The patient was supported in identifying specific self-talk that precipitates feelings of anxiety, fear, and depression.

16. Confront Catastrophizing (16)

A. The patient was confronted for catastrophizing the employment situation.

B. The patient was taught the effects of catastrophizing as leading to immobilizing anxiety.

C. The patient was taught that his/her catastrophizing is an overreaction to the actual employment situation.

17. Teach Realistic Cognitive Messages (17)

A. The patient was trained in more realistic, healthy cognitive messages that relieve anxiety and depression rather than precipitate it.

B. The patient was supported as he/she identified specific healthy, realistic cognitive messages that promote harmony with others, self-acceptance, and self-confidence.

C. The patient was reinforced for implementation of positive self-talk that has resulted in improved feelings associated with the employment situation.

18. Assign a Journal of Self-Defeating Thoughts (18)

A. The patient was assigned to keep a daily record of self-defeating thoughts.

B. The patient's record of self-defeating thoughts was reviewed, including those that reflected hopelessness, worthlessness, fear of rejection, catastrophizing, and negative predictions of the future.

C. The patient was challenged on his/her self-defeating thought tendencies and taught to replace each dysfunctional thought with one that is positive and self-enhancing.

D. The patient was strongly reinforced for implementing positive, realistic thoughts rather than self-defeating thoughts.

19. Explore Employment Termination Causes (19)

A. The possible causes for the patient's termination from employment were explored.

B. The patient was helped to understand that there may have been several causes for his/her termination that were beyond his/her control and, therefore, not his/her responsibility.

C. The patient was reinforced for verbalizing and understanding the circumstances that led up to his/her being terminated from employment, including those that may have been beyond his/her control.

20. Reinforce Realistic Self-Appraisal (20)

A. The patient was assisted in being realistic regarding appraising his/her successes and failures at employment.

B. The patient was supported for recalling employment successes and terminating self-disparaging comments that were based on perceived failure at employment.

21. Explore Vocational Stress Effects (21)

A. The patient was helped to explore the effects that his/her vocational stress has had on himself/herself and relationships with significant others.

B. The patient was supported for acknowledging that vocational stress has had a serious negative effect on himself/herself and relationships with others.

C. The patient was helped to develop a plan to reduce vocational stress through a change in employment actions or change of employment.

22. Facilitate Family Therapy (22)

A. A family therapy session was held in which feelings of family members were aired and clarified regarding the vocational situation.

B. Family members were supported as they verbalized their feelings of anxiety about the negative employment situation and expressed support for the patient.

C. Family members were given the opportunity to confront the patient regarding his/her responsibility for the current employment conflicts.

23. List Accomplishments and Support System (23)

A. The patient was assisted in listing his/her positive traits, talents, and accomplishments.

B. The patient was asked to list all those who care for, respect, and value him/her and who are there for him/her as a part of an ongoing social support network.

C. The patient was encouraged to view himself/herself as capable, likable, and of value, based upon previous successes and current affirmations from a social support network.

24. Teach Alternate Evaluation of Self (24)

A. The patient was taught that an individual's ultimate worth is not measured in material or vocational success, but in service to others and/or to a higher power.

B. The patient was encouraged to list ways to evaluate his/her worth apart from vocational success.

25. Develop Job Search Plan (25)

A. The patient was assisted in developing a written plan for attainable objectives in a job search.

B. The patient was supported and reinforced for implementation of a job search plan.

C. The patient was encouraged to share his/her feelings of fear, frustration, and disappointment as he/she has engaged in the job search process.

26. Teach Job Search Networking (26)

A. The patient was taught to utilize want ads and networking with friends and family to seek out job opportunities.

B. The patient was encouraged as he/she began the job search process and utilized a networking procedure.

27. Assign Job Search Support Classes (27)

A. The patient was assigned to attend a class that teaches skills and job searching.

B. It was recommended to the patient that he/she attend a resume writing seminar.

C. The patient was supported and reinforced for following through with attendance at classes that build job search skills.

28. Monitor Job Search Process (28)

A. The patient was supported and encouraged as he/she engaged in the job search experience.

B. The patient was encouraged to share his/her feelings of anxiety, frustration, anger, and failure as the job search experience continued.

C. The patient was confronted on not being consistent in the job search activity and redirected to pursue this more diligently.